Implementing Early Intervention

IMPLEMENTING EARLY INTERVENTION

From Research to Effective Practice

Edited by

DONNA M. BRYANT, PhD
Frank Porter-Graham Child Development Center
University of North Carolina at Chapel Hill

MIMI A. GRAHAM, EdD
Center for Prevention and Early Intervention Policy
Florida State University

Foreword by Samuel J. Meisels

THE GUILFORD PRESS
New York   London

© 1993 The Guilford Press
A Division of Guilford Publications, Inc.
72 Spring Street, New York, NY 10012

Printed in the United States of America

This book is printed on acid-free paper.

Last digit is print number: 9 8 7 6 5 4 3 2 1

Library of Congress Cataloging-in-Publication Data

Implementing early intervention: from research to effective practice
/ edited by Donna M. Bryant, Mimi A. Graham; foreword by Samuel J. Meisels.
     p.   cm.
  Includes bibliographical references and index.
  ISBN 0-89862-247-6
  1. Developmentally disabled children—Services for—United States.
2. Family social work—United States.   I. Bryant, Donna M., 1951–
II. Graham, Mimi A.
HV894.I47   1993
362.1'968—dc20   93-30813
                                                    CIP

Contributors

Sandra Adams, PhD, OTR/L, Child Development Center, Sarasota, Florida

Catherine C. Ayoub, RN, EdD, Harvard Medical School, Boston, Massachusetts, and Harvard Graduate School of Education, Cambridge, Massachusetts

Stephen J. Bagnato, EdD, Department of Pediatrics, University of Pittsburgh School of Medicine, Children's Hospital of Pittsburgh, Pittsburgh, Pennsylvania

Donald B. Bailey, Jr., PhD, Frank Porter Graham Child Development Center, University of North Carolina at Chapel Hill, Chapel Hill, North Carolina

Debra Beckman, MS, CCC-S/LP, Easter Seal Society, Orlando, Florida

Rita Benn, PhD, Merrill Palmer Institute, Wayne State University, Detroit, Michigan

Kathleen Y. Bernier, MEd, Frank Porter Graham Child Development Center, University of North Carolina at Chapel Hill, Chapel, Hill, North Carolina

Donna M. Bryant, PhD, Frank Porter Graham Child Development Center, University of North Carolina at Chapel Hill, Chapel Hill, North Carolina

Richard M. Clifford, PhD, Carolina Institute for Child and Family Policy, Frank Porter Graham Child Development Center, University of North Carolina at Chapel Hill, Chapel Hill, North Carolina

Susan M. Duwa, MA, Family Systems Design Associates, Crystal Beach, Florida

Barbara F. Foster, PhD, SERVE (Regional Education Laboratory for the Southeast), Florida State University, Tallahassee, Florida

Ray E. Foster, PhD, Improvement Concepts, Inc., Tallahassee, Florida

Kim Galant, MS, CCC-S/LP, Department of Special Education, Florida State University, Tallahassee, Florida

James J. Gallagher, PhD, Frank Porter Graham Child Development Center, University of North Carolina at Chapel Hill, Chapel Hill, North Carolina

Mimi A. Graham, EdD, Center for Prevention and Early Intervention Policy, Florida State University, Tallahassee, Florida

Anita Zervigon Hakes, PhD, Center for Prevention and Early Intervention Policy, Florida State University, Tallahassee, Florida

John C. Hall, MSW, Florida TaxWatch, Tallahassee, Florida

Mary Frances Hanline, PhD, Department of Special Education, Florida State University, Tallahassee, Florida

Laura W. Henderson, PhD, Frank Porter Graham Child Development Center, University of North Carolina at Chapel Hill, Chapel Hill, North Carolina

Thomas T. Kochanek, PhD, Department of Special Education, Rhode Island College, Providence, Rhode Island

Paula Lalinde, MA, Parent Resource Organization of Florida, Miami, Florida

Helen Masin, PhD, PT, Mailman Center for Child Development, University of Miami, Miami, Florida

Susan M. Munson, PhD, Department of Special Education, Duquesne University, Pittsburgh, Pennsylvania

John T. Neisworth, PhD, Department of Educational and School Psychology and Special Education, Pennsylvania State University, University Park, Pennsylvania

Julius Richmond, MD, Department of Social Medicine, Harvard Medical School, Boston, Massachusetts

Linda Stone, PhD, Early Development Consulting, Winter Park, Florida

Ronald L. Taylor, EdD, College of Education, Florida Atlantic University, Boca Raton, Florida

Elsie R. Vergara, ScD, OTR/L, Department of Occupational Therapy, University of Florida, Gainesville, Florida

Douglas W. Wager, BA, Florida TaxWatch, Tallahassee, Florida

Michael Walsh, BA, Florida TaxWatch, Tallahassee, Florida

Conni Wells, Family Systems Design Associates, Tallahassee, Florida

Acknowledgments

We are often reminded that the need for a better understanding of early intervention is more than just a recommended platitude. Recently we regained contact with an old friend and learned of his family's trauma after the birth of a son with Down syndrome. Nurses and social workers repeatedly advised giving up the "retarded child" for adoption or institutionalizing him. The family was given no referrals for services. We might have expected such a situation in a small town years ago, but not in the major American city in which this child lived in 1992. Thus, we dedicate this book to Alexander and his family, with hope that tomorrow's families will be supported and have real, informed choices about early intervention, that the quality of lives of children will be enriched, that policy makers and providers will be better able to serve children effectively, and that society will benefit through improved cost-effectiveness of services.

We acknowledge our many colleagues who authored the chapters in this book. We appreciate the administrative support of the Florida State University Center for Prevention and Early Intervention Policy and the University of North Carolina at Chapel Hill's Frank Porter Graham Child Development Center. We owe a special thanks to Marie Butts, whose skill and constant positive attitude encouraged our efforts, and to Kathi, Debbie, Chris, and Ned, who helped with logistics.

Finally, we appreciate the encouragement and patience of our friends and family, especially Don and Alan.

DONNA M. BRYANT
MIMI A. GRAHAM

Preface

Motivated by broad concern for the state of our nation's children and by the enormous cost of delivering public services in an uncoordinated and fragmented fashion, both private and public institutions are urging reform in the way in which we serve children. The passage of Public Law 99-457, Part H, has been the impetus for major philosophical shifts in attitudes regarding early intervention—a renewed focus on prevention, emphasis on interagency linkages, a stronger push for inclusion, a focus on the need for more holistic services, and, most importantly, a shift to family-centered early intervention. Incorporating these changes into our current models of service delivery will require adaptations to the ways in which we currently treat infants and young children with special needs, and, in many cases, the creation of new configurations of services.

In building statewide, coordinated, early intervention service delivery systems for infants, toddlers, and young children, each state has been challenged to integrate and operationalize the knowledge we have gained from theory, research, and practical experience in conducting programs. Transforming this knowledge into "best practices" in early intervention is a challenge for each individual program director, for effective practices have changed over the years and are continually evolving. Many diverse populations of children and families are now being served and their individual differences must be taken into account. Each year, research studies and exemplary programs generate new knowledge on which to base revised practices.

Motivated by the momentum of Part H and the hope for better service delivery systems, many of us have struggled to identify standards for quality early intervention and have asked the following questions:

- Can typical child care programs be enhanced to effectively serve children with special needs?
- How do services of paraprofessionals compare to those of accredited interventionists?

- Can home-based models effect change as well as center-based models?
- Are programs focused on both the child and the family more effective than primarily child-focused interventions?
- Are inclusive programs appropriate for all levels of disabilities?
- Are therapies integrated within the classroom more effective than pull-out therapies?

As we continued to implement Part H in our states, additional questions arose. Who should be served? How should delay be measured? How many children would be eligible? What service delivery models should be used? How much would it cost? How can we pay for the services?

Ideally, the knowledge gained from research and from the experiences of model programs currently being implemented will guide the design and implementation of new programs, but changes are happening quickly in this field. In addition, information transmittal is not always timely or centralized enough to affect the field. We intend this book to express *the most current thinking* of researchers who are experienced and knowledgeable in each of the major areas in early intervention. The book also provides the context for services (i.e., evolving theory, definitional issues), as well as more detailed information about specific and frequently conducted services (i.e., classroom strategies and learning environments in center-based programs), and offers suggestions for future policy, both state and federal.

We have previously directed early intervention programs and conducted research within those programs. In 1990, we were asked by a state agency to conduct an extensive review of the early intervention literature, interview experts, and conduct site visits at over 100 well-known state and national programs. The purpose of that work was to identify indicators of quality early intervention and synthesize this knowledge in the most up-to-date form. We sought the answers to many of the above questions. Because the concept of early intervention has rapidly evolved, and continues to evolve, nailing down "best practices" has often been an elusive task. This book is intended to fill the real need for a resource that summarizes research and translates it into effective practice. Many authors have included recommendations from the recently completed survey of best practices in early intervention from the Council for Exceptional Children, Division for Early Childhood.

ORGANIZATION OF THE BOOK

The book is organized into 15 chapters. The intent of each chapter is to provide the research or theoretical basis of the specific area, including briefly discussing major issues, providing guidelines for translating research into practice, giving state-of-the-art examples of best practices in the specific area, and identifying the challenges that remain to be addressed.

Chapter 1 begins with an extensive overview of the evolution of early intervention from its historical context through the present to challenges that must be met in the future (e.g., changes in services necessitated by improved medical technology and "new" etiologies of disabilities, such as substance-exposed and HIV-positive infants). This chapter draws on the extensive experience of Julius Richmond, founder of Head Start, and the integrative thought of both Richmond and Catherine Ayoub.

While we were struggling with the question of "Who should be served?" Samuel J. Meisels sent us a comprehensive report written for Michigan by Rita Benn. Benn has been studying the relationship between risk conditions and disabilities and those factors that best predict which children might need early intervention services. She agreed to author Chapter 2 and address issues surrounding definitions: Which children should be served? How should "developmentally delayed" or "at risk" be defined? These are especially relevant issues as states determine how far to stretch their early intervention dollars.

Thomas Kochanek has used large data sets from the National Collaborative Perinatal Project to examine various pre- and postnatal predictors of risk. His multivariate understanding of the precursors of risk is particularly relevant to the screening issue. Chapter 3 provides a review of effective methodologies for screening, a discussion of early identification as prevention, and application of Kochanek's extensive knowledge of screening to public policy and program design.

Once a state finally determines which children to serve (Florida is now on its 10th version of an eligibility definition), the next step is to project the numbers of children. State budget and policy makers are very particular about wanting to know exact numbers before committing to a new entitlement program. Accurate and recent prevalence and utilization data on disabilities and risk conditions of infants and toddlers are almost nonexistent. Chapter 4 offers practical information for determining how many children will be eligible for services (prevalence) and how many of those eligible will use services (utilization). This information is critical as states cautiously try to project the numbers (and subsequent cost) of children who will participate in Part H entitlements. Ray and Barbara Foster clearly explain the processes used in several states for determining prevalence and they provide methodologies that can be tailored to the unique needs of individual states.

When Congress passed Public Law 99-457 it clearly intended families to have a central role in the decision making concerning their children and in the ongoing early intervention. Everyone espouses family-centered programs, but what are the dimensions for true family-driven systems? Chapter 5 provides a wealth of ideas for applying family-centered practices for local programs to state policy making. The chapter is coauthored by Susan Duwa, a trainer for family-centered programming; Conni Wells, a parent of a child with multiple special needs; and Paula Lalinde, Florida's spokeswoman for parents of children with disabilities.

Part H requires that family-directed assessments be an available service, yet most programs have little experience with this component of intervention. In Chapter 6, Donald Bailey, Jr., a prolific author regarding family-centered programming, and his colleague, Laura Henderson, provide a helpful overview of techniques available for helping families to assess their concerns and priorities.

Although early interventionists have provided screening, assessment, and evaluations for infants and toddlers for decades, programs are still terribly misguided about how to conduct developmentally appropriate evaluations and how to select instruments appropriate to the population to be assessed. In Chapter 7, Stephen Bagnato, John Neisworth, and Susan Munson synthesize many sources to provide concise best practice guidelines. Ronald Taylor's extensive work in reviewing the instruments for infants and toddlers provides guidance for the practitioner in Chapter 8.

Part H requires a shift in the way services are delivered to young children and their families. Chapter 9 covers the fundamental question in building program models: Which services, provided in what setting, seem to be most effective for various children? We have been early intervention program directors ourselves and have visited many others. With these experiences as background, we review the literature pertaining to various models of service delivery. This chapter should help states in justifying their designs for early intervention service delivery systems.

Mary Frances Hanline has published extensively on the topic of classroom integration and is well known for her advocacy and research in inclusive environments for children with disabilities. In Chapter 10, Hanline and her talented doctoral candidate, Kim Galant, provide the research basis for full inclusion and offer many strategies for creating inclusive learning environments.

Because children with risks and special needs can benefit so substantially from quality center-based intervention, and because more and more infants and young children are receiving some type of center-based care, Chapter 11 provides recommendations for key aspects of the learning environment—the structure and layout of the classroom and outdoor environment, ratios and group size, integration of therapies into the normal routine, maintenance of health and safety, ways to assess and improve the overall learning environment, and the caregiver's role in facilitating social and emotional development. We provide a research basis for each recommendation.

Provision of therapies is an integral component of early intervention; however, there is little agreement about how therapies should be provided.

Chapter 12 describes and references trends in contemporary therapies with infants and toddlers and their families, including positioning and handling; integration of therapies; appropriateness of individual and group therapies; strategies for fine motor, gross motor, and oral motor development; and interventions for special populations (i.e., HIV-infected and cocaine-exposed). A multidisciplinary team of pediatric therapists have authored the chapter— a physical therapist, Helen Masin; an oral motor therapist, Debra Beckman; an occupational therapist, Sandra Adams; and the primary author, an occupational and physical therapist, Elsie Vergara.

During this period of fiscal retrenchment across the nation, reliable cost information is critical to policy makers considering a new entitlement program as required in Part H. Chapter 13 presents a unit cost methodology of forecasting costs. The authors are not your typical early intervention researchers—John Hall and his colleagues from Florida TaxWatch are conservative, well-respected economic analysts and watchdogs of public expenditures. They teamed up with researchers from Florida State University to conduct a major study on the cost of implementing Part H and synthesize their findings in this chapter.

Once states determine costs, the next struggle involves determining how to finance the program(s). Chapter 14 reviews potential funding sources for Part H, highlighting those that are available but underused (i.e., Medicaid). Richard Clifford has written prolifically on finance issues in early intervention and has recently completed a study of financing options that are being or could be used for early intervention. Clifford and Kathleen Bernier together provide a helpful array of funding strategies.

A tremendous need exists for coordinated federal and state policies concerning early intervention, yet diverse state conditions affect the level of policy prescribed by the federal government. Federal agencies have tended to leave to the states most of the important issues concerning early intervention: definitional issues, interagency agreements, personnel preparation, standard setting, and many others. Chapter 15 summarizes the policy issues around Part H and the implications from both a state and national perspective, including unique commentary on the impact of diversity. A former director of special education in Washington and current director of the Carolina Policy Studies Program, James Gallagher, and colleagues have published over 30 reports in the past year about the states' progress in implementing Public Law 99-457. Gallagher provides insight into state and national policies surrounding Part H.

We believe that the contributors to this book are in the forefront of early childhood intervention, some in research, some in service delivery, some in policy development and analysis, and many in multiple arenas. We hope that these chapters will be useful for professionals, policy makers, and students preparing for these roles. Ultimately, we hope that our accumulated knowledge will benefit the children and families we strive to serve.

Donna M. Bryant
Mimi A. Graham

Foreword

Part H of Public Law 99-457 has almost completed its infancy, as legislation goes, and is beginning to take on the complex, demanding, and often frustrating challenges of toddlerhood. When first introduced in 1986, Public Law 99-457 was legislatively exciting, intellectually gratifying, and potentially revolutionary from a human services perspectives, although like all good ideas it kept up many of those who conceived it until late at night. Now it has been reauthorized, renamed (as Part H of the Individuals with Disabilities Education Act), given greater funding, and begun to be implemented. The potential of this legislation is immense, but still unrealized.

The early struggles confronting Part H were daunting. They included defining recipients, analyzing costs, understanding family involvement, developing interdisciplinary cooperation, determining how to respond to cultural and linguistic differences in service recipients and service providers, maximizing program flexibility, controlling program intrusiveness, developing personnel, and facilitating transitions to programs for older children. All of these tasks had to be addressed prior to implementation. Moreover, since no federal mandate could fit all 50 states, each state—relying on the common expertise of the field—had the responsibility of devising the most appropriate solution for its particular situation.

Creating a statewide service system is not a simple task. As the chapters in this book attest, all of the issues mentioned above have numerous variations, subtleties, and complexities. For example, the activities or services that can be classified as "early intervention" include phone monitoring, information and referral, periodic reassessment, brief home visits, activity centers, parent support groups, home-based intervention, center-based intervention, parent counseling, and specialized therapy. Nothing less than this whole spectrum constitutes early intervention. Obviously, there is tremendous diversity in this field, diversity that represents both a strength and liability. It is a strength because it enables services providers, policy makers, researchers, and parents to create individually relevant programs for infants and toddlers who differ significantly from one another. It is a liability because the inherent multiplicity of early intervention services, service providers, policies, and agencies makes planning and managing these programs extremely difficult.

Today, we see striking diversity in early intervention programs, but this was not always the case. Thirty years ago, when early intervention was first studied systematically, it was focused primarily on children from low-income families. These programs could be described as hierarchical in structure, child-focused in program, cognitive in curriculum, professional in service providers, and federal in funding. Today, the picture is very different. Rather than a hierarchy of authority and management, intervention programs in the 1990s rely upon multiple lines of authority and multiple child- and family-serving agencies. Our programs today are not focused just on the child; they are directed to the entire family situation in its "ecological niche." Curriculum is similarly less constrained, attending to infant mental health and parental empowerment, as well as to child outcome in multiple domains of development. Service providers too have changed to include a wide range of professionals, lay professionals, and indigenous community members. And funding is more often obtained from state and local sources than from the federal government. Many of these transformations are described in this volume; indeed, the authors and editors of this book have helped to bring about some of these changes. However, just as early developmental changes are ongoing and emergent, so the policy and practical changes that are being implemented must be seen as in process rather than established.

Of all the challenges lying ahead, perhaps none is greater than that of finding ways to harness the diversity of programs and people involved in the early intervention arena. We see this as parents try out new voices for themselves, while professionals begin to realize that their voices must change so that parents can be heard. We see this also as expectations of service planners and providers are changed to reflect the multiplicity of cultures and child-rearing practices of our diverse communities. But nowhere is this challenge more acute than in terms of the need for cooperation among the various agencies that manage the fiscal and policy infrastructure of early intervention. Issues of differing boundaries, mandates, technical language, and funding sources continue to pose barriers to the provision of needed services to children and families, as they did long before this legislation was conceived. Part H has sought to remedy these problems through its regulations and its requirements, but more problems than solutions have emerged. This is an area that calls for greater thought, energy, and commitment. Only after we have brought harmony and common purpose to the diverse strengths and resources of this field, can be begin to have confidence that the developmental trajectory of early intervention will be ensured into the next generation.

Samuel J. Meisels
University of Michigan

Contents

Implementing Early Intervention

CHAPTER 1

Evolution of Early
Intervention Philosophy

JULIUS RICHMOND
CATHERINE C. AYOUB

A review of the historical evolution of early intervention philosophy offers a perspective into both the accomplishments and the challenges that face the field today. An examination of where we have been—both of the successes and disappointments—can guide our course for an expanded concept of early intervention. Such a concept includes both a preventive orientation and a continuum of services ranging from tracking and family supports to complex medical out-of-home care.

Despite the almost universal notion that infants and young children deserve support, the field of early childhood intervention has been neither embraced uniformly nor supported consistently (Meisels & Shonkoff, 1990). It has experienced battles over program philosophy and models, goals, target populations, and service providers (Bricker & Slentz, 1988; Ferry, 1981). Yet in the last three decades, there have been dramatic advances that are now resulting in opportunities unimagined by the early pioneers in the field.

Early intervention concepts of the 1990s represent the accumulation and integration of these varied ideas and their transformation into practice across disciplines. Contributors to the field range from the academic child developmentalist to the pragmatic pediatric planner to the parents of the young disabled and at-risk child. Consequently, an exploration of historical roots includes theories and practices developed over the last two centuries in early childhood education, child development, pediatrics, and social welfare. Each of these areas represents a strand of theory and practice that is being woven into the early intervention philosophy. This chapter will explore the philosophical roots of early intervention, including the influence of early child-

1

hood education, health, support for children with disabilities, and the state of early intervention programs today.

PHILOSOPHICAL ROOTS OF EARLY INTERVENTION

The recognition of childhood as a unique period in life is a relatively new one; prior to the 17th century, children in Western Europe were viewed as miniature adults (Aries, 1962). However, once childhood was acknowledged as a qualitatively different developmental state from adult life, the intellectual roots of early childhood education and a view of the modern child began to develop.

European philosophers of the 17th and 18th centuries, such as Locke (1632–1704) and Rousseau (1712–1778), were strong advocates of the concept of the unspoiled nature of the child. Children were seen as natural, that is, without reason or sophisticated judgment. Thus, children depended upon kind, firm management, with reasoning and morality to evolve as they grew. The consequence of these beliefs was a movement toward a developmental approach to childhood that allowed for the unfolding of natural talents.

These beliefs are contrasted with the child-rearing practices in America during the 1700s and 1800s, practices that were dominated by a harsh puritan influence that focused on spiritual salvation and recommended rigid discipline in education to counter the "sinful" tendencies of the young child (Greven, 1973). Our current philosophical approach to young children contains elements of both of these contrasting sets of beliefs.

THE INFLUENCE OF EARLY CHILDHOOD EDUCATION

The early childhood educational movement was one of the major contributors to the concepts and practice of early intervention. The development of formal kindergartens by Friedrich Froebel in Germany in the mid-1800s was a landmark beginning for early childhood educational programs. Froebel's philosophy was based on traditional religious values and a commitment to the importance of learning through supervised play (Osborn, 1980). He believed in the use of play as the natural activity of the young child and directed the child toward symbolic development by providing him carefully designed "gifts" (toys) and "occupations" (activities) with which to play. Kindergartens offered a form of early education that was to appeal to the middle class. These Froebelian ideas stimulated the growth of experimental kindergartens first across Germany and then throughout the United States in the late 19th century.

By the turn of the century there were over 5,000 kindergartens in the

United States (Osborn, 1980). This growth in early education was part of a complex series of social changes through which the social system for rearing children was renegotiated in the 19th century (White & Buka, 1987). A number of professions emerged dealing with young children and their growth, education, and well-being. Some of them began studies of children and formed a grass-roots movement toward child study.

In the early 1900s, early childhood researchers, such as G. Stanley Hall and John Dewey, proposed an alternative developmental approach to the Froebelian kindergarten, one that searched for empirically derived principles based on systematic observations, data collection, and analysis (White & Buka, 1987). Educational centers for young children became sites for the study of childhood itself and a number were founded for this purpose. The debate between the goals of kindergarten as the center for academic achievement versus the site for the nurturing of noncompetitive social and emotional development was begun. Eventually, Dewey's progressive kindergarten replaced many of the Froebelian kindergartens; the progressive approach emphasized the need for the child to reproduce home and neighborhood through play in order to learn to enter society.

The other early educational contribution to the development of early intervention was the concept of the nursery school. Like kindergartens, nursery schools originated in Europe. The emphasis of these early programs was on providing comprehensive preventive services to meet the social, physical, emotional, and intellectual needs of young children (Meisels & Shonkoff, 1990; White & Buka, 1987). The first nursery school in London, established by the MacMillians in 1910, began with a health clinic. Many nursery schools, particularly those developed by Maria Montessori in Rome, were aimed at poor, mentally retarded, urban children; her method, based on nongraded classrooms, individualization of instruction, sequential ordering of materials, sensory and motor training, and the abolition of punishment, soon was applied to nondisabled children as well (Goodman, 1974).

By the early 1930s, as many as 200 nursery schools existed in the United States (Osborn, 1980). Over half were associated with colleges and universities and housed some of the most productive child development laboratories of the time; the other half of the programs were run as private schools or were sponsored by child welfare agencies. By the mid-1900s, three groups of early childhood programs had developed: (1) family-oriented preschools, largely middle class, aimed at providing group experiences for children and child study for parents; (2) welfare-oriented preschools, directed toward working-class families with a central concern with family functioning, but a spoken interest in providing educational and other social services to children; and (3) research-oriented preschools, largely housed in universities, pursuing studies that were at times within and at times outside of the interests of American nursery school children (White & Buka, 1987).

In the 1930s and 1940s, there were several large, publicly supported nursery school projects. During the Great Depression, the United States government funded the Work Projects Administration (WPA) Nursery for children 2 to 6 years of age. The 3,000 nursery schools across the country had two purposes: to offer financial support for unemployed teachers, and to support the well-being of the children of unemployed parents. During World War II, the Lanham Act Nursery Schools assisted women working to contribute to the war effort. Neither program had as its primary goal meeting the needs of children, but rather assisting adults to work outside the home in times of economic and national crisis. Consequently, the end of the Depression and the end of the war signaled the end of each of the respective nursery school programs.

THE INFLUENCE OF MENTAL HEALTH AND PSYCHOLOGY

Education and mental health have been linked since the early 20th century. Special education, in particular, brought physical and mental well-being and learning into the same arena. Seguin's work in Paris in the early 1800s emphasized the importance of early intervention and teaching in the lives of disabled children (Kanner, 1960). Seguin migrated to the United States and influenced the development of residential institutions for the mentally retarded at the turn of the century. A number of Seguin's principles still serve as a foundation for intervention today. These include his beliefs that children learn from real things, that perceptual training should precede training for concept development, and that even the most disabled child has some capacity for learning; he believed in giving attention to the whole child and to the notion that observation of the child was the cornerstone of the child's education. How familiar these principles seem today.

However, the development of special education programs in public schools was slow and served only a few children. It was not until after World War II that the interest in developmentally vulnerable youngsters became a national concern. In 1946, the United States Office of Education developed the Section for Exceptional Children. By the late 1950s, both state and federal legislation were beginning to promote better access to special education for the population at large.

One impetus for the development of systems of care for both physically and socially vulnerable young children was the developmental studies of the 1950s and 1960s. After World War II, developmental theorists expanded the view of childhood and of the potential negative consequences of early difficulties. The works of Harlow and his colleagues (1959), Spitz (1945), and Provence and Lipton (1962) focused attention on the adverse consequences of deprivation in early human relationships. John Bowlby's (1959) empirical findings set the stage for a series of continuing studies on young children and their attachments (Ainsworth, 1969; Ainsworth, Blehar, Waters, & Wall, 1978; Crittenden & Ainsworth, 1989).

At the same time, the notions about normative development were also changing. The nature versus nurture debate continued among child developmentalists, such as pediatrician and psychologist Arnold Gesell (1929), a strong believer in the primacy of biologically determined maturation, and John Watson, an eloquent spokesperson for the behavioral counterargument. The elaboration of this debate by both sides pointed out the differences between maturing children and their adult counterparts. The 1950s and early 1960s ushered in the "cognitive revolution" of Jean Piaget, which helped to delineate the cognitive transformations of thought in childhood (Piaget, 1952). In addition, theorists including Erik Erikson and Harry Stack Sullivan were elaborating on stages of emotional development in childhood (Erikson, 1950; Sullivan, 1953). As a result, infancy and early childhood were beginning to be perceived as a unique and important time in the human life cycle.

THE INFLUENCE OF HEALTH PROGRAMS

At the turn of the century, in another important arena those concerned with the physical health of children began to focus on infant mortality, poor physical health, and the welfare of children, particularly the poor. However, in contrast to educational systems, an accepted responsibility of the state and federal government, health care services were and still remain a conglomeration of public and private resources and service delivery networks. In spite of this fact, the American political system has, through legislation, indicated that the care and protection of children is a public responsibility. The Children's Bureau, established by Congress in the Department of Labor in 1912, was mandated to attend to the welfare of children, particularly those "who were abnormal or subnormal or suffering from physical or mental ills" (Bradbury, 1962, cited in Lesser, 1985).

For the first time, the Children's Bureau acknowledged a federal responsibility for children and laid the foundation for what was to become a series of federal programs assisting children. The Children's Bureau conducted studies in a number of areas relevant to early intervention including child care, health in preschool children, care of children with disabilities, mental retardation, and institutional care (Lesser, 1985). These data helped highlight the unmet needs of children and, as a result, the 1930 White House Conference that focused on child health and protection recommended that federal funds be made available to states to establish "crippled children's" programs. These programs were to reflect cooperation among medical, educational, social welfare, and vocational rehabilitation agencies. Conference recommendations set in motion a multidisciplinary model with the potential to provide a comprehensive array of services to disabled children.

The Social Security Act of 1935 reinforced the responsibility of the federal government to assure the well-being of children and their mothers. Title V of the Social Security Act specifically mandated three resource allocation and program development components that form the foundation of the national health policy still active today.

Part I of Title V authorized financial assistance to states to develop services to promote the general health of mothers and children. This legislation supported immunization and well-baby clinics, school health programs, public health nursing services, and nutrition and health education. Part II created the first federal–state partnership through matching funds aimed at delivering medical services to prevent and ameliorate "crippling" diseases. Each state was required to promote cooperative systems between health and social welfare institutions in order to implement comprehensive case finding, diagnosis, treatment, and follow-up. Part III authorized funding to state welfare programs to develop systems of care and protection for children who were homeless, dependent, neglected, and at risk of delinquency.

Despite the 1935 legislation, prior to the 1950s there were virtually no studies of children growing up in poverty (Richmond, 1989). It was not until 1967 that provisions were made to improve the quality and accessibility of medical services for poor children through the Early and Periodic Screening, Diagnosis, and Treatment program (EPSDT). As part of the Medicaid provisions of the Social Security Act, this legislation was designed to assure early identification of preventable problems among the nation's poor youth. One of the primary aims of EPSDT was to break the cycle of poverty.

The last three decades have seen incredible changes in the conceptualization and implementation of programs for vulnerable infants and young children. Early childhood intervention entered the modern era in the 1960s with three central themes: (1) a belief in the responsibility of society to provide care and protection for young children; (2) a commitment to the special needs of children who are particularly vulnerable due to a chronically disabling condition or as a consequence of growing up in poverty; and (3) a sense that prevention is better than treatment and that earlier intervention is more effective than later remediation (Meisels & Shonkoff, 1990). The times ushered in the optimistic pursuit of the goal of creating genuine change in the life of the young child.

THE INFLUENCE OF HEAD START

In 1964, Caldwell and Richmond conducted an empirical test of the possibility that an enriched group-care environment might enhance the development of infants and toddlers. In 1965, the most far-reaching experiment of the decade, Head Start, began as an 8-week pilot for children in 2,500 communities. The authorizing legislation, the Economic Opportunity Act of 1964, did not mention Head Start (Richmond, Stipek, & Zigler, 1979); however, Sargent Shriver, director of the Office of Economic Opportunity, appointed a committee to advise him on what programs for poor children should look like. In early 1965, the committee submitted a seven-page report recommending a Head Start program for disadvantaged preschool children. By June 1965, 2,400 Head Start programs had been approved, to serve 500,000 4- and 5-year-old children (Richmond, 1966; Richmond et al., 1979).

Head Start pioneered the practice of intervention aimed at both the child and family. In addition to significant benefits for children, many parents worked their way from poverty to self-sufficiency through the parent involvement component of the Head Start program. Head Start was designed as a comprehensive service program that relied upon the expertise of a broad array of professionals and paraprofessionals to provide health, education, and social services in a coordinated system. Although Head Start was funded federally, it was implemented locally through direct funding to communities (Richmond & Beardslee, 1988). Almost from the outset, Head Start was concerned that the program started too late in the life of the young child. The founders of Head Start knew that a 6-week program or even a 1-year program aimed at young children could not eliminate the impact of continuing poverty on the child.

Initially, Head Start did not serve children with disabilities; it was not until the early 1970s that 14 pilots were initiated to mainstream children with disabilities. Head Start's success in serving disabled children eventually contributed to the inspiration of the 1986 Amendments to the Education of the Handicapped Act (Public Law 99-457). In particular, the concepts of parental involvement and family support evolved from Head Start (Zigler & Muenchow, 1992).

Head Start programs have survived and grown throughout the last three decades in spite of some relatively negative evaluations in the 1960s and the early 1970s (White, Day, Freeman, Hantman, & Messenger, 1972). Later, Lazar and Darlington (1982) cast a more positive light on Head Start by finding long-term benefits in early education when assessed in a more ecological framework.

Early Head Start evaluations were limited studies of the cognitive (IQ) functioning of children examined over time through meta-analysis of many varied Head Start programs. The result was a narrow and linear interpretation of the effects of Head Start programs. The controversy over the goals and design of such evaluations and ensuing discussions have served to guide later programs (Besherov & Hartle, 1987; Kotelchuck & Richmond, 1987). Some of the lessons learned through the evaluations of Head Start in the last two decades include (1) the need for multiple measurements that examine program effects on health, nutrition, cognitive development, social services, and parental involvement; (2) the acknowledgment of the diversity of programs and populations; and (3) the development of methodological and statistical techniques to assure a multifaceted, ecological approach to assessment. The findings that health, diet, parent education, and child self-esteem and cognitive abilities can improve through Head Start exemplify the importance of intervention across a range of domains (McKey et al., 1985; Zigler & Valentine, 1979). In spite of these findings, the 1960s goal to create a single program to eliminate welfare dependency, academic failure, delinquent behavior, and other social consequences of poverty, is an unrealistic one. However, Head Start was and remains the evolving prototype for the delivery of services to preschool children and serves as a model for program development with both younger and older children.

POLICY AND RESEARCH AFTER 1970

Out of the optimism and idealism of the 1960s emerged the 1970s focus and commitment to the needs of children with disabilities. Federally supported demonstration and outreach programs grew at rapid rates through both the Bureau of Education for the Handicapped and the Division of Maternal and Child Health. Early childhood special education became a higher priority and departments of education in many states began to develop guidelines for certification for teachers of special-needs children (Stile, Abernathy, Pettibone, & Wachtel, 1984). In 1972, Head Start centers were mandated to save at least 10% of their enrollment for children with identified disabilities through Public Law 92-424. The Division for Early Childhood was established in 1973, and by 1974, the government had designated separate funding for state implementation grants to assist states in developing services for preschool children with disabilities.

The Education for All Handicapped Children Act (Public Law 94-142), passed in 1975, established the right to free and appropriate public education for school-age children, regardless of the presence of a disability. The far-reaching legislation spelled out the mandate for Individualized Education Plans (IEPs) and delineated the principles of due process in the planning and implementation of these educational services. The enactment of this law placed responsibility for rehabilitative services for children soundly within the public education system. However, in the 1970s there was no sweeping mandate to extend such services to the very young. Although Public Law 94-142 allowed services from birth to age 21, it only mandated services from ages 5 through 18 years. Funds could be drawn down for services for younger children (birth to age 5), if desired.

In addition, the 1970s brought a new focus on child protection and child abuse prevention. By 1974, all states had mandatory child abuse reporting laws, and state welfare departments began to develop systems for identification and intervention for maltreated children, most of whom were under age 5. Early research in the field appeared in 1977 just as the first small group of perinatal prevention programs were founded (Ayoub & Pfeifer, 1977; Gabinet, 1979; Gladstone, 1975). Gray, Cutler, Dean, and Kempe (1977) provided support for the effectiveness of early intervention by demonstrating that not only were delivery room and postpartum observations accurate predictors of subsequent high-risk parenting behavior, but also that intervention tended to reduce the frequency of abusive incidents in at-risk families. Together, the two movements, one for early intervention with disabled infants and the other advocating supportive intervention for infants and toddlers in socially vulnerable families, paved the way for the expanded efforts of the 1980s.

Prior to the 1970s, the majority of existing theoretical models used as the basis for research in risk and resilience were linear/main effects models that explored links between single risk factors and outcomes. In 1975, Sameroff and Chandler proposed a psychobiological model of development that was transactional; it took into account the interrelationships among multiple dynamic systems—biological, psychological, interpersonal, family, community—and the compensatory processes that might counter potential risks to the child's health or well-being arising in any one of these subsystems. Such a transactional or ecological model viewed the multiple transactions among environmental forces, caregiver, and child as dynamic, reciprocal contributions to the events and outcomes of child development.

In the 1980s, this theoretical model was applied to understanding the interaction between risk factors and outcomes for a number of different risk groups, including children who are both physically vulnerable and those who are at increased social risk (Cicchetti, 1989; Rutter, 1990). This ecological approach gave impetus to the notion that service delivery systems that targeted the child alone were missing the rich and complex interactions between child, parents, extended family, and the larger community that together influenced outcomes over time. The movement to reframe the role of the family and to embrace the concepts of multidisciplinary, multisystem integration of services so strongly put forth late in the 1980s is grounded in these theoretical concepts of risk and resiliency.

The ecological model was further supported by the findings of several longitudinal population studies (Block & Block, 1980; Broman, Nichols, & Kennedy, 1975; Garmezy, Masten, & Tellegen, 1984; Werner & Smith, 1982) that explored the interaction between a multiplicity of risk factors and resiliency across the life span. These studies further confirmed the importance of the child–family–community interactions in determining child outcomes.

However, in contrast to this expanding conceptualization of risk and the benefit of intervention early in the life of the vulnerable child, the federal government retrenched during this decade. Politically conservative forces worked to reduce investment of federal resources in social programs and to shift the responsibility for such efforts, including the financial burden, to the states. A number of domestic programs for children and families began to be dismantled and others were restructured in light of reduced funding (Schorr, 1988). Funds for states were consolidated into block grants. For example, eight programs whose previous support was independent were combined into a single block grant to include crippled children, maternal and child health, and genetic and disease services; prevention programs for lead poisoning, sudden infant death, and adolescent pregnancy; hemophilia treatment; and Supplemental Security Income for children with disabilities.

This consolidation pitted categorical programs against each other in a struggle for their share of the federal dollar and resulted in the very splitting and fragmentation of service providers that the ecological approach sought to reduce. The survival of early childhood intervention programs in spite of the federal policies of the 1980s attests to the depth of early intervention's political and social strength and the breadth of its constituency groups. It is quite extraordinary that programs like Head Start survived and grew, and that the basic principles of early intervention for vulnerable children and their families gained national support as conceptualized in the Education for All Handicapped Children Act Amendments of 1986 (Public Law 99-457).

CHALLENGES OF THE 1990s

Public Law 99-457 is the most important legislation enacted for the developmentally vulnerable young child. It called for a statewide, comprehensive, coordinated, multidisciplinary, interagency program of early intervention for all handicapped infants and their families. These discretionary services for infants and toddlers are not mandated by law, but all states elected to participate in planning activities.

The key components of this federal initiative that have framed the present early intervention efforts into the 1990s are the operationalizing of the central role of the family through Individualized Family Service Plans (IFSPs); the interagency coordination and collaboration of health and education services; and a multidisciplinary, holistic approach to services for infants, toddlers, and their families. Although states have considerable leeway in defining the population of children to be served, there is little financial incentive for creating an entitlement program. Although there was a 22% increase in funding from 1992 to 1993, states must still assume the lion's share of the cost. Services are required to be delivered by the highest-level professional, ruling out paraprofessional, less costly service delivery models. Procedural safeguards for families create an adversarial, legalistic aspect, yet another disincentive for states.

The reauthorization of this initiative in the 1990s brings with it both hope and frustration. Zervigon-Hakes (1991) summarized the current state of affairs:

> Part H of P.L. 99-457 challenges basic policy structures because it requires that services be coordinated; however, services are defined by program bound budgets, laws and delivery systems. It also required services to be comprehensive, but currently eligibility is categorical, focusing on a single risk dimension (e.g., poverty, type of disability). Interagency collaboration is called for, but legal barriers exist making the blending of funds and programs across agencies very difficult. This situation is exacerbated by agency culture barriers and fiscal and resource differences which perpetuate turf guarding. A multidisciplinary approach to child and family evaluation and service delivery is essential to best practices, but historically, early intervention has largely been delivered as a medical model or sometimes an educational model. Cross disciplinary training is required but training, certification, and standards are discipline specific. Few university courses or professional standards focus on infants, toddlers, and their families. Early intervention services are supposed to be available but programs for infants and toddlers are not readily available statewide and many states are experiencing a fiscal recession. (p. 2)

Intervention models for the 1990s must account for a greater diversity and integration of needs. Part H assumed that early intervention services would be overlaid onto existing service delivery systems. However, considerable variation exists in the infrastructure of services and in the amount of integration that has actually occurred. States in which service delivery systems for child care, health care, housing, or foster care are weak have demanded that connecting service delivery systems be reconceptualized, augmented, or reconstructed in tandem with the Part H system.

It is not surprising that almost a dozen states are reluctant to commit to 5th year entitlement services and have requested a second extended 4th year of participation in Part H. The prescriptive nature of the federal entitlement, during a recession and without implementation dollars, leaves many states in a quandary about how to act.

We enter the 1990s with the knowledge that there continue to be tremendous health and social issues that must be considered in any plan for systems of service delivery for vulnerable young children. Among the most salient influences on the early intervention philosophy in this decade are a group of health needs often labeled the "new morbidities" of childhood (Vanderpool & Richmond, 1990); these include health issues that are intrinsically linked to environmental and sociodemographic factors such as issues of poverty, homelessness, lack of health care and related services, and the emergence of violence and drug abuse as major social problems in the society at large.

Of these, poverty continues to be the most potent and potentially mitigating factor contributing to poor outcomes (Vanderpool & Richmond, 1990). Children under age 5 are more likely to be poor than any other group (U.S. Census, 1990). Poverty increases the probability that a pregnancy will end in the delivery of a low-birth-weight baby (Wise & Meyers, 1988), and poverty is correlated with decreased prenatal care (Wise & Meyers, 1988), teenage pregnancy, and increased incidence of AIDS (Sealing, 1989), violence, and child abuse (Pelton, 1978). Not only is the poverty rate higher in female-headed, single-parent families, but poverty lasts much longer in these homes than it does in two-parent families (Ellwood, 1988).

The implications of poverty for children of the 1990s are tremendous. The youth of tomorrow are likely to be poorly educated, non-English-speaking, and located in metropolitan areas. A larger percentage of children will be of minority group background, due to high birth rates and immigration. Children will be more likely to be raised in a single-parent family and increasingly large numbers of children will spend large amounts of time outside their homes in child care facilities. These predictions make the need for high-quality, family-focused programs for young children imperative. At a time when need is increasing and resources are being reduced, communities must work together to coordinate services for vulnerable children.

In addition, multiple risk conditions exist in populations of young children with established conditions conservatively targeted for core early intervention services, for example, congenital disorders, neurological abnormalities, sensory impairments, severe prematurity, and documented moderate developmental delay. A study by Zervigon-Hakes (1991) found that of the infants and toddlers with established conditions in Florida, 66% had additional biological risks, 39.6% had further environmental risks, and 36% had family stressors above and beyond their identified handicapping condition. This multiplicity of problems, coupled with poverty, has tremendous implications for the design and implementation of early intervention systems for the future. Delivering effective interventions within complex family and community systems is difficult, but must be accomplished to best meet the needs of vulnerable children. The development of service delivery models over the next decade will demand a dedication to young children at biological and environmental risk. In addition, systems will require flexibility that enables the coordination of multiple services and the sensitivity to develop an individually tailored network of interventions for each child and family.

SUMMARY

Five major shifts have occurred in early intervention philosophy and practice over the last several decades that will help support our efforts in the 1990s.

The first is a movement from a focus on rehabilitation to a demand for prevention. This new conceptualization of service delivery requires basic changes in the structure and philosophy of developing early intervention systems. It directs agencies to move from a categorical approach to disability toward an understanding of the transaction of multiple risk conditions. Although a number of states have accepted this philosophy in principle, it has been more difficult in practice to serve children with HIV or substance abuse exposure unless a disability is present and identified.

Prevention by its very nature requires that more children be included in service offerings. However, it also affords the opportunity to coordinate separate but similar systems of care. For example, child abuse prevention programs and early intervention programs, often separated both physically and conceptually by narrow categorical focus, could share knowledge and resources. The cost–benefit data for the development of these kinds of partnerships is persuasive, but both federal and state governments are slow to commit resources to what appears to be an expanded endeavor.

The second major philosophical shift has been from a focus on interventions by discipline to a more holistic perspective on the child and family. Now instead of dividing the child according to a single need or specific service—medical, educational, psychological—there is a movement to operationalize integrated service delivery. Head Start was one of the first programs to conceptualize this type of programing, integrating education, child care, health services, and parent education (Zigler & Muenchow, 1992). Zigler's concept of the full-service school, a central institution that could serve as the hub of all core services for children and families in the 21st century, is a key example of an expansion of the Head Start philosophy. Caldwell (1991) has called this integration "educare" to clearly denote a vision of the meshing of education, nurturance, and health care for future generations.

This integrative shift has provided the foundation for a third important change in early intervention practices—the movement from single agency service to coordinated systems of service delivery. For example, schools used to be the primary educational institutions for the nation. Now community-based federal initiatives such as Head Start and Part H of Public Law 99-457, child care block grant, EPSDT, Title XX, and Chapter 1-funded prekindergarten programs for the disadvantaged are delivering services in most communities. Coordinating these service systems will continue to be a challenge.

Fourth, the family–professional partnership is replacing the child-focused model of early intervention. This expanded emphasis on family is based on the ecological and family systems philosophy that the child's needs are connected to those who are central in his/her care and nurturance. Federal initiatives such as Even Start, Head Start, and Healthy Start are examples of family-focused endeavors. Part H has also been a catalyst for the family-centered movement; however there are still obstacles to its expansion across other programs. For example, although birth to age 3 services are required to be family-focused, once they are under the umbrella of Public Law 94-142, the family focus is not ensured and the child again becomes the center of the service delivery system.

Finally, there has been a slow, but important movement away from a linear, single focus on cognitive outcomes and a tendency to use methodologies that offer only a summative synthesis of information toward evaluation methods that use broad outcome measures. Again, Head Start research and evaluation is a good example of the progression from early, IQ-driven meta-analyses to more ecological models of the examination of multiple facets of health, emotional, developmental, and educational outcomes (Kotelchuck & Richmond, 1987). Although such evaluation methodology requires the management of more variables and complex statistical methods, it has begun to yield varied and promising results.

The next generation of early intervention models for the 1990s must provide greater flexibility for a wider diversity of both needs and service delivery strategies. Although states want to invest in prevention and early intervention efforts, the financial responsibility of an ever-increasing at-risk and disabled population through entitlement is daunting. Federal assistance and flexibility regarding the entitlement could serve as tremendous incentives to proceed with the gradual development of comprehensive and integrated early intervention systems.

The roots of the concepts of early intervention extend back through the humanistic, scholarly, social, and political philosophies of the last 200 years. In recent decades, the planning and implementation of systems of service delivery have been accelerated through the culmination of these various systems of beliefs and development of bases of empirical knowledge. The application of this knowledge has been targeted at building service delivery systems. Early intervention philosophies are concepts that continue to evolve because of a commitment to reducing the vulnerability of young children in our society.

REFERENCES

Ainsworth, M. (1969). Object relations dependency and attachment: A theoretical review of the mother–infant relationship. *Child Development, 40,* 969–1025.

Ainsworth, M., Blehar, M., Waters, E., & Wall, S. (1978). *Patterns of attachment: A psychological study of the strange situation.* Hillsdale, NJ: Erlbaum.

Aries, P. (1962). *Centuries of childhood: A social history of family life* (R. Baldick, Trans.). New York: Random House.

Ayoub, C., & Pfeifer, D. (1977). The prophylaxis of child abuse and neglect—An approach. *Child Abuse and Neglect, 1,* 71–75.

Besherov, D., & Hartle, T. (1987). Head Start: Making a popular program work. *Pediatrics, 79,* 440–441.

Block, J. H., & Block, J. (1980). The role of ego-control and ego resiliency in the organization of behavior. In W. A. Collins (Ed.), *Minnesota symposia on child psychology* (Vol. 13, pp. 39–101). Hillsdale, NJ: Erlbaum.

Bowlby, J. (1959). *Attachment and loss: Vol. I. Attachment.* New York: Basic Books.

Bricker, D., & Slentz, K. (1988). Personnel preparation: Handicapped infants. In M.C. Wang, M. Reynolds, & H. Walberg (Eds.), *Handbook of special education: Research and practice* (Vol. 3, pp. 319–345). Elmsford, NY: Pergamon Press.

Broman, S., Nichols, P., & Kennedy, W. (1975). *Preschool IQ: Prenatal and early developmental correlates.* Hillsdale, NJ: Erlbaum.

Caldwell, B. (1991). Educare: New product, new future. *Developmental and Behavioral Pediatrics, 12*(3), 199–204.

Caldwell, B., & Richmond, J. (1964). Programmed day care for the very young child—A preliminary report. *Journal of Marriage and Family, 26,* 481–488.

Cicchetti, D. (1989). How research on child maltreatment has informed the study of child development: Perspective from developmental psychopathology. In D. Cicchetti & V. Carlson (Eds.), *Child maltreatment* (pp. 377–431). Cambridge, MA: Cambridge University Press.

Crittenden, P., & Ainsworth, M. (1989). Child maltreatment and attachment theory. In D. Cicchetti & V. Carlson (Eds.), *Child maltreatment* (pp. 432–464). Cambridge, MA: Cambridge University Press.

Ellwood, D. (1988). *Poor support: Poverty in the American family.* New York: Basic Books.

Erikson, E. (1950). *Childhood and society.* New York: W. W. Norton.

Ferry, P. (1981). On growing new neurons: Are early intervention programs effective? *Pediatrics, 67,* 38–41.

Gabinet, L. (1979). Prevention of child abuse and neglect in an inner-city population: II. The program and the results. *Child Abuse and Neglect, 3*(3/4), 809–817.

Garmezy, N., Masten, A., & Tellegen, A. (1984). The study of stress and competence in children: A building block for developmental psychopathology. *Child Development, 55,* 97–111.

Gesell, A. (1929). *Infancy and human growth.* New York: Macmillan.

Gladstone, R. (1975). Preventing the abuse of little children: The parent's center project for the study and prevention of child abuse. *American Journal of Orthopsychiatry, 45*(3), 372–381.

Goodman, L. (1974). Montessori education for the handicapped: The methods—the research. In L. Mann & D. Sabatino (Eds.), *The second review of special education* (pp. 153–191). Philadelphia, PA: JSE.

Gray, J., Cutler, C., Dean, J., & Kempe, H. (1977). Prediction and prevention of child abuse and neglect. *Child Abuse and Neglect, 1*(1), 45–53.

Greven, P. (Ed.). (1973) *Child rearing concepts 1628–1861.* Itasca, IL: F. E. Peacock.

Harlow, H., & Zimmerman, R. (1959). Affectional response in the infant monkey. *Science, 130,* 421–432.

Kanner, L. (1960). Itard, Seguin, Howe—Three pioneers in the education of retarded children. *American Journal of Mental Deficiency, 65*(2), 2–10.

Kotelchuck, M., & Richmond, J. (1987). Head Start: Evolution of a successful comprehensive child development program. *Pediatrics, 79*(3), 441–444.

Lazar, I., & Darlington, R. (1982). Lasting effects of early education: A report from the Consortium for Longitudinal Studies. *Monographs of the Society for Research in Child Development, 47* (2–3, Serial No. 195).

Lesser, A. (1985). The origin and development of maternal and child health programs in the United States. *American Journal of Public Health, 75,* 590–598.

McKey, R., Condelli, L., Ganson, H., Barrett, B. J., McConkey, C., & Plant, M. C. (1985). *The impact of Head Start on children, families, and communities: Final report of the Head Start evaluation synthesis and utilization project* (U.S. Department of Health and Human Services Pub. No. [OHDS] 85-31193). Washington, DC: U.S. Government Printing Office.

Meisels, S., & Shonkoff, J. (Eds.). (1990). *Handbook of early childhood intervention.* New York: Cambridge University Press.

Osborn, D. (1980). *Early childhood education in historical perspective.* Athens, GA: Education Associates.

Pelton, L. (1978). Child abuse and neglect: The myth of classlessness. *American Journal of Orthopsychiatry, 48,* 608–617.

Piaget, J. (1952). *The origins of intelligence.* New York: International Universities Press.

Provence, S., & Lipton, R. (1962). *Infants in institutions.* New York: International Universities Press.

Richmond, J. (1966). Communities in action: A report on Project Head Start. *Pediatrics, 37*(6), 905–912.

Richmond, J. (1989). Early education. *Bulletin of the New York Academy of Medicine, 65,* 307–318.

Richmond, J., & Beardslee, W. (1988). Resiliency: Research and practical implications for pediatricians. *Journal of Developmental and Behavioral Pediatrics, 9*(3), 157–163.

Richmond, J., Stipek, D., & Zigler, E. (1979). A decade of Head Start. In E. Zigler & J. Valentine (Eds.), *Project Head Start: A legacy of the war on poverty* (pp. 135–152). New York: Free Press.

Rutter, M. (1990). Psychosocial resilience and protective mechanisms. In J. Rolf, A. Masten, D. Cicchetti, K. Nuechterlein, & S. Weintraub (Eds.), *Risk and protective factors in the development of psychopathology.* New York: Cambridge University Press.

Sameroff, A., & Chandler, M. (1975). Reproductive risk and the continuum of caretaking causality. In F. Horowitz, M. Hetherington, S. Scarr-Salapatek, & G. Siegel (Eds.), *Review of child development research* (Vol. 4, pp. 187–244). Chicago, IL: University of Chicago Press.

Schorr, L. (1988). *Within our reach.* New York: Doubleday.

Sealing, P. (1989). *Profile of child health in United States.* Alexandria, VA: National Association of Child Hospital and Related Institutions.

Spitz, R. (1945). Hospitalism: An inquiry into the genesis of psychiatric conditions in early childhood. *Psychoanalytic Study of the Child, 1,* 53–74.

Stile, S., Abernathy, S., Pettibone, T., & Wachtel, W. (1984). Training and certification for early childhood special education personnel: A six-year follow-up study. *Journal of the Division for Early Childhood, 11,* 66–73.

Sullivan, H. S. (1953). *The interpersonal theory of psychiatry.* New York: W. W. Norton.

U.S. Bureau of the Census. (1992). *Workers with low earnings 1964–1990.* Washington, DC: U.S. Department of Commerce.

Vanderpool, N., & Richmond, J. (1990). Child health in the United States: Prospects for the 1990s. In G. Omenn (Ed.), *Annual review of public health 1990* (Vol. 11, pp. 185–205). Palo Alto, CA: Annual Reviews.

Werner, E., & Smith, R. (1982). *Vulnerable but not invincible: A longitudinal study of resilient children and youth.* New York: McGraw-Hill.

White, S., & Buka, S. (1987). Early education: Programs, traditions, and policies. In E. Rothkopf (Ed.), *Review of research in education* (Vol. 14, pp. 43–91). Washington, DC: American Educational Research Association.

White, S., Day, M. C., Freeman, P. A., Hantman, S., & Messenger, K. (1972). *Federal programs for young children: Review and recommendations* (3 vols.). Washington, DC: U.S. Government Printing Office.

Wise, P., & Meyers, A. (1988). Poverty and child health, *Pediatric Clinics of North America, 35*(6), 1169–1186.

Zervigon-Hakes, A. (1991). *Florida's cost implementation study for P.L. 99-457, Part H, infants and toddlers: Phase II findings: Executive summary.* Tallahassee, FL: Center for Prevention and Early Intervention Policy, Florida State University, and Florida Department of Education.

Zigler, E., & Muenchow, S. (1992). *Head Start: The inside story of America's most successful educational experiment* (pp. 1–27; 211–246). New York: Basic Books.

Zigler, E., & Valentine, J. (Eds.). (1979). *Project Head Start: A legacy of the war on poverty.* New York: Free Press.

CHAPTER 2

Conceptualizing Eligibility for Early Intervention Services

RITA BENN

Defining the potential population of children and families who are to benefit from early childhood services is one of the most arduous tasks facing states today. Policymakers need extensive knowledge to define the target group(s) for prevention and early intervention services. Each state must decide whether to include *primary prevention strategies*, targeted for infants and toddlers at risk of delay or disability, or to pursue only *secondary prevention strategies*, focused on those currently experiencing delays or disabilities. Eligibility decisions have tremendous implications for a state's entire early intervention service delivery system and, ultimately, the welfare of a generation of children. Consequently, the conceptualization of eligibility requires serious deliberation, especially for states currently trying to operationalize definitions for entitlement under Part H of the Individuals with Disabilities Education Act (IDEA).

CONSTRUCTING AN ELIGIBILITY DEFINITION

Typically, intervention policies and programs have focused on three groups of children: those with established conditions, developmental delays, and risk factors. The task of constructing a broad definition (as proposed through Part H) requires each state to analyze several key issues, for example, their policy toward primary and secondary prevention; the statewide incidence of risk and established conditions; the fiscal climate and availability of resources; the predictive value of various risk factors; and the ability to measure and operationalize definitions for each of the potentially eligible conditions or risks. Each individual state will need to balance the information derived from these facets of study in order to target an eligible population who might benefit from early intervention services.

Because a state's eligibility definition is ultimately the vehicle for implementing a state's prevention/early intervention policy, it is first and foremost important to understand the state's priorities with regard to prevention. Serving *at-risk* children reflects a primary prevention strategy that has as its goal the reduction in the incidence of children later identified as having developmental delay. Serving children with *established conditions* or *developmental delays* suggests a focus on secondary prevention that has as its goal the reduction in severity of outcomes of the identified conditions. The decision to provide services to populations under a definition of eligibility depends initially on the philosophy of prevention in the state, and then on the resources available to actualize this philosophy.

After a state addresses its commitment to prevention and intervention, a second step might entail examination of the feasibility of implementation for the proposed eligible populations. How many children and families would be included under each of the categories of established risk, developmental delay, and at risk? What intervention programs and services currently are in place to meet the needs? What are the anticipated state expenditures for the delivery of a coordinated, interagency, comprehensive early intervention service system? Analyses of these questions enable states to incorporate realistic projections into policy decisions on eligibility. A state with limited resources, or a low incidence of high-risk populations, might restrict eligibility for any of these categories.

The issue of risk as it relates to the categories of developmental delay and established conditions, and to developmental outcome in general, is critical to the construction of an early intervention policy. Many states, such as Michigan and Florida, have conducted extensive reviews of relevant research, highlighting the interrelationships of risk factors with other risk factors and conditions, and the relative needs for intervention within each factor. Several of the conclusions reached from these analyses (Benn, 1991) have implications for early intervention eligibility policy. First, developmental outcomes for many established or biological risk conditions are not as severe as those that result from the confluence of many environmental risks. Second, many established conditions cannot clearly be differentiated from biological risk markers. Third, single risk factors are never unitary risks in and of themselves. Fourth, the presence of certain protective factors within the family can frequently mitigate developmental risk. States need to consider whether a multiple risk eligibility policy might better predict who needs or would benefit from early intervention services than one that focuses on selected single risk populations.

Operationalizing constructs is one of the final steps to be accomplished in the development of an eligibility policy. Measurable definitions are needed for policymakers to plan how many infants and toddlers may be eligible, to find the children and families to serve, to ensure equity for service delivery within and across agency programs, and to produce sound outcome data that can be tied to a consistently identified population of children within a state. Without measurable definitions, it will be difficult to effectively evaluate the impact of a state's prevention and early intervention policy, or, to determine what kinds of early intervention services would be of most benefit to what types of children and families and under what conditions.

Often, public policy is hastily developed, emotionally charged, and not grounded in research. Policymakers can make decisions for eligibility for early intervention services based on a research perspective that systematically addresses each of the issues presented above. The purpose of this chapter is to illustrate how a research perspective can be applied to formulate concrete eligibility definitions. A framework for defining an eligible birth to age 3 Part H population is presented which incorporates findings derived from studies on infant assessment and development, family systems, and the prediction of risk and developmental delay. In this chapter, information derived from the scientific literature that led to this conceptual framework for eligibility is described for each of the three categories of infants and toddlers to be served.

DEVELOPMENTAL DELAY

The purpose of a precise definition for developmental delay is to specify which infants and toddlers who demonstrate some level of delay may receive early intervention services. States are required to establish criteria for eligibility that specify the extent of the developmental delay necessary in order to be eligible for services and to outline the acceptable procedures with which to document the delays. The process of determining developmental delay is inextricably tied to a description of the criteria that constitute a developmental delay.

The federal regulations suggest that *psychometric criteria*, such as a cut-off point in standard deviation units on standardized measures or a percent delay, and/or *informed clinical opinion* can be used as the basis for identifying children with developmental delays. Although no single procedure is permitted to be used as the sole criterion for determining a child's eligibility, states may consider the use of two standardized tests to suffice, rather than two different assessment approaches.

A 1991 content analysis of Part H state definitions revealed that of the states with documented criteria ($n = 42$), 38% included test data as the only criterion, 11% the use of professional judgment, and 51% a combination of both these measures (Harbin & Maxwell, 1991). For states using test data as the basis for eligibility, there was little uniformity. Different cutoff levels and metrics were used. Similarly, professional judgment varied in terms of its definition and the conditions under which this criterion was to be applied. Information on the types of procedures states used to arrive at decisions of eligibility for developmental delay was not reported.

From a research perspective, the first and foremost issue for states to address is whether it is appropriate to utilize a psychometric cutoff score based on a standard deviation or percent delay; and if this choice is made, the designation of which quantitative metric(s), and what amount of deviation or percent delay. The other significant issue to address is the role of clinical opinion.

The Use of a Quantitative Metric

Most standardized tests yield scores along a continuum; the standard deviation is the extent to which scores deviate from the mean of a normative sample. Based on population statistics, 68% of a normative sample falls within one standard deviation of the mean on any given standardized test. Those who score between one and two standard deviations below the norm make up 13.6% of the population and are typically considered "delayed." About 2% of the population will score lower than two standard deviations below the mean and would be considered "disabled."

The use of a standard deviation as qualifying criteria for eligibility assumes that children of similar ranges in developmental abilities can be identified. The regulations permit the use of different standardized tests for evaluation for developmental delay provided they are appropriate to the area of developmental concern. Different tests may have different means and standard deviations. Consequently, the scores that are considered outside the normal range may vary between tests. Setting an arbitrary cutoff score for eligibility as the criterion for delay may be in conflict with the cutoff score recommended for those particular tests (Harbin, Gallagher, & Terry, 1991).

> If a state requires that a child must score less than 1.5 standard deviations below the mean in two or more areas of development on standardized tests in order to be eligible for services, and more than one such standardized test of development is permitted to be used, it is possible that children of greatly differing abilities may all be considered eligible. Even when mean abilities are equal, distributions of these abilities may vary. This is the case when two separate groups are administered the same test, and it is even more likely when different tests that have not been standardized on each other are used. (Meisels, 1991, p. 31)

Use of a common standard deviation as a criterion for eligibility for developmental delay across a variety of measures would not be appropriate, and may result in over- or underidentification of children for services.

Some standardized tests yield scores only in terms of age levels (e.g., tests of language development). Developmental age scores are divided by children's chronological ages to compute a percentage of discrepancy between an observed performance and expected behavior when compared to a norm group. For instance, a 12-month-old infant whose developmental age is 8 months can be reported as functioning 33% below chronological age.

Percent delays, however, cannot be assumed to be equivalent across developmental abilities (Meisels, 1991). A 25% delay in motor development has very different implications for service delivery and developmental outcome than a 25% delay in language development. In addition, research indicates that current developmental scales have not been constructed with sufficient reliability to be accurate enough to make fine age distinctions across developmental levels (Meisels, 1991). Similarly, to attribute equivalent meaning to delays in domains across the age levels is misleading. The severity of delay of a 3-year-old who is functioning 25% below age level cannot be equated with that of a 1-year-old infant who is functioning 25% below chronological age.

Because standardized tests yield different units of measurement, the equivalency of the extent of delay across these tests cannot be reliably assessed. Defining eligibility for developmental delay based on scores that are two standard deviations below the mean *or* 25% below normative levels on instruments that yield scores in months (as some states do), combines two metrics representing different levels of delay. Infants and toddlers of widely different capacities could be served in the same eligibility category.

The literature on assessment of young children provides further rationale for not relying solely on scores derived from psychometric instruments to identify the need for services. First, some types of delays are difficult to detect and document using only standardized assessment tools. Scores based on standard developmental tests or scales do not reflect the qualitative differences observed in the behavior and motor performance of certain groups of children with disabilities or at high risk for delay. For example, the tonal abnormalities, unusual postures, sensory processing difficulties, and attentional problems frequently observed in low-birth-weight babies are not reflected in Bayley scores, which are largely within normal limits at 13 months (Anazole, 1988). Second, many of the infant tests have been normed on samples that have purposively excluded high-risk groups; hence, the scores obtained for these groups are not necessarily valid or easily interpretable (Meisels & Provence, 1989). Third, test scores provide little information about the underlying processes that contribute to the infant or toddler's developmental status or about individual differences in patterns of development—critical information that is necessary for the development of an Individualized Family Service Plan (IFSP). Fourth, few standardized infant and toddler evaluation tools exist that capture and quantify aspects of young children's socioemotional development, coping capacity, or quality of the parent–infant relationship (see Cicchetti & Wagner, 1990). Identification of children with delays in this domain of development would not be possible if only psychometric scores based on standard instruments were used as eligibility criteria.

Finally, the use of test scores for determining eligibility criteria can be challenged because existing assessments have limited predictive value. Research indicates that standard infant tests have poor predictive power for determining later developmental outcome (McCall, 1981). The dynamic changes, nonlinearity, and fluidity of development during the first 3 years of life complicate accurate prediction of developmental outcome based on a single quantitative index.

At best, the use of psychometric instruments may help document the presence, type, and extent of some delays in some young children in comparison to the general population. Testing enables professionals and parents to observe systematically the specific behaviors and capabilities of a child under standard conditions and over time. Different approaches and criteria, however, must be considered for determining more clearly and equitably eligibility for service provision for children considered to be developmentally delayed.

The Use of Clinical Opinion

Informed clinical opinion is a major component in determining developmental delay. Part H federal policy indicates its use as an initial criterion *and* in the process of evaluating continuing eligibility for services. The process for arriving at a clinical opinion of developmental delay, however, has not been spelled out. Although informed clinical opinion of developmental delay may be based on interpretation of standardized developmental test scores, other sources are essential for formulating a clinical opinion of the infant/toddler's developmental status and developing an appropriate plan of service.

Best practice with infants and toddlers requires a multidimensional approach to assessment from which clinical opinion is derived. A multidimensional approach to assessment can be defined as one that employs multiple measures, derives data from multiple sources, and surveys multiple domains (Neisworth & Bagnato, 1988). The federal regulations list several basic elements in the determination of delay: informed clinical opinion; more than one procedure, including a review of medical records; and evaluation of each of the developmental domains. Based on a synthesis of qualitative and quantitative information derived from a multidimensional assessment, highly trained professionals can arrive at an informed clinical opinion about the developmental appropriateness of a young child's abilities (Biro, Daulton, Szanton, & Garner, 1991). Including clinical opinion as the qualifying criterion for identification of developmental delay reduces the weight placed on a standardized test score.

The procedures on which to base clinical opinion need to reflect the dynamic, interactive context of development in the first 3 years of life and elucidate the processes that may be contributing to the infant/toddler's developmental abilities in a number of areas. An infant/toddler's capacities and vulnerabilities within and across multiple domains cannot be understood apart from the individual family and cultural context in which the young child is raised (Greenspan, 1990; Cicchetti & Wagner, 1990). Consequently, any evaluation of developmental status needs to be interpreted within this framework and to be based on procedures that reflect this interactive context (Gibbs & Teti, 1990).

Assessment of development during the early years has largely relied on an inferential process (Meisels, 1992). The inferential process that results in clinical opinion of a delay or dysfunction is nonetheless based on information derived from several key components of a diagnostic evaluation: (1) information gathered from the parents about the child's development and health as well as caregiving patterns (Greenspan, 1990; Meisels & Provence, 1989); (2) qualitative observations of the child and of parent–child interaction (Cytryn, 1976; Fraiberg, 1980; Greenspan, Nover, & Scheuer, 1987); (3) an appraisal of the child's health status (Cytryn, 1976); and (4) scores based on standardized infant assessment instruments. Together, data obtained from these multiple sources contribute to the integration of information that leads professionals to formulate a clinical opinion of delay (Cytryn, 1976; Gibbs & Teti, 1990; McCune, Kalmanson, Fleck, Glazewski, & Sillari, 1990).

In a developmental history, descriptive information provided by the parents sets the preliminary context for professional understanding of the main areas of developmental concern. The parents' perception of the child 's developmental capacities, patterns of development, and accomplishment of significant milestones in all developmental areas (cognitive, emotional, motor, and health) is essential. An account of the pregnancy, birth, and perinatal history; daily caregiving activities; experience of parenting the child; and significant or stressful family life events, *as related by the family*, helps to further frame the context in which to see how the child's developmental capacities are enhanced or blocked (see Greenspan, 1990). Additional information regarding the family's current and past health history, available resources, and networks of social support collected as part of the developmental history reveals the dynamic forces shaping the child's growth within both the individual and cultural context of the family.

Direct observation of infants in their natural environment permits the professional to understand development across multiple lines and within the context of their caregiving environment (Cytryn, 1976; Gibbs & Teti, 1990; Greenspan, 1990). Observation of the child's behavior and parent–child interaction during caretaking or play activities, as well as during other naturalistic interactions (e.g., during the course of the informal conversation with the family, etc.), provides the professional with a method for identification of (1) the child's developmental capabilities under optimal conditions—at home and with the child's caregivers; (2) the child's style of interaction with family members and play things; and (3) the unique capacities that the primary caregivers demonstrate in taking care of their child.

A health appraisal provides another very important source of information about the child's developmental status (Cytryn, 1976). A comprehensive health examination that addresses the physical and neurodevelopmental status of the child is necessary in order to connect the child's past and current physical development with observed developmental abilities. Data available solely in medical records may not be sufficient to accomplish this purpose.

A clinical approach to identification of developmental delay relies on the utilization and integration of information derived from these multiple procedures. The accuracy of this process in predicting developmental delay is ultimately based on the skill and experience of intervention professionals. With less skilled interventionists, some of the same criticisms leveled against the use of psychometric criteria can be applied to the measure of clinical opinion (e.g., over- or underidentifying children due to variability of judgment, etc.). However, informed clinical opinion that makes use of multiple data sources as well as a multidisciplinary team of professionals to arrive at the determination of developmental delay would safeguard against misidentification, enhance the accurate prediction of developmental outcome, contribute to a more appropriate understanding of the context and processes underlying the developmental capacities of the child, and result in a more useful, multifaceted IFSP (Cicchetti & Wagner, 1990; Gibbs & Teti, 1990; McCune et al., 1990).

Recent Proposals for Defining Eligibility under Developmental Delay

Different emphasis for defining an eligible population of infants and toddlers to be served have been offered in the research literature. Harbin et al. (1991) proposed that an eligibility policy include the use of standardized tests as the primary means for determining eligibility, with the use of professional judgment based on observation allowed for those atypical children whose delays may not be detectable through standardized assessment instruments. Their suggested criteria for developmental delay included test performance using the instruments' established cutoff scores when available, test procedures that yield scores of two standard deviations below the mean for tests scored in this manner, or scores indicative of 25% delay on instruments so quantified.

As presented earlier, the use of percent delay or standard deviation as the only or primary criterion for eligibility would not be the most appropriate choice. In addition, although it is agreed that professional judgment needs to be based on observation, this should not be the sole criterion for determining atypical developmental delays. Qualitative observation is essential to the inferential diagnostic process as a means for interpreting the clinical significance of test scores, and the developmental processes that may be influencing these scores; however, multiple measures of the infant and toddler assessed within the context of the individual family are also critical contributing components. Furthermore, best clinical practice would involve observation as part and parcel of all evaluations for any infants and toddlers (Cytryn, 1976; Fraiberg, 1980; Weatherston & Tableman, 1988), not only for those children whose delays cannot be measured through standard test procedures.

Shonkoff and Meisels (1991) suggest that confirmation of delayed development based on a valid and reliable diagnostic instrument should be sufficient to confirm eligibility for services, without designating an arbitrary cutoff score. Furthermore, they suggest that the clinical significance of test scores based on information provided about the current abilities and resources of the child and family, not merely statistical significance of test scores, constitute the basis for determining eligibility of significant delays.

Recommended Method of Defining Developmental Delay

The definition of developmental delay summarized in Table 2.1 goes a step further than that initially suggested by Shonkoff and Meisels (1991) by (1) outlining the process and context within which to interpret the clinical significance of test scores; (2) describing the procedures from which an informed clinical opinion is derived; and (3) presenting informed clinical opinion as the preferred criterion on which to base identification for developmental delay for children birth to age 3. Interpretation of a very young child's abilities and available family resources needs to be based on a systematic, multidimensional clinical evaluation process that involves gathering developmental information on the child within the context of the family. The significance of test data needs to be weighed along with data obtained from three other critical components of the process—a developmental history as interpreted by the parents, direct observations of the child and parent together, and a health status appraisal. An informed clinical opinion of the developmental capacities of the infant or toddler can then reliably be derived.

ESTABLISHED CONDITIONS

Some diagnosed mental and physical conditions have a very high probability of resulting in developmental delay. The established conditions category allows infants and toddlers who show no observable developmental delay at the time

TABLE 2.1. Recommended Definitions of Eligibility for Early Intervention Services under Part H of IDEA

Developmental delay
Eligibility is based on four sources of information—a parent(s) report of a developmental history, observation of the parent(s) and child together, health status appraisal, and developmentally appropriate formal evaluation measure—that are used together to arrive at an informed clinical opinion of a delay in one or more areas of developmental functioning.

Established condition
Eligibility is based on a diagnosed physical or mental condition related to a(n):
   Chromosomal anomaly/genetic disorder (e.g, fragile X, trisomy 18, etc.)
   Neurological disorder (e.g., cerebral palsy, neurofibromatosis, etc.)
   Congenital malformation (e.g., patent ductus arteriosis, de Lange syndrome, etc.)
   Inborn error of metabolism (e.g., Hunter syndrome, maple syrup disease, etc.)
   Sensory disorder (e.g., amblyopia ex anopsia, retinopathy of prematurity, etc.)
   Severe attachment and atypical developmental disorder (e.g., autism; reactive attachment disorder, including child abuse; etc.)
   Severe toxic exposure (e.g., fetal alcohol syndrome, maternal pheylketonuria, etc.)
   Chronic illness (e.g., technology dependent, cancer, etc.)
   Severe infectious disease (e.g., cytomegalovirus, meningitis, HIV-positive, etc.)

At risk
Eligibility is based on the presence of four or more risk factors that may interfere with the caregiving, health, or development of the child. Risk factors include (1) any serious concern expressed by parent(s) or professionals regarding a child's development, parenting style, or parent–child interaction; and/or those related to (2) the prenatal period (i.e., severe prenatal complications, maternal prenatal substance abuse/use, limited prenatal care), (3) the perinatal period (i.e., severe perinatal complications, asphyxia, small for gestational age, very low birth weight), (4) the postnatal period (i.e., atypical infant behavioral characteristics, recurrent accidents, chronic otitis media), (5) demographics (i.e., poverty, teenage mother, four or more preschool-aged children under age 6, single parent and/or parent education less than high school and/or parent unemployed), (6) ecology (i.e., family has inadequate health care, lack of stable residence, physical or social isolation and/or lack of adequate social support, parent–child separations), and/or (7) family's health, caregiving, and interaction (i.e., parent with severe chronic illness, parent with chronic/acute mental illness/developmental disability/mental retardation, parent with drug or alcohol dependence, parent with a developmental history of loss or abuse, family medical/genetic history characteristics, acute family crisis, and chronically disturbed family interaction).

Note. This framework for eligibility was originally developed for the State of Michigan under a Part H grant awarded by the State Board of Education. The use of the term "parent" implies the primary caregiver of the child.

of referral to be eligible for services because their diagnosed condition is highly assumed to result in delay. Because the term "high probability of delay" has not been operationalized in the federal regulations, some states may choose to serve only infants and toddlers whose conditions have a 90% inevitability of delay; for other states, a 65% probabilistic indicator for developmental vulnerability would be sufficient. Whereas some traditionally diagnosed disorders (e.g., Down syndrome, etc.) are associated with firmly established probabilistic outcomes of moderate to severe developmental delay, there are several for which there is no such information. Furthermore, clear-cut probabilistic markers are available neither for disorders with a low incidence of occurrence nor for newer identified biological risks.

The two categories of risk, established and biological, were initially proposed in Tjossem's tripartite classification (Tjossem, 1976) and were based on potential etiological factors. Infants and toddlers whose developmental delays were presumed to result from diagnosed medical disorders were classified as having established risk whereas infants and toddlers whose perinatal or prenatal conditions predisposed them to higher probability for delay were considered at biological risk. The delineation of conditions that would fit under established or biological risk categories has been subject neither to rigorous research nor to consensual validation by medical specialists. In reality, these categories are not mutually exclusive. A 1-year-old who is identified with an established diagnosis of cerebral palsy may have experienced severe asphyxiation at birth. The mother of a preschooler with AIDS may have been HIV-infected when pregnant. If a state elects to serve infants and toddlers with certain biological risks under the established condition category, it may serve many infants who would never exhibit developmental difficulties. However, if a state excludes biological risk from its definition of Part H eligibility and elects not to serve the at-risk group, many children who might benefit from early intervention services will not receive them until they exhibit clear symptoms of developmental dysfunction.

The condition of Failure to Thrive (FTT) illustrates the conceptual difficulty that states face in delineating eligibility under the proposed Part H categorical system. Although FTT is listed in the 1989 Federal Regulations as an example of a condition to be subsumed under established risk, this condition is not uniformly accepted in the scientific literature as an established medical disorder (Drotar, 1989; Rosenn, Loeb, & Jura, 1980). There is no unanimously accepted definition of FTT; the term itself has been used in numerous contexts to refer to infants whose poor weight gain is without apparent physical cause (nonorganic failure to thrive), and/or a by-product of a more disturbed parent–child interactional process (Drotar, 1984; Tibbits-Kleber & Howell, 1985). Although there is wide agreement that FTT is an indication of high-risk status in the developing infant (Drotar, 1984; Singer, Drotar, Fagan, Devost, & Lake, 1983), in many cases, it can be a symptom of an underlying organic problem and not a diagnosis in and of itself. Limitations of methodology in longitudinal studies, moreover, preclude arriving at any definitive conclusions about developmental outcomes. What can be extracted from the research is that FTT is a risk condition prevalent in about 1–3% of the population (Bithoney & Newberger, 1987; Tibbits-Kleber & Howell, 1985). To include all infants and toddlers with FTT under an established risk definition may result in providing comprehensive services to many families whose children exhibit normative patterns of development.

A review of the research on the effects of HIV infection provides another very important example of the difficulties states may encounter when trying to differentiate the delivery of services to populations based on a categorical system of established versus biological risk. Findings suggest that children with HIV appear to be at considerable risk for a wide range of central nervous system and developmental abnormalities, in addition to the most serious outcome, AIDS (Belman et al., 1988; Diamond, 1989; Epstein & Sharer, 1988; Epstein et al., 1985; Kastner & Friedman, 1988; Ultmann et al., 1985). Nonetheless, there are no clear-cut predictors of risk to an infant born to an HIV-infected mother. Mothers can transmit HIV in one pregnancy, but not in the next. The rate of perinatal transmission of HIV is approximately 40–50%. Antibodies to HIV are invariably detected in the bloodstream of babies born to HIV-infected mothers and persist in HIV-infected as well as uninfected infants for as many as 15 months after birth. Current estimates suggest that 20–60% will go on to have the real disease after this age, whereas uninfected babies may become serologically negative (Novello, Wise, Willoughby, & Pizzo, 1989; Rubinstein, 1986). If states consider maternal HIV as a biological risk condition and not as established risk, large number of families and children may not be provided with early intervention services until their children exhibit developmental difficulties.

Part of the problem in defining established risk arises because there are so many disorders that may be included in this definition, and there is wide variation in underlying etiology and developmental outcome (Meisels & Wasik, 1990). Not surprisingly, there is no national data base on the incidence and prevalence of these disorders specifically for children birth to age 3 (Meisels & Wasik, 1990). Estimates provided from the U.S. Department of Education vary from 1 to 12%, depending on the breadth of the definition of established disabilities (Meisels & Wasik, 1990; Benn, 1991). These inadequate databases, in addition to inconsistencies in research methodology for investigating short- and long-term developmental outcomes across a wide variety of medical risk conditions, may lead states to consider under the category of established conditions many children with biological risk conditions and medical disorders that will not eventuate in developmental delay (Harbin et al., 1991).

One way to differentiate a biological risk from an established risk condition would be to determine the degree to which a developmental delay can be remediated with intervention. An established condition could be defined as a condition where the delays might be improved through intervention but never eradicated (Murphy, Nichter, & Linden, 1982). For biological risk conditions, delays may conceivably be prevented and/or normative functioning attained. Using this framework, there is ample evidence to suggest that specific conditions related to chromosomal defects (e.g., Down syndrome, etc.), neurological problems (e.g., cerebral palsy, etc.), atypical developmental disorders (e.g., autism), central nervous system damage (e.g., sensory disorders, etc.), chronic medical illness (e.g., cystic fibrosis, etc.), and infectious diseases (e.g., cytomegalovirus, etc.) can be considered under established risk. For several other medical or biological risk conditions (e.g., FTT, low birth weight, or cocaine exposure, etc.), there are not sufficient data on which to base a decision for categorical placement. States will need to turn to other sources, (e.g., statewide prevalence data, existing programmatic resources, etc.) for determining eligibility and mandating services to certain populations of infants and toddlers and their families.

Recent Proposals for Defining Eligibility under Established Conditions

Harbin et al. (1991) suggest that until expected prevalence ranges for each of the established conditions are gathered and systematic research is available that addresses the identification of disorders having the most serious developmental consequences for children and families, states elect to serve under established risk both traditional biological categories (i.e., chromosomal anomalies/genetic disorders; inborn errors in metabolism; neurological disorders; congenital malformations; sensory disorders; severe attachment and other atypical disorders), and newer biological risks (i.e., toxic exposure, including cocaine-exposed infants; and infectious diseases, including maternal HIV). These same classifications are recommended by Shonkoff and Meisels (1991). Shonkoff and Meisels further suggest that a multidimensional evaluation of the infant and family may provide the basis for determining the level and/or intensity of the intervention services that will be helpful to the growth of the child within the context of the family.

Recommended Method of Defining Established Conditions

The use of Harbin et al.'s (1991) taxonomy for established risk appears sound, with the addition of the population of infants and toddlers who have disorders related to chronic medical illness. A review of the research on chronic medical illness suggests that young children with such disorders as cancer, renal or heart disease, cystic fibrosis, or other "medically fragile" or "technology dependent" conditions, have a very high probability of experiencing developmental delays across a variety of domains (Fletcher & Copeland, 1988; Geary & Haka-Ikse, 1989; Rotundo et al., 1982; Rovet, Ehrlich, & Hoppe, 1988; U.S. Congress, Office of Technology Assessment, 1987). Because these delays can be ascribed to established medical disorders (albeit compounded by related hospitalizations and/or medical treatment effects), and they cannot totally be remediated with intervention, it would seem most appropriate to include this group of infants and toddlers and their families in the established risk category.

Note that the category of severe attachment and atypical developmental disorders that is outlined under the established risk classification in Table 2.1 includes children who have experienced physical and sexual abuse. Criteria for the diagnosis of reactive attachment disorder listed in the third revised edition of the *Diagnostic and Statistical Manual of Mental Disorders* (DSM-III-R) (American Psychiatric Association, 1987) reflect the clinical picture of many infants and toddlers who experience child abuse, such as a disturbed social relatedness in most contexts and grossly pathogenic parental care (e.g., overly harsh punishment by a caregiver, consistent neglect, persistent disregard of the child's basic physical needs). The research on child abuse is consistent in demonstrating adverse developmental outcomes, particularly with regard to socioemotional development and attachment to primary caregivers (Costner, Gersten, Beeghly, & Cicchetti, 1989; Crittenden, 1985, 1988, 1989; Dietrich, Starr, & Weisfeld, 1983; Egeland & Sroufe, 1981; Farber & Egeland, 1987; Hoffman-Plotkin & Twentymen, 1984; Schneider-Rosen, Braunwald, Carlson, & Cicchetti, 1985; U.S. Congress, Office of Technology Assessment, 1988).

Families with infants and toddlers who have established risk conditions will differ tremendously with respect to both the immediacy with which they may want early intervention services and the intensity and scope of the services. An IFSP can best be determined, as Shonkoff and Meisels (1991) suggest, only from a multidimensional assessment of the infant and family's resources, strengths, and vulnerabilities. To accomplish this end, it is recommended that states follow the same clinical approach described for assessing developmental delay.

AT RISK

Typically children are considered to be at risk of developmental delay if they have been exposed to a recognized high-risk biological or environmental condition (e.g., preterm birth, mentally ill mothers). Children birth to age 3 at substantial risk for developmental delay are eligible for services at the discretion and definition of individual states. Although the benefits of early intervention and prevention have been repeatedly documented, policy makers may be concerned that too many families may qualify for entitled services and exert a financial drain on existing resources. Thus, states have cautiously approached the inclusion of the at-risk population in their definitions of eligibility.

States may choose to define the at-risk population in a variety of ways: in terms of a discrete risk group (e.g., teenage mothers, Medicaid-eligible families, etc.); the presence of a single biological or environmental risk factor (e.g., low birth weight, lack of prenatal care, etc.); or a combination of risk conditions (e.g., small for gestational age and poverty affected). The manner in which each of these individual risk groups or factors are further defined will affect the number of children and families eligible for services. For instance, depending upon a state's definition of the risk factor "teenage mother," services may be offered to all adolescent mothers under the age of 20, regardless of marital status, or only to single adolescents under the age of 17. Systematic examination of research related to determining developmental outcomes for young children birth to age 3 based on specific risk conditions can enable states to decide on the scope and definition of the population and whether or not to serve the at-risk population.

Single versus Multiple Risk

An extensive review of research related to 27 biological and environmental risk conditions was undertaken to determine criteria for eligibility in the State of Michigan (see Benn, 1991). In general, this review revealed no definitive information as to which risk factors, in and of themselves, were most predictive of developmental delay. Biological risk factors, such as prematurity, asphyxia, and low birth weight, were rarely found to have a lasting developmental impact on the child independent of the caregiving environment. Investigations (e.g., Meisels & Plunkett, 1988; Sameroff & Seifer, 1983) indicated that the early characteristics of the child typically become overpowered by factors in the child's environment. For environmental factors, there appeared to be more severe short-term effects related to several risk factors; however, the long-term effects were more questionable. Investigations of the effects of parental mental illness, poverty, parental substance abuse, and homelessness demonstrated more serious developmental consequences for children birth to age 3 than other factors, such as parental divorce during this time period, teen parenthood, or parental unemployment. An overview of the findings related to a sample of these risk conditions is presented in Table 2.2.

The higher probability of developmental delay resulting from any of these single risk conditions needs to be interpreted with caution. For the most part, studies on specific risk conditions have been poorly designed, relying on unsophisticated statistical analysis and inconsistently defined samples. Furthermore, as shown in Table 2.2, outcomes related to all risk conditions are not independent of other risk factors. Developmental effects were found to be highly associated with other risks inherent either in the caregiving environment or in the biological status of the child. For example, investigations of the development of low-birth-weight babies are confounded by other naturally occurring risks, such as multiple birth complications, a history of no prenatal care, or maternal youth. Because of the highly intercorrelated sets of risks, developmental outcomes associated with any single risk factor cannot be identified; they are, in essence, a result of multiple risk indices.

Empirical investigation of the combination of factors that are most predictive of developmental outcomes has been scant and also subject to methodological problems. Whereas some researchers have developed risk indices consisting of various combinations of multiple factors in order to select at-risk children for intervention, typically these indices have been developed only on specific groups of children, and therefore are not generalizable to the population at large (Meisels & Wasik, 1990). There is no way to know how effective such scales are in predicting later outcome for all children. In addition, assigning different predictive weights to single risk factors as a basis for determining developmental outcomes would not necessarily have conceptual or consensual validity. Should prematurity, for example, have an equivalent or higher predictive weight for risk of delay than adolescent parenthood in such an equation?

Throughout the research on individual risk factors, the impact of family stress, socioeconomic status (SES), and social support were raised as mediators of developmental effects (see Kochanek, Chapter 3, this volume). The context of the family's environment was seen as either impeding or fostering the growth of the young child (Sameroff & Fiese, 1990). Developmental outcomes were shown to be determined not only by the presence of risk factors alone but by the balance among risk factors (both biological and environmental), stressful life events, the capacities of the child, and the quality of the child's caregiving environment (Ramey & MacPhee, 1986; Werner, 1986). The degree of risk for developmental delay, similar to the evaluation of developmental delay, needs to be interpreted within the individual family and cultural context. It is only through consideration of the balance between risk and protective factors within the individual context of a child's caregiving environment that the most accurate picture of risk can emerge (Werner, 1986).

TABLE 2.2.   **Examples of Related Risks, Developmental Effects, and Observable Age Periods of Developmental Effects Associated with Selected Risk Conditions**

Risk condition	Related risk	Developmental areas	Age periods
Adolescent mother	Demographics—age, education Maternal mental health—depression, stress Parent–child interaction and parenting style Poverty Prenatal care Social support	Cognitive—IQ, reading, and school achievement Physical—birth weight Social–emotional—temperament, attention, cooperation, compliance, aggression, affect, social relations	Preschool and school age Birth–3 All ages
Lack of prenatal care	Adolescent mother Demographics—single parent, primiparous, education, race Maternal mental health Maternal prenatal substance abuse Medical insurance Perinatal complications Poverty	Physical—birth weight, infant mortality, growth	Birth–3 and preschool
Maternal mental illness (i.e., uni- and bipolar depression, psychosis, schizophrenia)	Demographics—SES, single parent, severity of illness Family interaction—marital quality Parent–child interaction and parenting style Poverty Social support	Cognitive—developmental status, language, school achievement Physical—birth weight, neurological status Social–emotional—affect, attachment, social relations	Birth–3 and school age Birth–3 All ages
Maternal prenatal substance abuse (i.e., smoking, drinking, use of cocaine, methadone, opiate, heroin)	Demographics—single parent, race Established risk—Fetal Alcohol Syndrome Prenatal toxic exposure Polydrug use Poverty Prenatal care	Cognitive—developmental status, IQ Physical—birth weight, congenital malformations Social–emotional—temperament, activity level, attention	All ages Birth–3 Birth–3 and school age
Parent–child separations (i.e., divorce, incarceration)	Demographics—SES, single parent, race Family interaction Parent–child interaction Poverty Social support	Social–emotional—affect, aggression, cooperation, social relations	Preschool and school age

(continued)

TABLE 2.2   (*continued*)

Risk condition	Related risk	Developmental areas	Age periods
Perinatal complications (i.e., asphyxia, intraventricular hemorrhage, low birth weight, prematurity)	Demographics—SES, age Established risk—chronic medical illness (e.g., cerebral palsy) Parent–child interaction and parenting style Parent–child separation— hospitalization Perinatal complications— severity of intraventri- cular hemorrhage, respiratory illness Prenatal care Social support	Cognitive—developmental status, IQ Physical—illness, motor, neurological status Social–emotional— attachment, affect	All ages All ages Birth–3
Poverty	Adolescent mother Demographics—single parent, race Established risk—child abuse Homelessness Maternal mental health— depression, stress Parent–child interaction and parenting style Perinatal complications Prenatal care Social support	Cognitive—IQ, school achievement Physical—infant mortality, illness, low birth weight Social–emotional— aggression	Preschool and school age All ages School age
Small for gestational age	Demographic—education, SES Family history of small for gestational age Maternal prenatal substance abuse Perinatal complications— prematurity	Cognitive—developmental status, IQ, speech delays Physical—growth Social–emotional— temperament	All ages Birth–3 and preschool Birth–3

Cumulative Effect of Risk

The results of several risk studies show that as risk factors multiply, their combined effect is greater than the effect of any one single factor alone. Rutter (1983) reported no relationship between single factors and developmental outcome; however, the presence of two risk factors increased the likelihood of an adverse outcome fourfold, and the presence of four risk factors increased it tenfold. In their longitudinal study of almost 700 children in Kauai, Werner and Smith (1982) found adverse developmental outcomes at age 10 evident only when children had experienced a minimum of any 4 of the 12 biological and environmental risk factors that were examined. (Some of their biological factors, however, were those that might be considered established risk.)

Similarly, Sameroff, Seifer, Barocas, Zax, and Greenspan (1987) have demonstrated that it was the number rather than the nature of any combination of risk factors that predicted adverse outcomes. These researchers assessed a set of ten environmental variables, some of which were correlates of SES (e.g., maternal education, chronicity of mental illness, minority status, family support, maternal–infant interaction, etc.) in a longitudinal study of 215 children. When these factors were related to socioemotional and cognitive competence scores at age 4, major differences were found between those children with low multiple risk scores and those with high scores. In terms of intelligence, for instance, children with no environmental risks scored more than 30 points higher than children with eight or nine risk factors. None of the single factors in and of themselves were related to either good or poor outcomes, and similar outcomes resulted from different combinations of risk factors. The cumulative effect of risk was, however, the critical determinant of severity of delay. Moreover, it was only with the inclusion of the fourth risk factor that substantial decrements in performance were observed.

Recent Proposals for Defining an At-Risk Population of Infants and Toddlers

In accordance with the cumulative notion of risk, Harbin et al. (1991) proposed that the presence of three risk factors constitute eligibility for early intervention services, without specification as to which biological or environmental risk factors to include. The risk research suggests that four factors might be a more appropriate criterion. In order to minimize duplication of risk factors and maximize uniformity of standards, it is critical that eligibility policies based on a multirisk model define and operationalize the risk factors under consideration. Omission of these definitions from a multirisk eligibility policy may result in overidentification of children and families for services.

Shonkoff and Meisels (1991) provide definitions of biological and environmental risk with examples and suggest that eligibility be determined on a case-by-case basis, through comprehensive child and family evaluation that takes into account the risks and resources inherent in the family and child's history and environment. This individualized, multidimensional approach to at-risk eligibility is similar to their proposed method for determining eligibility under developmental delay. Using this framework for at-risk eligibility, however, states may encounter a very large number of potential recipients requiring diagnostic evaluations, and an already overburdened service delivery system may be more heavily taxed. It would seem that preliminary to this case-by-case assessment should be the implementation of a more restricted, multifactorial screening for eligibility (Meisels, 1992).

Recommended Method of Defining At Risk

The multirisk conceptualization of at-risk eligibility proposes four risk factors as the defining criteria from among the specified list of factors that is presented in Table 2.1. Selection of risk factors included in this framework was based on the significance of risk accorded by the clinical and research literature (Benn, 1991). Each factor is defined in the Appendix. A multidimensional assessment (such as the one described in the earlier section on developmental delay) is recommended for the purposes of developing an appropriate IFSP once a child and family have been identified with four risk factors.

This multirisk framework for eligibility should enable service provision to the population of infants and toddlers and their families who are in greatest need of service, and it should not result in a huge influx of service recipients. To investigate this assumption and incidence of risk, a pilot study was undertaken in Michigan using most of the risk factors defined in the Appendix (Benn, 1991). Based on the hospital records of 2,186 live births in a midsize, demographically representative city in Michigan, it was found that 19% of the families were characterized by one risk factor, 16% with two risk factors, 5% with three risk factors, and 3% with four or more risk factors. As risk factors increased, the potential pool of eligible families decreased substantially.

Because children can move into and out of risk status over the course of their development, the actual prevalence rate for children aged birth to 3 who are at environmental and/or biological risk is an unknown. Negative outcomes that may be projected at an early age may improve with changes in maturation or family circumstances. It is only through a prospective, longitudinal study of a birth cohort that reliable estimates of prevalence may be ascertained.

The multirisk definition of eligibility that has been presented in this chapter may be identified as an established condition under prospective rule-making changes proposed for Part H (Federal Register, 1992). Under the newly proposed rules, "a combination of risk factors that taken together makes developmental delay highly probable" (p. 18995), such as low birth weight and poverty, may be considered as "a diagnosed physical or mental condition that has a high probability of resulting in developmental delay." This conceptual change in federal policy will allow states to specify a constellation of risk factors as an established condition.

SUMMARY

The definitions of early intervention service eligibility derived from a research perspective can enable states to identify families with children aged birth to 3 who are most in need of early intervention services based on a common set of evaluation procedures that reflect (1) the dynamic, interactive context and principles of early child development and (2) the clinical, qualitative process of assessment. Although the categories of eligibility in this framework can be conceptually delineated from each other, the procedures with which to evaluate the infant/toddler's development and the design of an IFSP cut across these categorical distinctions.

The definitions for the three categories of eligibility discussed in this chapter can provide direction to other states as they construct their early intervention service delivery system. Eligibility for service provision under the category of developmental delay is recommended to be based on clinical opinion and derived from four sources of information: a parent report, parent–child observation, health status appraisal, and formal evaluation measure. Eligibility under established risk is recommended to include children who do not necessarily demonstrate a developmental delay upon service delivery but whose diagnosed physical or mental condition is related to one of nine conditions: (1) chromosomal anomalies/genetic disorders; (2) inborn errors of metabolism; (3) neurological disorders; (4) congenital malformations; (5) sensory disorders; (6) severe attachment and atypical developmental disorders; (7) chronic medical illness; (8) severe toxic exposure; and (9) severe infectious diseases. Eligibility for services under the category of at risk is recommended for families who present with four risk (biological and/or environmental) factors that may interfere with the caregiving, health, or development of the child. Risk factors are identified from a specific list of defined prenatal, perinatal, postnatal, demographic, and family factors.

The ultimate utility of this eligibility framework for the service delivery system and the recipient client population will need to be evaluated. Evolving social policies are not unlike the processes underlying family interaction, infant development, and clinical intervention; they are dynamic and ongoing. Changes in definitions for eligibility may be needed as new scientific data emerges on developmental outcomes, assessment tools, and risk conditions, and as planning for Part H results in actual implementation of coordinated, comprehensive early intervention services.

APPENDIX: RISK DEFINITIONS FOR MULTIRISK INDEX OF ELIGIBILITY[1]

Acute Family Crisis. This risk factor refers to any sudden and extremely stressful family event that substantially disrupts the equilibrium of the family and impacts on the caregiving of the child. A death of a spouse or a child, a sudden hospitalization of a family member, or an eviction from the home are examples of acute family crisis that may impact on the stability of the family and resulting care or the development of the child.

Adolescent Mother. This risk factor refers to any mother who is under the age of 20 years at the time of the birth of her child.

Asphyxia. This risk factor refers to a particular cluster of clinical signs that indicate that a reduction in the oxygen level below the physiological requirements of the neonate has occurred. The clinical signs of asphyxia include fetal distress (e.g., fetal heart rate during the first stage of labor that is lower than 120 or above 160, abnormal heartbeat patterns, and/or the passage of meconium) and neonatal distress (e.g., poor color, poor muscle tone, failure to breathe spontaneously as typically assessed by Apgar scores). To interpret a low Apgar as indicative of asphyxia, other signs known to occur during intrapartum asphyxia must also be present (e.g., fetal distress, passage of meconium, etc.). Symptoms in the neonate that indicate that asphyxia occurred are lethargy (abnormal state of consciousness), seizures, abnormal muscle tone, poor feeding, and abnormal reflexes.

Atypical Infant Behavioral Characteristics. This risk factor refers to specific behavioral characteristics of the neonate and infant, such as excessive irritability, crying, or tremulousness, that are not responsive to usual comforting measures. These characteristics may be related to the infant's inability to self-regulate transitional behavioral states, physiological immaturity, and/or temperament. The presence of this risk factor should be differentiated from *regulatory disorders* (an atypical developmental disorder categorized as an established condition) that may be characterized by these same behavioral symptoms. Regulatory disorders are defined by distinct behavioral patterns coupled with sensory, sensory–motor, or organizational processing difficulties that affect daily adaptation, interaction, and/or relationships.

---

[1]This framework for eligibility was orginally developed for the state of Michigan under a Part H grant awarded by the State Board of Education. The use of the term "parent" implies the primary caregiver of the child. The factors related to acute family crisis, atypical infant characteristics, atypical accidents, and otitis media were not coded from the hospital records for the pilot study on incidence of risk reported in this chapter.

Atypical or Recurrent Accidents Involving the Child. This risk factor refers either to unusual accidents of the type not commonly experienced by the child's developmental age (e.g., broken leg) and to recurrent accidents that could imply the existence of physical disease, environmental neglect, or child abuse.

Chronic Otitis Media. Otitis media refers to infection of the middle ear and resulting effusion (development of fluid) in the middle ear cleft behind the tympanic membrane. Chronic otitis media refers to blockages/infections that do not drain in a timely fashion and are resistant to typical drug treatment procedures. A history of recurrent bouts of acute otitis media (i.e., at least six times in a year's period) often implies a condition of chronic otitis media.

Chronically Disturbed Family Interaction. This risk factor refers to persistent, chaotic, and disorganized family patterns of interaction or family interaction characterized by a history of domestic violence or threats of violence.

Demographic Characteristics. This risk factor refers to one or more of three specific demographic indices that are typically found to be highly interrelated: families where either parent has less than a high school education or equivalent certificate, families where neither parent is currently employed, or families where there is only a single (i.e., separated, widowed, divorced, never married) parent.

Family Has Inadequate Health Care or No Health Insurance. This risk factor refers to families who have no regular health care maintenance for their child, or to families who have no private medical insurance.

Family Income Up to 185% of Federal Poverty Guidelines. This risk factor refers to families who are eligible for federal assistance programs, such as ADFC, Medicaid, or WIC. The poverty line, which varies by family size, is the income level that agencies within the Federal government set to approximate the amount of money that will allow a frugal family to pay for its most essential needs, which include food, shelter, and clothing.

Family Medical/Genetic History Characteristics. This risk factor refers to characteristics in the medical history of the biological parents that may directly relate to the developmental status of the child. A family history of sensory impairment, a previous birth of a handicapped child, or a death of a baby due to Sudden Infant Death Syndrome are examples of family medical history characteristics that are included under this risk factor.

Lack of Stable Residence, Homelessness, or Dangerous Living Conditions. This risk factor refers to the absence of permanent housing resulting in the need to be housed in temporary shelters, or welfare hotels; transient living situations due to frequent shifts in residence; or dangerous living conditions, which include houses or neighborhoods characterized by crime and violence or homes that are physically unsafe and/or have been condemned.

Limited Prenatal Care. This risk factor refers to pregnant mothers who have had four or fewer obstetric visits prior to their 34th week of pregnancy, or whose prenatal care was not initiated until the third trimester.

Maternal Prenatal Substance Abuse/Use. This risk factor refers to regular maternal use of tobacco, alcohol (more than one drink per day), or illicit and prescription drugs known to affect the developing fetus during pregnancy. Information on drug use may be obtained through self-report or results from urine analysis procedures.

Parent Has Four or More Preschool-Aged Children. This risk factor refers to families with four or more children under the age of 6, or families where the mother is pregnant and has three children under the age of 6.

Parent with Chronic or Acute Mental Illness/Developmental Disability/Mental Retardation. This risk factor refers to parents with a formal diagnosis of mental illness, developmental disability, or mental retardation.

Parent with a Developmental History of Loss and/or Abuse. This risk factor refers to either a history of perinatal loss, miscarriages, or sexual or physical abuse that a parent has experienced, or the death of a parent, spouse, or child as reported by a parent.

Parent with Drug or Alcohol Dependence. This risk factor refers to a parent who is known or has been observed to regularly abuse drugs (e.g., barbituates, marijuana, cocaine, heroin, etc.) or alcohol (i.e., more than three drinks per day). This risk factor is to be differentiated from the category found under established conditions that refers to infant toxic exposure resulting from drug or alcohol ingestion.

Parent with Severe Chronic Illness. This risk factor refers to a parent who has a terminal or severe chronic illness (e.g., cancer, multiple sclerosis, etc.) and has experienced the debilitating emotional or physical effects related to medical treatments (e.g., drug therapies, etc.) or to the progression of the disease.

Parent–Child Separation. This risk factor refers to significant, extended, or recurrent separations of the parent from the child. Examples of such events might include parent or child hospitalizations, divorce, parental separations, parental incarceration, parental military duty, or foster care placements.

Physical or Social Isolation and/or Lack of Adequate Social Support. This risk factor refers to families who are geographically or emotionally isolated such that there is very limited connection to personal or community networks. This risk factor may also refer to the isolation experienced by families who are non-English speaking.

Serious Concern Expressed by a Parent or Professional Regarding a Child's Development, Parenting Style, or Parent–Child Interaction.[2] This risk factor refers to any serious developmental concern that is raised in relation to the child's development (e.g., child's physical health status, emotional well-being, atypical development, etc.) by a parent or professional. The concern may be specifically child-focused, related directly to the child's developmental status, or parent–child focused, related to the nature of parent–child interaction. If the concern raises considerable anxiety on the part of the parent or professional, the presence of this concern should be interpreted as a risk factor.

Severe Perinatal Complications. This risk factor refers to severe complications in the birth and postpartum period, such as prematurity, respiratory distress syndrome,

---

[2]This risk factor should be used to represent only risks not included in another category in this multirisk index.

and so forth. This risk factor should not be used in conjunction with the risk factor "very low birth weight" unless there are severe perinatal complications other than prematurity or respiratory distress that describe the infant's condition.

Severe Prenatal Complications. This risk factor refers to complications during pregnancy that are known to potentially compromise neonatal outcomes. Examples of such complications include moderate to severe toxemia, placenta previa, abruptio placentae, more than one infant in a single pregnancy (e.g., twins, etc.), or such prenatal maternal illness, as diabetes, rubella, and so forth.

Small for Gestational Age. Small for gestational age refers to premature or full-term infants whose birth weights are abnormally small for their gestational age. Researchers have been very consistent in defining "abnormally small" as having a birth weight below the 10th percentile for gestational age on one of several sets of sex-specific norms for that population.

Very Low Birth Weight. This risk factor refers to premature infants whose birth weight is less than 1,500 grams (approximately, 3.3 pounds).

REFERENCES

American Psychiatric Association (1987). *Diagnostic and statistical manual of mental disorders* (3rd ed., rev.). Washington, DC: Author.

Anazole, M. (1988). Neonatal outcome: From clinical result to research. *Developmental Disabilities: Special Interest Section Newsletter, 11,* 1–3.

Belman, A. L., Diamond, G., Dickson, D., Horoupian, D., Llena, J., Lantos, G., & Rubinstein, A. (1988). Pediatric acquired immunodeficiency syndrome. *American Journal of Diseases of Children, 142,* 29–35.

Benn, R. (1991). *A state wide definition of eligibility under P.L. 99-457, Part H: A final research report.* Detroit, MI: Merrill-Palmer Institute, Wayne State University.

Biro, P., Daulton, D., Szanton, E., & Garner, C. (1991). Informed clinical opinion, *NEC*TAS NOTES: A Periodic Topical Publication, 4,* 1–4.

Bithoney, W. G., & Newberger, E. H. (1987). Child and family attributes of failure-to-thrive. *Developmental and Behavioral Pediatrics, 8*(1), 32–36.

Cicchetti, D., & Wagner, S. (1990). Alternative assessment strategies for the evaluation of infants and toddlers: An organizational perspective. In S. J. Meisels & J. P. Shonkoff (Eds.), *Handbook of early childhood intervention* (pp. 246–277). New York: Cambridge University Press.

Costner, W. J., Gersten, M. S., Beeghly, M., & Cicchetti, D. (1989). Communicative functioning in maltreated toddlers. *Developmental Psychology, 25,* 1020–1029.

Crittenden, P. M. (1985). Maltreated infants: Vulnerability and resilience. *Journal of Child Psychology and Psychiatry, 26,* 85–96.

Crittenden, P. M. (1988). Relationships at risk. In J. Belsky & T. Nezworski (Eds.), *Clinical implications of attachment* (pp. 136–174). Hillsdale, NJ: Erlbaum.

Crittenden, P. M. (1989). Teaching maltreated children in the preschool. *Topics in Early Childhood Special Education, 9*(2), 16–32.

Cytryn, L. (1976). Methodological issues in psychiatric evaluation of infants. In E. N.

Rexford, L. W. Sander, & T. Shapiro. *Infant psychiatry, a new synthesis* (pp. 17–25). New Haven, CT: Yale University Press.

Diamond, G. W. (1989). Developmental problems in children with HIV infection. *Mental Retardation, 27*(4), 213–217.

Dietrich, K. N., Starr, R. H., & Weisfeld, G. E. (1983). Infant maltreatment: Caretaker–infant interaction and developmental consequences at different levels of parenting failure. *Pediatrics, 72*, 532–540.

Drotar, D. (Ed.). (1984). *New directions in failure to thrive: Implications for research and practice.* New York: Plenum Press.

Drotar, D. (1989). Behavioral diagnosis in nonorganic failure-to-thrive: A critique and suggested approach to psychological assessment. *Developmental and Behavioral Pediatrics, 10*(1), 48–55.

Egeland, B., & Sroufe, L. A. (1981). Attachment and early maltreatment. *Child Development, 52*, 44–52.

Epstein, L. G., & Sharer, L. R. (1988). Neurology of human immunodeficiency virus infection in children. In M. L. Rosenblum, R. M. Levy, & D. E. Bredesen (Eds.), *AIDS and the nervous system* (pp. 79–101). New York: Raven Press.

Epstein, L. G., Sharer, L. R., Joshi, V. V., Fojas, M. M., Koenigsberger, M. R., & Oleske, J. M. (1985). Progressive encephalopathy in children with acquired immune deficiency syndrome. *Annals of Neurology, 17*, 488–496.

Farber, E. A., & Egeland, B. (1987). Invulnerability among abused and neglected children. In E. J. Anthony & B. J. Cohler (Eds.), *The invulnerable child* (pp. 253–288). New York: Guilford Press.

Federal Register. (1992, May 1). *Early Intervention Program for Infants and Toddlers with Disabilities; Proposed Rulemaking* (U.S. Department of Education [34 CFR Part 303]). Washington, DC: U.S. Government Printing Office.

Fletcher, J. M., & Copeland, D. R. (1988). Neurobehavioral effects of central nervous system prophylactic treatment of cancer in children. *Journal of Clinical and Experimental Neuropsychology, 10*(4), 495–538.

Fraiberg, S. (Ed.). (1980). *Clinical studies in infant mental health: The first year of life.* New York: Basic Books.

Geary, D. F. & Haka-Ikse, K. (1989). Neurodevelopmental progress of young children with chronic renal disease. *Pediatrics, 84*(1), 68–72.

Gibbs, E. D., & Teti, D. M. (Eds.). (1990). *Interdisciplinary assessment of infants: A guide for early intervention professionals.* Baltimore, MD: Paul H. Brookes.

Greenspan, S. I. (1990). Comprehensive clinical approaches to infants and their families: Psychodynamic and developmental perspectives. In S. J. Meisels & J. P. Shonkoff (Eds.), *Handbook of early childhood intervention* (pp. 150–172). New York: Cambridge University Press.

Greenspan, S. I., Nover, R. A., & Scheuer, A. (1987). A developmental diagnostic approach for infants, young children and their families. In S. I. Greenspan, S. Wieder, R. Nover, A. Lieberman, R. Lourie, & M. Robinson (Eds.), *Infants in multi-risk families: Case studies in preventive intervention* (pp. 431–498). Madison, CT: International Universities Press.

Harbin, G. L., Gallagher, J. J., & Terry, D. V. (1991). Defining the eligible population: Policy issues and challenges. *Journal of Early Intervention, 15*(1), 13–20.

Harbin, G. L., & Maxwell, K. (1991). *Progress toward developing a definition for devel-*

opmentally delayed: Report #2. Chapel Hill, NC: University of North Carolina at Chapel Hill, Carolina Institute for Child and Family Policy.

Hoffman-Plotkin, D., & Twentymen, C. T. (1984). A multimodal assessment of behavioral and cognitive deficits in abused and neglected preschoolers. *Child Development, 55,* 794–802.

Kastner, T., & Friedman, D. (1988). Pediatric acquired immune deficiency syndrome and the prevention of mental retardation. *Developmental and Behavioral Pediatrics, 9*(1), 47–48.

McCall, R. (1981). Early predictors of later IQ: The search continues. *Intelligence, 5,* 141–147.

McCune, L., Kalmanson, B., Fleck, M. B., Glazewski, B., & Sillari, J. (1990). In S. J. Meisels & J. P. Shonkoff (Eds.), *Handbook of early childhood intervention* (pp. 219–245). New York: Cambridge University Press.

Meisels, S. J. (1991). Dimensions of early identification. *Journal of Early Intervention, 15*(1), 26–35.

Meisels, S. J. (1992). Early intervention: A matter of context. *Zero to Three, 12*(3), 1–6.

Meisels, S. J., & Plunkett, J. W. (1988). Developmental consequences of preterm birth: Are there long-term effects? In P. B. Baltes, D. L. Featherman, & R. M. Learner (Eds.), *Life span development and behavior* (Vol. 9, pp. 87–128). Hillsdale, NJ: Erlbaum.

Meisels, S. J., & Provence, S. (1989). *Screening and assessment: Guidelines for identifying young disabled and developmentally vulnerable children and their families.* Washington, DC: National Center for Clinical Infant Programs.

Meisels, S. J., & Wasik, B. A. (1990). Who should be served? Identifying children in need of early intervention. In S. J. Meisels & J. P. Shonkoff (Eds.), *Handbook of early childhood intervention* (pp. 605–632). New York: Cambridge University Press.

Murphy, T. F., Nichter, C. A., & Linden, C. B. (1982). Developmental outcomes of the high-risk infant: A review of methodological research. *Seminars in Perinatology, 6,* 353–364.

Neisworth, J. T., & Bagnato, S. J. (1988). Assessment in early childhood special education: A typology of dependent measures. In S. L. Odom & M. B. Karnes (Eds.), *Early intervention for infants and children with handicaps: An empirical base.* Baltimore, MD: Paul H. Brookes.

Novello, A. C., Wise, P. H., Willoughby, A., & Pizzo, P. A. (1989). Final report of the United States Department of Health and Human Services Secretary's Work Group on Pediatric Human Immunodeficiency Virus Infection and Disease: Content and implications. *Pediatrics, 84*(3), 547–555.

Ramey, C. T., & MacPhee, D. (1986). Developmental retardation: A systems theory perspective on risk and preventive intervention. In D. C. Farran & J. D. McKinney (Eds.), *Risk in intellectual and psychosocial development* (pp. 61–82). Orlando, FL: Academic Press.

Rosenn, D. W., Loeb, L. S., & Jura, M. B. (1980). Differentiation of organic from nonorganic failure to thrive syndrome in infancy. *Pediatrics, 66*(5), 698–704.

Rotundo, A., Nevins, T. E., Lipton, M., Lockman, L. A., Mauer, S. M., & Michael, A. F. (1982). Progressive encephalopathy in children with chronic renal insufficiency in infancy. *Kidney International, 21,* 486–491.

Rovet, J. F., Ehrlich, R. M., & Hoppe, M. (1988). Specific intellectual deficits in children with early onset diabetes mellitus. *Child Development, 59,* 226–234.

Rubinstein, A. (1986). Pediatric AIDS. *Current Problems in Pediatrics, 16,* 361–409.

Rutter, M. (1983). Stress, coping and development: Some issues and some questions. In N. Garmezy & M. Rutter (Eds.), *Stress, coping and development in children* (pp. 1–41). New York: McGraw-Hill.

Sameroff, A. J., & Fiese, B. H. (1990). Transactional regulation and early intervention. In S. J. Meisels & J. P. Shonkoff (Eds.), *Handbook of early childhood intervention* (pp. 119–149). New York: Cambridge University Press.

Sameroff, A. J., & Seifer, R. (1983). Familial risk and child competence. *Child Development, 54,* 1254–1268.

Sameroff, A. J., Seifer, R., Barocas, R., Zax, M., & Greenspan, S. (1987). Intelligence quotient scores of 4-year-old children: Social–environmental risk factors. *Pediatrics, 79*(3), 343–350.

Schneider-Rosen, K., Braunwald, K. G., Carlson, V., & Cicchetti, D. (1985). Current perspectives in attachment theory: Illustration from the study of maltreated children. In I. Bretherton & E. Waters (Eds.), *Monographs of the Society for Research in Child Development: Vol. 50. Growing points of attachment theory and research* (pp. 194–210). Chicago: University of Chicago Press.

Shonkoff, J. P., & Meisels, S. J. (1991). Defining eligibility for services under PL 99-457. *Journal of Early Intervention, 15*(1), 21–25.

Singer, L. T., Drotar, D., Fagan J. F., III, Devost, L., & Lake, R. (1983). The cognitive development of failure to thrive infants: Methodological issues and new approaches. In T. Field & A. Sostek (Eds.), *Infants born at risk: Physiological, perceptual, and cognitive processes* (pp. 211–242). New York: Grune & Stratton.

Tibbits-Kleber, A. L., & Howell, R. J. (1985). Reactive attachment disorder of infancy (RAD). *Journal of Clinical Child Psychology, 14*(4), 304–310.

Tjossem, T. D. (Ed.). (1976). *Intervention strategies for high risk infants and young children.* Baltimore, MD: University Park Press.

Ultmann, M. H., Belman, A. L., Ruff, H. A., Novick, B. E., Cone-Wesson, B., Cohen, H. J., & Rubinstein, A. (1985). Developmental abnormalities in infants and children with acquired immune deficiency syndrome (AIDS) and AIDS-related complex. *Developmental Medicine and Child Neurology, 27,* 563–571.

U.S. Congress, Office of Technology Assessment (OTA). (1987). *Technology-dependent children: Hospital v. home care—A technical memorandum* (OTA TM-H-38). Washington, DC: U.S. Government Printing Office.

U.S. Congress, Office of Technology Assessment (OTA). (1988). *Healthy children: Investing in the future* (OTA H-345). Washington, DC: U.S. Government Printing Office.

Weatherston, D., & Tableman, B. (1988). *Infant mental health services: Supporting competencies, reducing risks.* Lansing, MI: Michigan Department of Mental Health.

Werner, E. E. (1986). A longitudinal study of perinatal risk. In D. C. Farran & J. D. McKinney (Eds.), *Risk in intellectual and psychosocial development* (pp. 3–27). Orlando, FL: Academic Press.

Werner, E. E., & Smith, R. S. (1982). *Vulnerable but invincible: A longitudinal study of resilient children and youth.* New York: McGraw-Hill.

CHAPTER 3

Enhancing Screening Procedures for Infants and Toddlers
The Application of Knowledge to Public Policy and Program Initiatives

THOMAS T. KOCHANEK

Examining the lives of children and the health care and educational systems created to promote their well-being is a study that reveals enormous capacity yet distressing shortcomings. Viewed optimistically, the United States does indeed spend a greater share of its resources on health care than does any other nation. In 1960, these expenditures were approximately 5% of the Gross National Product (GNP). In 1989, they exceeded $600 billion, nearly 12% of the GNP. It is estimated that by the year 2000, health care spending will reach 15% of the GNP (Lazenby & Letsch, 1990; Lewit & Monheit, 1992).

Within the world of education, substantial investments are also evident. In fact, America ranks seventh worldwide in expenditures on public education (Children's Defense Fund, 1990). Furthermore, calls to education reform in the last decade (National Commission on Excellence in Education, 1983) have resulted in virtually every state increasing its appropriation to public education. Adjusting for inflation, expenditures increased by 25% from 1983 to 1986 (Odden, 1987). Despite such funding increases in both health care and education, the perilous conditions that confront children are enormous. More specifically, recent data (Children's Defense Fund, 1990) indicate that:

- The overall infant mortality rate lags behind 18 other nations; in fact, an African-American child born in Boston has less chance of surviving the first year of life than a child born in Panama, Korea, or Uruguay.

- Nonwhite 1-year-old children in America are less likely to be immunized against polio than are comparable children in Sri Lanka, Colombia, and Botswana.
- Of the infants born in the United States, 7% are low birth weight (LBW), and 28 countries, including Hong Kong and Central African Republic, have fewer LBW newborns.
- Of every 1,000 children, 13 die before their fifth birthdays, which places the country 22nd worldwide, behind nations such as Singapore and Japan.
- The United States has the highest adolescent pregnancy rate among seven industrialized nations (France, England, Wales, Canada, the Netherlands, and Sweden).

To a great extent, the failure of programs to reduce or eradicate the above afflictions is rooted in two overarching problems: (1) that our ability to define and identify those in jeopardy is imperfect; and (2) that our ability to match appropriate, risk-responsive interventions with hazardous events and rearing conditions is underdeveloped (i.e., what works, for whom, and under what circumstances). Although promising lines of inquiry and discovery are occurring in both areas, the purpose of this chapter is to focus on the first area, that is, early identification of disability and vulnerability. In this regard, the objectives are (1) to review and synthesize contemporary knowledge regarding screening and early identification; (2) to identify the extent to which this knowledge is reflected in public policy; and (3) to offer specific recommendations on methods for ensuring the appropriate utilization of current wisdom in policy formulation, model conceptualization, and program implementation.

By definition (Meisels & Provence, 1989), screening is a process intended to identify children who have a high probability of exhibiting delayed or abnormal development. Central to the creation of effective screening models is an understanding of risk research. Briefly, this line of inquiry is rooted in epidemiology and is concerned with the identification of factors that accentuate or inhibit disease or disability. These studies include an examination of biological and behavioral precursors, genetic and environmental influences, stressful experiences, and coping behaviors. Risk research requires an investment in children whose outcomes appear to fit predictions of subsequent vulnerability, and also in others who manifest unexpected strengths (Garmezy, 1985).

Crafting effective screening and early identification programs necessitates a clear understanding of the literature on both adverse as well as favorable outcomes in children, and the factors that are related to these outcomes. With regard to the relationship between risk factors and poor outcomes, a high-risk condition exists when a child has a greater than average chance of developing a disability. Risk is not a condition but rather a circumstance to indicate an elevated probability that a disorder will occur. Identifying, defining, and assessing these risk factors over time is an enormous challenge that requires the collaborative efforts of specialists in education, medicine, psychology, and epidemiology. Alternatively, the concepts of resilience and protective factors are the positive analogues to the constructs of vulnerability and risk factors (Werner, 1990). Whereas resilience is a characteristic of the individual, protective factors include both individual and environmental characteristics that buffer a child's response to constitutional risk factors or harmful life events (Masten & Garmezy, 1985). Protective factors can promote stable, healthy personalities for many children reared in chaotic, impoverished families or those who are born with multiple medical complications and conditions.

In conceptualizing screening models, both domains of factors are equally prominent in that the presence of risk factors and/or the absence of protective factors can operate, separately or interdependently, to produce poor outcomes. As such, both sets of factors must be accommodated in decision making and model formulation. A brief review of the literature reveals a rich and extensive knowledge base within each area.

RISK FACTORS AND ADVERSE OUTCOMES

Whereas early conceptual models of screening presumed that elevated risk for disability arose from a wide array of hazardous events surrounding the birth process and, moreover, were confined to the child independent of context, numerous studies (Bierman-van Eenderburg, Jurgens-van der Zee, & Olinga, 1981; Gottfried, 1973; Papile, Munsick-Bruno, & Schaefer, 1983; Stewart, Reynolds, & Lipscomb, 1981) have demonstrated that single-factor predictive models are plagued with error and misclassification. For example, compelling findings were reported from the National Collaborative Perinatal Project (Broman, Bien, & Shaughnessy, 1985; Nichols & Chen, 1981), which reported that at 7-year follow-up, significant causal factors reside not so much in the child's medical history as in the ecological context within which a child is reared.

Sameroff, Seifer, Barocas, Zax, and Greenspan (1987) have offered additional insight into multiple risk models by examining the impact of 10 factors on verbal IQ scores derived at 4 years of age. Specific risk factors included such conditions as maternal anxiety and mental health, stressful life events, family social support, occupation, educational levels, and mother–child interactive behaviors. Results indicated that as the number of risk factors increased, intellectual performance decreased, with the difference between the lowest and highest groups being approximately 30 points. Of greatest interest is that no child-centered information was entered into the multiple risk analyses.

Consistent with these findings, the Collaborative Project data set was used to conduct a follow-up study of project participants into adolescence (Kochanek, Kabacoff, & Lipsitt, 1987) by examining the usefulness of information gathered before 12 months of age in predicting the presence of a disability reported between 14 and 20 years of age. Major findings indicated that maternal characteristics (e.g., level of educational attainment) were more accurate predictors of adolescent status than child performance data gathered at infancy and at 4, 8, and 12 months of age. Moreover, addition of child-centered behaviors into the regression equation did not increase accuracy in identifying students with disabilities beyond that from maternal education alone. This study concluded that models of screening founded on child-centered data alone are of suspect validity.

As an extension of this study, analyses were also conducted related to the ability of child-centered data (from birth to age 7) and familial factors to predict the presence of disabilities in adolescence (Kochanek, Kabacoff, & Lipsitt, 1990). Of significance was that all prenatal and perinatal data (i.e., pregnancy history, maternal medical and reproductive history, labor and delivery information, birth presentation and trauma) failed to yield significant results with univariate analyses. Therefore, despite the substantial differences observed between disabled and nondisabled groups in adolescence, these groups, as a whole, were indistinguishable from each other during infancy.

When each variable cluster was viewed separately, the classification rates revealed important differences. More precisely, whereas parental traits (e.g., maternal education) were more accurate predictors of disabled adolescent status than the child's own behavior from birth to 3 years of age, child-centered skills assessed at 4 and 7 years of age proved to be better indicators of disabling conditions than maternal level of educational attainment. Moreover, even when environmental traits were considered with child performance data gathered at 4 and 7 years of age, the accuracy of group classification was not appreciably influenced. Therefore, while results underscored the initial role of ecological determinants of adolescent status, findings also suggested that the effects of these determinants were not consistent over time; in fact, individual factors (e.g., maternal education) contributed differently to group classification depending on the age at which child level of functioning was examined. It is also crucial to note that while no single child factor (e.g., anoxia, prematurity, neurological status) predicted outcome, it is also true that isolated environmental factors alone did not account for significant variance, and accordingly, should not be used exclusively in the development of screening and early identification models.

Overall, available studies indicate that although single factors alone do not inevitably produce poor outcomes, an accumulation of risk factors (both biological as well as environmental) substantially increases the odds of compromised success. Developmental outcome is determined by multiple variables (Sameroff et al., 1987) and the greater the number of risk factors, the poorer the outcome for the child. Developmental disabilities have their origins in biological conditions, familial characteristics, and primary caregiving behaviors; as such, all must be fully accommodated in screening initiatives.

Implications of Risk Research for Screening Models

Three significant implications for screening and surveillance systems can be derived from the above studies. First, screening processes for infants, toddlers, and preschool children must broaden in definition and scope. The degree of risk or the severity of potential developmental disability for infants cannot be accurately predicted by the occurrence of any one traumatic prenatal or neonatal event (Broman, Bien, & Shaughnessy, 1987; Sameroff & Chandler, 1975). Studies that have followed a "medical model" of disease, attempting to identify a linear relationship between cause and outcome, have produced disappointing results. In fact, evidence suggests that selecting children for programs based upon isolate factors (e.g., socioeconomic status) provides no assurance that those "most in need" will be served.

Second, screening programs must include sources of data beyond that presented by the child alone. Longitudinal studies report complex interactions between a child's physical, neurological, and developmental status and the environmental context within which the child is reared (Werner, 1989). The assessment of newborn and early developmental status is of equivalent importance to that of caregiver response and adaptation to the developing child. As Sameroff and Chandler (1975) indicated, "if developmental processes are to be understood, it will not be through continuous assessment of the child alone, but through a continuous assessment of the transactions between the child and his environment to determine how these transactions facilitate or hinder adaptive integration as both the child and his surroundings change and evolve" (p. 283).

Finally, surveillance programs should be serial in their operation. Because of the instability of findings reported in several studies, screening outcomes should not be binary in nature (i.e., refer for diagnostic testing, exit from system) but rather should be an ongoing process, with the frequency of examination determined by the type and extensiveness of special need revealed through multifactorial screening data. The developmental surveillance process (Dworkin, 1989) is a system that involves features of serial examination to discriminate between transient and permanent insults, and, in addition, takes into account the ongoing transactions between child and environment that affect developmental progress.

PROTECTIVE FACTORS AND RESILIENCY

Although understanding the complex manner in which risk factors interact to produce poor outcomes is critical to developing effective screening models, identification of factors that promote favorable outcomes is equally significant. The literature base on resiliency is both impressive and extensive. For example, investigations have been conducted on the resilient offspring of psychotic parents (Anthony & Cohler, 1987; Garmezy, 1987; Kaufman, Grunebaum, Cohler, & Gamer, 1979), children reared in abusive/neglectful environments (Farber & Egeland, 1987), children of divorced parents (Hetherington, Cox, & Cox, 1982), and children raised in acute and chronic poverty (Clark, 1983; Elder, Caspi, & Van Nguyen, 1985; Lewis & Looney, 1983). Furthermore, studies have also been completed on children who have experienced dramatic upheaval of their social context, such as children who have been abandoned and orphaned, or have experienced the horrors of the Nazi holocaust or of wars in Europe, Central America, the Middle East, and Southeast Asia (Boothby, 1983; Moskovitz, 1983; Sheehy, 1987). Such studies have allowed for the examination of the cross-cultural universality of protective factors. Three types of protective factors emerge from these diverse studies.

Child Temperament Characteristics

Studies that have focused on the roots of resiliency in infancy have reported a range of temperament characteristics that elicit positive responses from other people. More specifically, the majority of resilient children were characterized as cuddly, affectionate, good natured, and without sleeping and feeding disturbances (Werner, 1985). During the preschool years, resilient children are described as alert, self-confident, socially adept, and are more advanced in communication and self-help skills (Werner & Smith, 1982).

For the middle years and adolescence, stress-resistant children demonstrate several common traits including social maturity, a more positive self-concept, and an internal locus of control (Werner, 1985). Overall, protective factors in children appear to relate to behavioral characteristics (e.g., sociability, independence, adaptability, optimism, hopefulness) that permit a sense of confidence and self-fulfillment to occur and also elicit positive attention and support from other individuals. The good naturedness and pleasing personalities of these children assisted in the development of a wide network of caring adults, both within and outside of their families, which buffered them from the adversity in their lives.

Family Characteristics

Despite the constitutional or environmental adversity that resilient children encountered, all report having had the opportunity to establish a close bond with at least one other person who provided stability and emotional nourishment during the first year of life (Anthony, 1987; Farber & Egeland, 1987; Musick, Stott, Spencer, Goldman, & Cohler, 1987). In some families, the nurturing may be provided by alternative caregivers (e.g., grandparents and siblings) who emerge as buffers of stress. In more unique circumstances, this key role can be assumed by babysitters, nannies, or house mothers in orphanages or refugee centers (Ayala-Canales, 1984; Moskovitz, 1983; Sheehy, 1987).

Beyond the opportunity for a close relationship, high-risk resilient youths reported the expectation of "required helpfulness" in which they assumed responsibility for household chores and caring for younger siblings. Furthermore, families that were grounded in religious beliefs were those in which stress-resistant children were more likely to be present.

In summary, resilient children are those who have had the opportunity to establish a secure attachment to at least one stable caregiver who, in turn, created a context of caring, helpfulness, and assumption of responsibility.

Community Characteristics

Abundant data from numerous studies (Bryant, 1985; Werner & Smith, 1982) suggest that resilient children obtain a great deal of support from outside of their own family. Resilient children tend to be well liked by their peers and invariably report having one or more close friends (Garmezy, 1981; Kaufman et al., 1979; Werner & Smith, 1982). Furthermore, such children frequently report having had a favorite teacher who not only provided formal instruction, but also served as a role model and confidant. Overall, therefore, among the most potent protective factors in the lives of resilient children are friends, neighbors, and teachers who have provided emotional support, rewarded competence and achievement, and promoted self-esteem.

Implications of Resiliency Research for Screening Models

Thoughtful examination of the above literature yields several implications for screening procedures. First, vulnerability and resiliency have their origins in complex, dynamic interactions among constitutional factors, family characteristics, and significant life events and circumstances. As such, screening models must be comprehensive and ongoing and must accommodate the interplay among the child's competencies, family environment, and larger social context in which the child lives.

Second, intervention may be conceived as an attempt to shift the focus from vulnerability to resilience, either by decreasing exposure to risk factors or stressful life events, or by increasing the number of protective factors. Consequently, screening models must include information in both areas and, moreover, attend to factors (e.g., social competency and temperamental characteristics of children; social context and support network for children and families) that will provide important guidance for crafting interventions and services.

Third, screening models must be designed to identify children who appear vulnerable due to an absence of essential social bonds in their environment. Among these are survivors of neonatal intensive care, abusive/neglectful environments, alcoholic or psychotic parents, and migrant and refugee children without meaningful roots in a community or social context.

Fourth, research on resilient children has shown repeatedly that if a parent is incapacitated or unavailable, other significant individuals (e.g., grandparents, older siblings, child care providers, other kin) can assume an enabling role. Screening models should attempt to assess the presence and strength of connections between children, kin, and the community. Establishing and amplifying these connections, rather than professional interventionists assuming such a role, is an important goal and outcome of screening paradigms.

Finally, a common trait among all stress-resistant children is that they report having at least one person in their lives who accepted them unconditionally, regardless of their temperamental or constitutional idiosyncrasies. If intervention is to ensure that strong connections are formed between children and persons who provide them with a secure basis for trust and autonomy, then screening approaches must gather information that uncovers the presence and "goodness of fit" of connections between adults and children.

CORE INGREDIENTS OF EFFECTIVE SCREENING MODELS

Fortunately, recent publications (Meisels & Provence, 1989) have synthesized the above knowledge base, and accordingly, provide clear and insightful guidance regarding the core components of screening models. The ten essential concepts advanced are described here.

Screening as Services

The sole purpose of screening is not to exclude children and families from service systems. Alternatively, screening should be viewed as the initial step in service provision, and as such, is designed to gather information concerning child and family needs, and ensure linkage with appropriate community-based resources and programs.

Multiple Information Sources

Predictive validity studies (Broman, Bien, & Shaughnessy, 1985; Kochanek, Kabacoff, & Lipsitt, 1990; Sameroff et al., 1987) have indicated that early identification models that rely on single factors are replete with decision-making error. Consequently, valid screening systems must include information on the child (i.e., significant historical events and current level of functioning); family attributes, strengths, and significant life events; and the social context within which a child is reared.

Multiple Information Reporters

As previously indicated, both vulnerability and resiliency emerge from a complex interplay of factors that cannot be totally derived from child-centered, standardized measures. Although the appraisal of a child's developmental competency is an important ingredient in screening models, perceptions of the child's status and needs from family members and other significant adults and caretakers must assume equal weight in the decision-making equation.

Periodicity

Because of significant variation in child developmental pathways as well as ongoing changes in family status, all children and families should participate in screening on multiple occasions between birth and 5 years of age. Judgment regarding the need for further evaluation should be based upon evidence of jeopardy from individual time points as well as from determination of cumulative risk.

Multivariate Decision-Making Models

No single condition, risk factor, or protective factor leads irrevocably to a predictable outcome. Rather, both risk and protective factors are linked over time to produce a child's status, and therefore, screening models must allow for multiple sources of evidence to assume different weights in decision making over time.

Reliability and Validity

The psychometric properties of standardized instruments not only have a remarkable influence on the accuracy of decision making, but also determine the prevalence and type of children in need of follow-up. Tests used to make decisions on children and families should be rigorously evaluated for reliability, validity, sensitivity, and specificity. Comprehensive, contextually based screening models, if founded upon weak instruments, are harmful and discriminatory.

Families as Major Informants

An array of studies (Bricker & Squires, 1989; Glascoe & MacLean, 1990, 1991) exists that suggests that families are key informants regarding child and family status, needs, and goals. Screening procedures must be designed that fully engage families as not only reliable sources of information, but also as key members of the decision-making team.

Cultural Sensitivity

Current literature on cultural differences reveals that several important dimensions and traditions characterize the uniqueness of various cultural groups (Randall-David, 1989). Such factors include:

- Family structure, roles, and relations.
- Health beliefs, particularly related to chronic illness and disability.
- Religious beliefs and their interrelationship with health beliefs.
- Styles of communication and decision making, particularly those that impact on the goals and implementation strategies of service plans.

Although many attempts have been made to understand fragments of the above domains, very few screening models have been developed that engender a holistic perspective and attempt to understand disability and vulnerability in the context of a broader socioeconomic, religious, and cultural system. Given the heterogeneity of the population to be served within early intervention in the forthcoming decade, new models of screening must fully engage minority families in the conceptualization and design of early identification models rather than view such families as passive recipients of what are perceived as invaluable services.

Coordination with Other Screening Initiatives

Examination of Federal policy in health care (e.g., Title V), preventive services (e.g., Early Periodic Screening, Diagnostic, and Treatment Program [EPSDT]), and education (Individuals with Disabilities Education Act [IDEA]) reveals a rich history of commitments to children and families over the last 50 years, particularly with regard to early identification mandates. Despite the enormous potential of these initiatives, such programs have fallen short of their intended outcomes (Margolis & Meisels, 1987; Meisels & Margolis, 1987). New screening efforts must determine methods for capturing and coordinating the resources in these initiatives such that comprehensive, community-based, accessible, and universal screening may be available to all young children and families.

Training

The quality, effectiveness, and long-term impact of screening initiatives is inextricably tied to the competency of those who implement the process. Mandating that all individuals who conduct screenings are appropriately certified or licensed does not always ensure that they have independently gained access to current literature, instruments, and approaches to screening that are systems-based, psychometrically sound, and culturally relevant. As a result, screening programs must include provisions for ongoing training and clinical supervision, even for those who have already achieved the highest requirements in the state applicable to a professional or academic discipline.

CONGRUENCE BETWEEN SCREENING CONCEPTS AND STATE POLICIES IN EARLY INTERVENTION

Part H of IDEA requires states to (1) locate and identify all disabled children and, at the state's discretion, those at substantial risk for poor health and educational outcomes; and (2) coordinate such efforts with other programs (e.g., Title V and EPSDT) to identify eligible children. As a result of a 4-year planning and development period underwritten by a $300 million Congressional appropriation, 55 states and U.S. territories have received "fourth"-or "fifth"-year awards that include formal policies and procedures relating to the above mandate (Early Childhood Report, 1992). These policies will undeniably exert substantial influence over the course and content of early intervention services in the next decade.

In order to assess the extent to which these policies reflect the contemporary wisdom noted above, this author conducted an analysis of state child-find policies that have been approved by the U.S. Office of Special Education Programs. Within this analysis, policy documents were reviewed for 39 of the 55 states with approved policies.[1] Of these, two represented Year Five (i.e., entitlement) states, whereas the remainder were Year Four states with approved policies and procedures.

The evaluative criteria used to assess each state's policies were identical to the ten dimensions noted above, which are widely accepted as reflecting the current knowledge and perspective on screening and early identification. In assessing state policies, sections pertaining to screening, child find, evaluation, and assessment were reviewed in full for each state, and additionally, where relevant appendices were referenced, these documents were analyzed as well.

In order to assess policies in the context of the ten exemplary criteria, a 4-point rating scale was developed. Each state's policies were given a rating for each of the 10 criteria. Definitions and decision-making guidelines were as follows:

1. *Policy fully reflects current knowledge.* This rating was used when states' expressed policies fully reflected the knowledge base described earlier. Beyond the inclusion of key concepts, states receiving this rating were also distinguished by explicit procedures and quality assurance standards that would guide the implementation process.

2. *Policy partially reflects current knowledge.* This rating was given to states that included key concepts in expressed policies and reflected a clear understanding of the principles and values governing individual components of the screening process, but did not include specific procedures and implementation strategies.

3. *Policy is restricted to Part H statute only.* States that received this rating included those in which written policies were a mirror image of Part H language. For example, on the dimension relating to coordination with other screening initiatives, the statute explicitly names those programs (e.g., Title V, EPSDT, Head Start Act) that must be incorporated. States that simply adopted identical language without further embellishment were given this rating.

4. *Policy does not include information on this exemplary factor.* This rat-

[1]I gratefully acknowledge the support and generous cooperation of Pat Trohanis and Joan Danaher of the National Early Childhood Technical Assistance System (NEC*TAS) at the University of North Carolina at Chapel Hill for providing access to these documents.

ing was given to any state in which no information was provided that related to this exemplary or "best practice" factor.

Results of these ratings are presented in Figures 3.1 and 3.2. In Figure 3.1, the six exemplary factors that are included in Part H statutory language are represented. Figure 3.2 includes all factors that are consistent with the knowledge base, but are not included within Part H (e.g., periodicity, screening as intervention).

Within each figure, the distribution of ratings (i.e., percent of states within each of the four categories) is presented such that contrasts among exemplary indicators can be visually examined. Several interesting and noteworthy findings are evident in these portrayals.

Exemplary screening procedures are much more likely to appear in state policies if they are included in Part H rules and regulations. More specifically, while the proportion of states that did make reference to specific exemplary factors approximates 85% overall in Figure 3.1 (i.e., factor present in statute), Figure 3.2 (factor not present) indicates that states that included discretionary "best practice" factors ranged from 30 to 46%. In short, the inclusion of knowledge-based, exemplary components in federal regulations appears to be influential in state policies relative to early identification and child find.

Considerable variability is evident in Figure 3.1 with regard to the extent to which exemplary factors are represented in policies. While concepts that

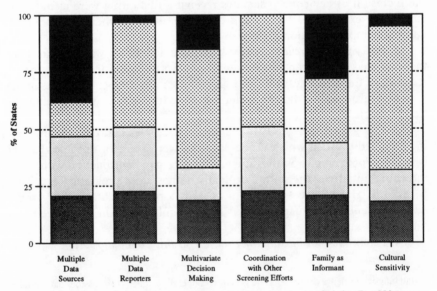

FIGURE 3.1. Status of state policies on six screening factors that are included in Part H language. (See Figure 3.2 for key.)

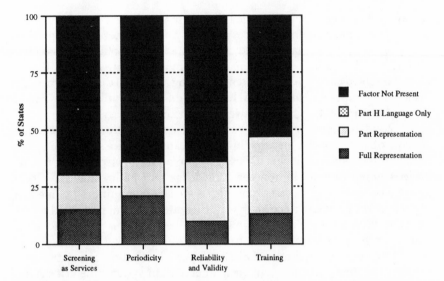

FIGURE 3.2.   Status of state policies on four screening factors that are not included in Part H language.

are explicit in federal regulations (e.g., coordination with other screening efforts, cultural sensitivity, no single factor used in decision making) are often included in state policies, concepts that are expressed in philosophical or values-oriented terms (e.g., families as major informants in the screening process) are less likely to be fully incorporated and embellished in state policy.

With regard to exemplary factors not included in Part H (Figure 3.2), very few states elected to include such concepts in written policies. Of concern is that in approximately two-thirds of the states reviewed, no reference is made to three significant concepts in screening: periodicity, the psychometric properties of screening instruments, and the fact that screening encounters should serve as the initial step in intervention. Furthermore, only one-half of the states presented a plan to ensure the ongoing training and clinical supervision of principal data collectors.

Despite the availability of a rich knowledge base in screening and early identification, only one out of five states have elected, thus far, to fully include this information in approved policies. In short, state policies appear to be more congruent with federal regulations than with contemporary literature and research findings, and very few states have crafted procedures that extend beyond the language of Part H.

Several important limitations to the above analyses must be noted. First, because there is considerable evidence in policy implementation literature of the disparities between policy and actual program operations (Elmore, 1978;

Lipsky, 1980), it cannot be assumed that these policies are an accurate portrayal of current screening practices nationally. Furthermore, although these data suggest underutilization of knowledge in written policies, actual community-based screening activity may be more consistent with the 10 principles presented earlier. Also, differences among states and disparities between principles and practices would likely yield a different profile if an examination of implementation practices were conducted.

Second, the above ratings are based upon a point-in-time (October 1991) analysis of state policies and documents. Because the process of policy formulation is ongoing and dynamic, it must also be acknowledged that the disparities noted previously between knowledge and policy may have been reduced or eliminated in recent months as a result of continuing refinement of policies within states. Accordingly, further attempts at appraising the presence and utilization of current knowledge in both written policy and actual clinical practice are strongly endorsed for the future.

Third, although written policies are a partial reflection of a state's commitment to, and portrait of, an early intervention system, the criteria and process used by the U.S. Office of Special Education Programs to approve state plans also significantly influences the language, content, and specificity of such policies. Although this study did not attempt to examine the influence of the policy-approval process on policy content, it must be acknowledged that this process is a powerful force. In short, if the policy-approval process did not fully reflect the 10 exemplary factors described earlier, this may also have influenced the content of approved policies.

Overall, analysis of state policies relative to screening and child find indicate that important voids are apparent in documents developed to date. As noted above, although the origins of these limitations are not discernible from this study, and furthermore, that actual practice in states may or may not be consonant with approved plans, current policies are cause for concern. The fidelity between policies and Part H regulations is high, but a serious concern is that the congruence between policies and current knowledge is considerably weaker. A major positive finding of this study is that the content of Part H regulations casts an influential framework on state policies. Clearly, the solution for the above concern rests with increasing the synchrony among Part H, state policy, actual clinical practice, and current knowledge.

ENHANCING DEVELOPMENTAL SURVEILLANCE CAPABILITY

In order to more effectively utilize existing knowledge in screening and early identification efforts, the following specific actions are recommended.

1. Evaluate rigorously the benefits and costs of existing screening initiatives in states. Programs that are ineffective should be discontinued. An urgent

need exists to identify the outcomes of the extant system, that is, what works and at what expense? Despite the apparent simplicity of this objective, surprisingly little is known about numerous highly significant programs and financial commitments. As an example, the EPSDT program, despite its existence for nearly three decades, has never been subjected to systematic evaluation or research inquiry (Meisels, 1984). The capability and expertise exist to determine the relative value of current programs; this determination should be initiated immediately.

2. Conceptualize screening models with knowledge as the centerpiece rather than federal rules and regulations. Our ability to identify and prevent disease and disability has dramatically increased in recent years. Research has identified factors that promote and support healthy development and equally clear factors that place children in jeopardy. Developmental pathways are contextually determined by a child's constitutional and temperamental factors, the characteristics of primary caregivers, and the broader community and social ecology within which a child is raised. Screening paradigms should be founded upon these well-established principles.

3. Design and implement screening systems that use an existing, well-developed initiative as its nucleus. It is not unusual to discover numerous, concurrent efforts in states to identify disabled and vulnerable children. However, assuming that such initiatives represent a comprehensive, coordinated, interagency approach to early identification is simply inaccurate. Such disparate programs are typically founded upon a different philosophical and values base; involve different items, protocols, and data collection schedules; and engender different decision-making algorithms. The net consequence is often inconsistency, unevenness, and in some instances, overt discrimination.

Despite considerable diversity across states with regard to the manner in which screening and developmental surveillance are conducted, each state sponsors at least one screening effort that is generally consistent with the exemplary principles noted earlier. Although this system may reside in the health care sector (e.g., Title V Maternal Child Health services or the EPSDT mechanism), in education (i.e., child-find stipulations in IDEA), or in other specialized programs, it is apparent that systems already exist which, if supported and amplified, could evolve into efficient, cost-effective, reliable, and valid procedures to conduct early identification mandates.

4. Develop more effective ways to synthesize and disseminate current knowledge to policymakers, clinicians, and families. The gaps in effective information dissemination exceed the limitations of our knowledge base. With regard to screening and early detection, an adequate research base exists upon which effective models can be formulated. The manner in which this information is aggregated and disseminated influences the extent to which it is used in decision making. The characteristics of the individual who distributes and interprets the information also affect its utilization and application.

More time and effort must be devoted to applying existing knowledge rather than generating new knowledge. This will require the collaborative efforts of research scientists and media specialists to jointly craft more effective techniques of knowledge compilation and dispersion.

5. Acknowledge the critical role that the human element assumes in systems development and implementation. Numerous impressive documents (Institute of Medicine, 1985, 1991; National Conference of State Legislatures, 1990; National Commission on Children, 1990) have recently been prepared that accurately summarize contemporary knowledge and perspectives on several important human service problems. Despite this knowledge base and, in certain instances, the political will for action, successful, large-scale implementation strategies have not been developed (Schorr, 1989). This is true, in part, because of the complexity of the human service system and its enormous, self-perpetuating capacity, but is also true because of the human beings who manage and implement these systems.

Major system change efforts must respect, plan for, and accommodate the divergent values, attitudes, assumptions, and competencies of the human beings responsible for such efforts. Despite well-formulated policies and full access to adequate funding, success is not guaranteed unless those individuals who carry out the policies feel confident, comfortable, and competent to do so. Understanding the complex, dynamic process of behavior change is an essential and often neglected component to implementing effective screening programs.

CONCLUSION

In spite of admirable intentions, the failure of service and support systems created to ensure well-being in children has never been more apparent. The focal problem is twofold: (1) poor access to existing programs and (2) continued reliance upon ineffective services. With regard to access, the EPSDT is a powerful example. EPSDT was launched in 1967 as part of a national commitment to enhance the health and welfare of families in poverty. Despite this impressive, fully funded commitment, studies indicate that only 25–30% of eligible children ever receive the benefits of EPSDT (Children's Defense Fund, 1990).

With respect to the efficacy of select existing services, the data are equally disconcerting. More precisely, extensive resources in many states are consumed by placements in residential treatment centers and psychiatric hospitals (National Mental Health Association, 1989). In fact, recent reports indicate that $261 million are being spent nationally in psychiatric hospitalization of children (Fox & Yoshpe, 1987). Despite such utilization, research on outcomes of such treatment is virtually nonexistent (Friedman & Street, 1985;

Institute of Medicine, 1989; Saxe, Dougherty, Cross, & Silverman, 1987). In current dollars, this investment would support approximately 65,000 children in early intervention programs.

Although ambitious solutions have been advanced regarding our commitments to children and families (National Commission on Children, 1990), given the current economic climate, only finite resources will be available in the future. As a result, the need for prudently expending scarce dollars will become more apparent. Valid screening initiatives, that is, identifying children and families most in need, must assume a prominent role in charting our future course. As indicated in this chapter, the manner in which this should be accomplished is not obscure. While new investments must be made in experimenting with alternative screening models, full and thoughtful utilization of the rich information base that already exists must also be rigorously and aggressively pursued.

REFERENCES

Anthony, E. J. (1987). Children at risk for psychosis growing up successfully. In E. J. Anthony & B. Cohler (Eds.), *The invulnerable child* (pp. 147–184). New York: Guilford Press.

Anthony, E. J., & Cohler, B. (Eds.). (1987). *The invulnerable child.* New York: Guilford Press.

Ayala-Canales, C. E. (1984). *The impact of El Salvador's civil war on orphan and refugee children.* Unpublished master's thesis in child development, University of California, Davis, CA.

Bierman-van Eenderburg, M., Jurgens-van der Zee, A., & Olinga, A. (1981). Predictive value of neonatal neurological examination: A follow up study at 18 months. *Developmental Medicine and Child Neurology, 23,* 296–305.

Boothby, B. (1983). The horror, the hope. *Natural History, 92,* 64–71.

Bricker, D., & Squires, J. (1989). The effectiveness of screening at-risk infants: Infant Monitoring Questionnaire. *Topics in Early Childhood Special Education, 3*(9), 67–85.

Broman, S., Bien, E., & Shaughnessy, P. (1985). *Low achieving children: The first seven years.* Hillsdale, NJ: Erlbaum.

Bryant, B. K. (1985). The neighborhood walk: Sources of support in middle childhood. *Monographs of the Society for Research in Child Development, 50* (30, Serial No. 210).

Children's Defense Fund. (1990). *Children 1990.* Washington DC: Author

Clark, R. M. (1983). *Family life and school achievement: Why poor black children succeed or fail.* Chicago: University of Chicago Press.

Dworkin, P. H. (1989). British and American recommendations for developmental monitoring: The role of surveillance. *Pediatrics, 84,* 1,000–1,010.

Early Childhood Report. (1992, May). Horsham, PA: LRP.

Elder, G. H., Caspi, A., & Van Nguyen, T. (1985). Resourceful and vulnerable children: Family influence on hard times. In R. Silbereisen & H. Eyferth (Eds.), *Development in context* (pp. 167–186). Berlin: Springer-Verlag.

Elmore, R. F. (1978). Organizational models of social program implementation. *Public Policy, 26,* 185–228.

Farber, E. A., & Egeland, B. (1987). Invulnerability among abused and neglected children. In E. J. Anthony & B. Cohler (Eds.), *The invulnerable child* (pp. 253–288). New York: Guilford Press.

Fox, H. B., & Yoshpe, R. (1987). *An explanation of Medicaid and its role in financing treatment for severely emotionally disturbed children and adolescents.* Washington, DC: Georgetown University Child Development Center.

Friedman, R. M., & Street, S. (1985). Admission and discharge criteria in children's mental health services: Review of the issues and options. *Journal of Clinical Child Psychology, 14,* 229–235.

Garmezy, N. (1981). Children under stress: Perspectives on antecedents and correlates of vulnerability and resistance to psychopathology. In A. I. Rabin, J. Aronoff, A. M. Barclay, & R. A. Zucker (Eds.), *Further explorations in personality* (pp. 196–269). New York: Wiley.

Garmezy, N. (1985). Stress-resistant children: The search for protective factors. In J. E. Stevenson (Ed.), *Journal of Child Psychology and Psychiatry: Book Suppl. No. 4. Recent research in developmental psychopathology* (pp. 213–233). Oxford: Pergamon Press.

Garmezy, N. (1987). Stress, competence and development: Continuities in the study of schizophrenic adults, children vulnerable to psychopathology, and the search for stress-resistant children. *American Journal of Orthopsychiatry, 57*(2), 159–174.

Glascoe, F. P., & MacLean, W. E. (1990). How parents appraise their child's development. *Family Relations, 39,* 280–283.

Glascoe, F. P., MacLean, W. E., & Stone, W. L. (1991). The importance of parents' concerns about their child's behavior. *Clinical Pediatrics, 30,* 8–11.

Gottfried, A. W. (1973). Intellectual consequences of perinatal anoxia. *Psychological Bulletin, 80,* 231–242.

Hetherington, E. M., Cox, M., & Cox, R. (1982). Effects of divorce on parents and children. In M. Lamb (Ed.), *Non-traditional families* (pp. 223–285). Hillsdale, NJ: Erlbaum.

Institute of Medicine. (1985). *Preventing low birthweight.* Washington, DC: National Academy Press.

Institute of Medicine. (1989). *Research on children and adolescents with mental, behavioral, and developmental disorders.* Washington, DC: National Academy of Sciences.

Institute of Medicine. (1991). *Disability in America: Toward a national agenda for prevention.* Washington, DC: National Academy of Sciences.

Kaufman, C., Grunebaum, L., Cohler, B., & Gamer, E. (1979). Superkids: Competent children of psychotic mothers. *American Journal of Psychiatry, 136,* 1398–1402.

Kochanek, T. T., Kabacoff, R. I., & Lipsitt, L. P. (1987). Early detection of handicapping conditions in infancy and early childhood: Toward a multivariate model. *Journal of Applied Developmental Psychology, 8,* 411–420.

Kochanek, T. T., Kabacoff, R. I., & Lipsitt, L. P. (1990). Early identification of developmentally disabled and at-risk preschool children. *Exceptional Children, 56,* 528–538.

Lazenby, H. C., & Letsch, S. W. (1990). National health expenditures, 1989. *Health Care Financing Review, 12,* 1–26.

Lewis, J. M., & Looney, J. D. (1983). *The long struggle: Well functioning working class black families.* New York: Brunner/Mazel.

Lewit, E., & Monheit, A. (1992). Expenditures on health care for children and pregnant women. In Packard Foundation, *The future of children.* Los Altos, CA: Packard Foundation.

Lipsky, M. (1980). *Street level bureaucracy.* New York: Russell Sage Foundation.

Margolis, L. H., & Meisels, S. J. (1987). Barriers to the effectiveness of EPSDT for children with moderate and severe developmental disabilities. *American Journal of Orthopsychiatry, 57,* 424–430.

Masten, A. S., & Garmezy, N. (1985). Risk, vulnerability, and protective factors in developmental psychopathology. In B. B. Lahey & A. E. Kazdin (Eds.), *Advances in clinical child psychology,* (Vol. 8, pp. 1–52). New York: Plenum Press.

Meisels, S. J. (1984). Prediction, prevention, and developmental screening in the EPSDT program. In H. W. Stevenson & A. E. Siegel (Eds.), *Child development research and social policy* (pp. 83–97). Chicago: University of Chicago Press.

Meisels, S. J., & Margolis, L. H. (1987). Is EPSDT effective with developmentally disabled children? *Pediatrics, 81,* 262–271.

Meisels, S. J., & Provence, S. (1989). *Screening and assessment: Guidelines for identifying young disabled and developmentally vulnerable children and their families.* Washington, DC: National Center for Clinical Infant Programs.

Moskovitz, S. (1983). *Love despite hate: Child survivors of the Holocaust and their adult lives.* New York: Schocken.

Musick, J. S., Stott, F. M., Spencer, C. K., Goldman, J., & Cohler, B. J. (1987). Maternal factors related to vulnerability and resiliency in young children at risk. In E. J. Anthony & B. J. Cohler (Eds.), *The invulnerable child* (pp. 229–252). New York: Guilford Press.

National Commission on Children. (1990). *Beyond rhetoric: A new American agenda for children and families.* Washington, DC: Author.

National Commission on Excellence in Education. (1983). *A nation at risk: The imperative for educational reform.* Washington, DC: U.S. Government Printing Office.

National Conference of State Legislatures. (1990). *Putting the pieces together: Survey of state systems for children in crisis.* Washington, DC: Author.

National Mental Health Association. (1989). *Report of the invisible children program.* Alexandria, VA: Author.

Nichols, P. L., & Chen, T. (1981). *Minimal brain dysfunction: A prospective study.* Hillsdale, NJ: Erlbaum.

Odden, A. R. (1987, March). *The economics of financing educational excellence.* Paper presented at the annual meeting of the American Educational Research Association, Washington, DC.

Papile, L., Munsick-Bruno, G., & Schaefer A. (1983). Relationship of cerebral intraventricular hemorrhage and early childhood neurological handicaps. *Pediatrics, 103,* 273–277.

Randall-David, E. (1989). *Strategies for working with culturally diverse communities and clients.* Bethesda, MD: Association for the Care of Children's Health.

Sameroff, A., & Chandler, M. (1975). Reproductive risk and the continuum of caretaking casualty. In F. Horowitz, M. Hetherington, S. Scarr-Salapatek, & G. Siegel (Eds.), *Review of child development research* (Vol. 4, pp. 187–244). Chicago: University of Chicago Press.

Sameroff, A., Seifer, R., Barocas, R., Zax, M., & Greenspan, S. (1987). Intelligence quotient scores of 4-year-old children: Social–environmental risk factors. *Pediatrics, 79,* 343–350.

Saxe, L. M., Dougherty, D. M., Cross, T., & Silverman, N. (1987). *Children's mental health: Problems and services.* Durham, NC: Duke University Press.

Schorr, L. B. (1989). *Within our reach.* New York: Doubleday.

Sheehy, G. (1987). *Spirit of survival.* New York: Bantam Books.

Stewart, A. L., Reynolds, E., & Lipscomb, A. (1981). Outcome for infants of very low birthweight: Survey of world literature. *Lancet, 1,* 1038-1041.

Werner, E. E. (1985). Stress and protective factors in children's lives. In A. R. Nichol (Ed.), *Longitudinal studies in child psychology and psychiatry* (pp. 335–356). Chichester, England: Wiley.

Werner, E. E. (April, 1989). Children of the garden island. *Scientific American, 260,* 106–111.

Werner, E. E. (1990). Protective factors and individual resilience. In S. Meisels & J. Shonkoff (Eds.), *Handbook of early childhood intervention* (pp. 97–116). Cambridge, England: Cambridge University Press.

Werner, E. E., & Smith, R. S. (1982). *Vulnerable but invincible: A study of resilient children.* San Francisco: McGraw-Hill.

CHAPTER 4

Definitional Issues
Prevalence, Participation, and Service Utilization

RAY E. FOSTER
BARBARA F. FOSTER

Whom shall we serve? How many people in a state or county would qualify for services if all were screened? How many people who qualify for services currently participate in a program? How many persons in a program are using particular services? These questions are asked by advocates, policy makers, planners, and program managers in considering the provision of services to a particular population in need of special support, assistance, care, or treatment. Answering these questions requires (1) the definition of a target population, (2) an estimation of prevalence of the target population within the general population, (3) a determination of current participation in existing programs, and (4) a summary of services used by program participants. Legislators often demand answers to these questions before they will consider the entitlement of a group of persons to receive a particular set of services to be paid at taxpayer expense. Without answers to these questions, there is no way to assess the fiscal impact of a government-sponsored program. Thus, the issues of prevalence, participation, and service utilization are fundamental to policy analysis and planning. This chapter explores the estimation of prevalence of developmental delay, disability, and risk status in a population of infants and toddlers in the context of planning early intervention services. Program participation and service utilization are discussed. Various approaches to the estimation and use of prevalence, participation, and utilization information by selected states are presented.

DEFINITION OF TERMS

Three terms used in this chapter require definition to provide the reader with an understanding of the manner in which they are used: prevalence, program participation, and service utilization. Figure 4.1 offers a graphic explanation of the definitions. As used here, *prevalence* refers to an estimate of the portion of a general population that is comprised by a specific target group of infants and toddlers who would be eligible for participation in a particular program. For example, children with a specific set of risk factors may comprise an estimated 6% of the general population of children the same age at a given point in time. Prevalence may be expressed as a rate (%) or as a number of children within a given population.

Program participation refers to the portion of the children in the target group who are identified and served in an early intervention program. For example, at a given point in time, 40% of the target population may be identified and served though a particular program. The remaining unidentified and/or unserved 60% of the target group are those for whom outreach and screening activities may be directed to increase program participation over time. Similarly, if participation is limited by resources available to provide needed services, then the unserved rate may be used to advocate for additional funds and resources. Participation may be expressed as a rate or number.

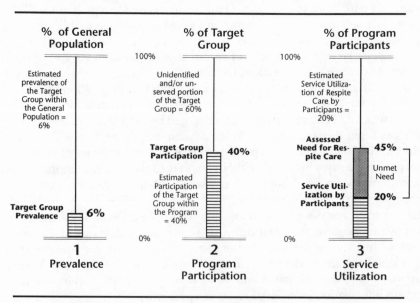

FIGURE 4.1.   Prevalence, program participation, and service utilization.

Service utilization refers to the proportion of current participants in a particular program using a given service, such as respite care. For example, 20% of the participants in a program may use respite care at a given point in time. Service utilization should be compared to assessed need among participants for that service to determine the extent to which service provision meets the actual need or demand. In the example shown in Figure 4.1, service utilization for respite care was 20% while the assessed need for that service was 45%, leaving a 25% gap between services received by program participants and the level of services recommended according to their needs.

Each of these three measures has a specific meaning and a different use in policy development, planning, and budgeting for early intervention programs and services designed for infants and toddlers.

CONSTRUCTING AN ELIGIBILITY DEFINITION

Policy makers require information to define, estimate, and identify the target group of children for whom prevention and early intervention services are to be directed. Targeting services through an eligibility definition involves the use of *determination factors,* which are descriptors of the distinguishing characteristics of the children of concern. For example, if policy makers wished only to target children who already have a developmental delay or disability, then a description of the conditions or attributes for distinguishing children in this group from other children would be developed. Descriptive categories, such as children having a congenital or genetic disorder associated with developmental delay or disability, are used to describe a group of children for whom early intervention services would be provided. Known conditions associated with each descriptive category (e.g., Down syndrome, cerebral palsy, or spina bifida) provide a set of determination factors by which the prevalence of the group can be estimated and an eligibility definition constructed. The same approach may be used to target, estimate, and identify children at elevated risk of developmental delay due to predisposing biological factors (e.g., low birth weight) and predisposing environmental factors (e.g., a victim of child abuse or a child of a teenage mother who did not complete her high school education). Thus, a set of determination factors is the basis for an eligibility definition used in the screening and identification of children in the group to whom early intervention services are to be targeted.

Constructing an eligibility definition for the infant and toddler target group usually involves a threefold approach. The first provision is the definition of developmental delay. This portion of the definition specifies the evidence-based criteria that must be met for the presence of developmental delay to be positively determined. Any person who presents evidence consistent with the definition is deemed eligible for early intervention services. The second provision in the definition is a listing of categories of established conditions that are known to cause developmental delay and disability. A person presenting any one condition that matches any category on the established condition list is considered eligible for services, regardless of whether a measured delay is present at the time of screening. The third provision is a list of predisposing biological and environmental risk factors with a threshold number of risks that must be present in a child's life before sufficient risk is believed to be present to warrant further consideration or determination of eligibility. If a staged screening process is used, one risk factor may be sufficient to warrant further assessment, but two, three, or even four risk factors may be necessary for actual eligibility determination (see Benn, Chapter 2, this volume).

In conclusion, an eligibility definition for early intervention services should be considered a targeting mechanism for implementing a state's prevention/early intervention policy. Serving at-risk children involves primary prevention strategies aimed at reducing the number of children later identified as having developmental delay. Serving children with established conditions involves secondary prevention strategies designed to mitigate the effects and lessen the complications of those conditions in the children's lives. A state's eligibility definition answers the question of whom we shall serve.

APPROACHES USED TO ESTIMATE PREVALENCE AMONG INFANTS AND TODDLERS

Use of determination factors set forth in a state's eligibility definition is necessary for estimating the proportion of children in the general population of a state who meet an eligibility definition fashioned by planners and policy makers. Such an estimate of proportion is referred to as prevalence and may be expressed as a rate or a number of cases based on an estimated rate within a given population. For example, the estimated prevalence of infants and toddlers in a given state at a point in time might be 6% of the general population when using a definition focused on both developmental delay and established risk conditions. In a state with 100,000 infants and toddlers, this prevalence rate would yield 6,000 children in that state who could qualify for services. Thus, a prevalence estimate answers the question of how many persons could qualify for services if all persons meeting the definition were screened at a single point in time. Prevalence defines the size of the target group.

Because individual rates of occurrence of the determination factors used to define a target population may increase or decrease over time, estimates of prevalence also may vary over time. In times of economic hardship, for example, children's nutrition and health care may suffer; access to health care for expectant mothers may become limited, resulting in an increase in low-birthweight infants; and unemployment and alcoholism may increase, leading to greater family stress and increased rates of child abuse. Conditions such as these would be likely to contribute to an increase in the prevalence of developmental delays and disabilities among infants born into these circumstances. Prevalence rates may be expected to vary through time as a function of presenting social and economic conditions that accompany the conception, gestation, birth, survival, and the early life of a child.

A prevalence rate may be thought of as a theoretical upper limit of the portion of a general population that presents the types and numbers of determination factors necessary to meet an eligibility definition at a fixed point in time. In a sense, a prevalence rate is a relative value that can be estimated, not an absolute value that can be measured exactly. Although a certain portion of a population may be eligible for certain services, not all of those who qualify will be identified or present themselves for service all at once. For example, it might be estimated that 6% of all infants and toddlers (birth to 36 months of age) in a state would meet a particular eligibility definition, but only 3% of the population might be identified over the time period that a given group of children were of eligible age to receive early intervention services. Thus, the participation of children identified may be significantly less than estimated prevalence. Of those who are identified as eligible for services, not all will choose to make use of particular services offered. Actual service utilization by eligible persons taken into a service system may be substantially less than the number of persons identified as eligible and participating in an early intervention program. Estimates of prevalence, participation, and service utilization are important information in planning for adequate system capacity to serve the number of children likely to need and use particular services at given points in time. Service utilization rates, actual or estimated, are often used as a basis for analyzing and projecting service costs for planning and budgeting.

Given an eligibility definition, how should prevalence be estimated? In conducting their Public Law 99-457 Part H planning activities, states have taken a number of different approaches to estimating prevalence. This section describes the approaches taken by six states and discusses their advantages and limitations. States have estimated prevalence rates in various ways, including establishing a rate based on nationally derived estimates, synthesizing existing state and local data sources to produce a localized prevalence estimate, and conducting either small-scale or large-scale surveys of the population to obtain prevalence estimates based on direct measures of the population of concern. In most cases, states have used a combination of methods as will be described below. The first step in estimating prevalence is the review of the determination factors associated with the definition to be used for service eligibility. The procedures selected should allow the state to estimate how many persons, on the basis of the determination factors identified, would meet the eligibility definition.

The most accurate, costly, labor-intensive, and least likely to be adopted approach to determining prevalence would be to conduct a census of every child in a state or county using the identified determination factors provided in the eligibility definition. The portion of children identified as meeting the definition would set the prevalence rate for that point in time. The portion of children meeting the definition and having contacted the system for services would set the participation rate. For each service of interest, the portion of children meeting the definition and having used that particular service would set the utilization rate for that service. States have neither the staff nor the finances necessary to conduct a census study of all children. Other options and strategies used by a sample of states are explored below.

Use of Nationally Derived or Reported Estimates

One step most states have used is a review of nationally derived or reported estimates for individual determination factors. For example, Benn (1990) conducted an extensive review of the literature concerning 27 risk factors. Her review examined national incidence or prevalence data of each risk factor, results pertaining to the short- and long-term developmental effects, their association with other risk factors or demographics, and information about prevention/intervention programs that have been suggested or actually implemented to minimize adverse developmental outcomes.

Another frequently used source of information related to prevalence of disabling conditions is found in nationally conducted health surveys. Federally sponsored, the National Center for Health Statistics (NCHS), located in Hyattsville, Maryland, has conducted the National Health Interview Survey (NHIS) on an annual basis and publishes the *Vital and Health Statistics* series (National Center for Health Statistics, 1962). This survey is a well-designed and ongoing nationwide probability sample of households in the United States. Only the civilian, noninstitutionalized population is interviewed, excluding persons living in nursing and convalescent homes, institutions, and group living arrangements that are not defined by the NCHS as households. The data collected in the surveys are used to produce prevalence estimates for the United States and large geographic regions. Because the data are based on surveys, the national prevalence estimates are subject to sampling error, the extent to which the results from surveying the sample would be different from the results that would be obtained from the entire population. The national prevalence estimates are also subject to measurement error, in that the results of the survey could be attributable to causes other than those being measured. In the case of the NHIS, the sample is not large enough to generalize the findings directly to each state. In order to reduce sampling error, NHIS data can be combined over several years, due to the stability in the content in the core questionnaire and the sampling design (Newacheck, 1991).

Through a procedure known as *synthetic estimation* for demographic analysis, it is possible to create state-level estimates using these national data adjusted to reflect state population characteristics (Newacheck, 1991; Therapeutic Concepts, Inc., 1991). Synthetic estimation is a statistical technique that provides the capability to take data from a sample and, based on common classification characteristics, synthetically generate estimates for either a larger or smaller population. For example, synthetic estimation can be used to take large-area, nationally derived estimates and calculate estimates for a smaller area such as for a region or state. Similarly, synthetic estimation can be used to take estimates based on a county and calculate estimates for the entire state. Synthetic estimation has both cost and convenience advantages, compared to the resource intensiveness of conducting a state-level survey. The accuracy of the estimation technique depends upon the extent to which the statistician is able to adjust the initial estimates according to relevant characteristics at the state level that may influence prevalence.

Gortmaker and Sappenfield (1984) published 1980 estimates and ranges of prevalence estimates of chronic diseases and conditions in children, ages birth through 20 years. These estimates were provided for disorders such as arthritis, asthma, autism, central nervous system injury, cerebral palsy, chronic renal failure, cleft lip/palate, congenital heart disease, cystic fibrosis, diabetes mellitus, Down syndrome, hearing impairment, hemophilia, acute lymphocytic leukemia, mental retardation, muscular dystrophy, spina bifida, phenylketonuria, sickle cell disease, seizure disorder, and visual impairment. To derive these estimates and ranges of estimates, Gortmaker and Sappenfield used the results of multiple NHIS surveys and extensive reviews of rates found in the literature. Some states have reviewed and drawn prevalence rate information from these studies.

Using synthetic estimation based on NHIS survey data spanning the period 1985–1989, Newacheck (1991) developed regional- and state-level estimates of the prevalence of activity-limiting chronic conditions for the 50 states and the District of Columbia. To create the synthetic estimates, two demographic variables, age and race, were used to adjust the data from national estimates to state-level estimates. During the survey, conditions were classified as either main or secondary causes if more than one was reported. In order to keep the data unduplicated, only conditions reported as main causes of activity limitation were counted. Newacheck's tables provide estimates of the number of children and youth with a condition (combining three levels of limitation—mild, moderate, and severe) in each of 17 condition categories, including impairment of vision, hearing, and speech; mental retardation; deformities; orthopedic impairments; endocrine, nutritional, metabolic, blood, mental, or nervous system disorders; diseases of the eye, ear, respiratory system, digestive, or musculoskeletal system; genitourinary disorders; pregnancy; and childbirth. Newacheck limited his study to conditions that limited activity.

The NCHS publishes annual prevalence estimates at the national level for a select list of chronic conditions that do not cause limitation of activity but may be related to developmental delay. Additionally, the extent to which variables other than age and race actually influence prevalence and were not used in the synthetic estimation process would result in estimates that were biased. Newacheck (1991) advises that states view his synthetic estimates as provisional estimates of the prevalence of chronic conditions causing limitation of activity and that they use the estimates as an initial approximation until more accurate and reliable prevalence estimates can be obtained from other sources.

The decision whether to use existing estimates in the literature or from national surveys depends upon the goodness-of-fit between the determination factors used to derive these estimates and the determination factors selected by a state as part of the eligibility definition. A limitation to collecting estimates from a variety of sources exists because it is difficult to avoid duplicating the counts. Also, the user must judge the extent to which the conditions and populations studied in the literature reflect the population interests of the state considering the use of the data. Because persons may have more than one condition, which may not be reflected in the survey results, rates for individual conditions cannot be added together to estimate prevalence. Given that many states are concerned with a variety of diverse conditions and risk factors, no single existing survey will cover them all. This leaves planners with incomplete information for prevalence estimation.

Strategies Used by Selected States

What could a state do with so much disparate information, gleaned from the literature, national estimates, statewide databases, and local and state surveys? States have taken a variety of approaches in using these data to estimate prevalence. Minnesota used a combination of nationally derived estimates and state-level data to estimate the prevalence rate of children with special health care needs in the state (D. J. Peterson, personal communication, April 6, 1992). Massachusetts tailored its estimation methodologies to the definitions of the groups under consideration, using a combination of vital statistics data and consensus estimations from a review of the literature (J. Shimer, personal communication, June 5, 1992). California applied a variety of techniques, using nationally derived data as a foundation and augmenting these data through the use of information obtained from the literature, existing state databases, and local surveys (Human Services Research Institute, 1989). Florida's prevalence estimates relied on data obtained from statewide databases, local surveys, and case studies (Therapeutic Concepts, Inc., 1991). Virginia combined the use of state-level vital statistics data and local survey data collection to develop prevalence estimates (Virginia Department of Mental Health, Mental Retardation and Substance Abuse Services, 1992). Further details about the approaches used by various states are provided below.

Minnesota

In its 1991 Maternal Child Health (MCH) Services Block Grant application, the state of Minnesota used a variety of state and nationally derived estimates to set a prevalence rate of children with special health care needs in the state. Data were selected from several sources: national prevalence estimates for 1990 extrapolated from Gortmaker and Sappenfield's 1980 data (1984); state-level diagnosis data based on enrollments in Services for Children with Handicaps (Title V CSHN), Special Education, and Head Start; and state-level synthetic estimates from Newacheck's analyses (1991). The condition groups are the same as those studied by Newacheck. Prevalence rates were estimated based on the programmatic or political purpose of an activity (D. J. Peterson, personal communication, April 6, 1992). Of the population of children, 2% were estimated to be medically fragile or technology-dependent; 5% were estimated to have conditions that limit their activity, and 10% were estimated to have conditions that interfere with normal growth and development, which would include chronic illnesses that neither limit activity nor hamper normal functioning. This 10% constitutes the eligible population for the MCH program.

Massachusetts

In 1986, the state of Massachusetts convened a Needs Assessment Working Group to conduct a needs assessment for early intervention services. Three policy option groups were identified for study:

- Established Problem: children whose early development is influenced by diagnosed medical disorders of known etiology bearing relatively well-known expectancies for developmental outcome within varying ranges of developmental delay, or children who manifest developmental delays during the first 2 years of life even though the etiology is unknown.
- Biological Risk: children with a history of prenatal, perinatal, neonatal, or early developmental events suggestive of biological insults to the developing central nervous system that, either singly or collectively, increase the probability of later atypical development.
- Environmental Risk: children who are biologically sound, but whose early life experiences, including maternal and family care, health care, nutrition, opportunities for expression of adaptive behaviors, and

patterns of physical and social stimulation are limiting to the extent that they impart high improbability for delayed development.

Based on these group definitions, three estimates were made, one for each group, with each using different strategies for estimation. For Biological Risk, 3 years of birth files were reviewed for 1984–1986. The number of babies with very low birth weight surviving past their first 28 days of life was then used to estimate the 1990 prevalence. This was a rate of 54.9% of very-low-birth-weight babies. For the Established Problem group, a rate of 6.5% of the infant and toddler population was used to determine the number of such children with an established risk. The rate was based on a literature review by the Early Intervention Needs Assessment Working Group. This rate was multiplied by the population aged birth to 2 years. The number of Biological Risk children were subtracted from this product to estimate the 1990 prevalence. Because of a lack of available documentation, the deliberations of the group cannot be described further. For Environmental Risk, a literature review was conducted to identify factors that related to developmental delay. From this list, four factors were identified that were uniformly available on birth certificates: children born to young teenage mothers (<18 years), children born to older teenage mothers (18–19 years) with at least one previous live birth, children born to mothers with less than a high school education, and children with birth weights between 1,501 and 2,500 grams. The number of children at environmental risk of developmental delay in 1990 was determined by multiplying the percent of high-risk births by the estimated population aged birth to 2 years, excluding those accounted for in the other two groups.

According to J. Shimer (personal communication, June 5, 1992), Massachusetts ultimately elected to discontinue use of the prevalence estimates derived above. One limitation that contributed to this decision was that the strategies used did not account for those children whose handicapping conditions appeared after birth, sometimes as late as 2 years of age. Additionally, the methods for deriving birth counts changed and other counts were based on the 1980 census. These limitations, changes, and concerns about lack of documentation of qualitative analyses led the state to discard the estimates as initially developed. For program implementation purposes, the state included all three groups into the definition of eligibility and relied on an upper limit imposed by funding constraints instead of prevalence or estimated utilization rates.

California

The approach used by the state of California synthesized prevalence information from the literature, national surveys, and local and state databases. In 1989 and 1990, California conducted a series of planning efforts concerning early intervention that entailed six projects:

- A study of individual and family service planning.
- An evaluation of the definition of developmental delay.
- An examination of personnel development and standards.
- A study of early intervention program public awareness and outreach.
- An exploration of client data and management information systems.
- A cost evaluation project to examine the existing system of service delivery and funding for early intervention services and to develop estimates of the funding that would be required in order to participate in Part H in the fourth and succeeding years of the program.

As part of these planning efforts, the Human Services Research Institute (HSRI) conducted a prevalence study (Human Services Research Institute, 1989). The study produced four sets of estimates, statewide and by county, for the number of:

- Persons with developmental disabilities by age, as defined by California law.
- Persons with developmental disabilities by age, as defined by the federal government;
- Persons with developmental disabilities by age, as defined by the state and adjusted to reflect the distribution of persons with developmental disabilities in developmental centers, nursing homes, and community care facilities in California.
- Children at risk of mental retardation, epilepsy, cerebral palsy, and autism (conditions named in the state's definition of developmental disabilities) and brain injury based on the expected incidence of causal conditions observed at birth and in early childhood.

In order to derive these estimates, the HSRI used a 3-year aggregation of the data from the NHIS, along with a number of other national and state data sources. The HSRI report provided estimated prevalence rates per 100,000 population, by main cause of limitation for infants and toddlers birth through age 2 who were unable or limited in their ability to perform major life activities. The main causes of limitation identified in the report included autism; brain injury; cerebral palsy; digestive, circulatory, and respiratory disorders; epilepsy; mental illness; mental retardation; orthopedic impairments; paralysis; spina bifida; and visual impairments. The combined use of these rates provided a basis for estimating prevalence of the eligible group as set forth in the state's definition.

Florida

To support the work of the Florida Interagency Coordinating Council for Infants and Toddlers (FICCIT), the Florida Department of Education funded a threefold study effort that included (1) a prevalence and service utilization study; (2) service delivery and design studies; and (3) a cost-analysis and funding study. The prevalence and service utilization study used a variety of study methods (Therapeutic Concepts, Inc., 1991). A panel consisting of in-state and out-of-state experts was formed to assist with planning and conducting the study. A literature review was conducted that identified factors to be used in the study. Prevalence surveys were conducted in a county representative of the state. State and local databases were used to obtain unduplicated population counts and to measure the extent to which multiple services were used by infants and toddlers. These data were used for sampling and analysis of utilization data.

Three policy option groups were identified for study because they represented the range of children who potentially could be entitled to early intervention services under Public Law 99-457 Part H:

- Established Conditions: infants and toddlers having established handicapping conditions and/or manifested developmental delays—estimated at a prevalence rate of 6.9%.
- Three or More Risk Factors: infants and toddlers having three or more biological and/or environmental risks but not having an established handicapping condition or manifested developmental delay—estimated at a prevalence rate of 4.2%.
- One or Two Risk Factors: infants and toddlers having one or two biological and/or environmental risks but not having an established handicapping condition or manifested developmental delay—estimated at a prevalence rate of 17% of Florida's children.

Established conditions included congenital/genetic disorders, neurological abnormalities, congenital/acquired infectious diseases, atypical developmental disorders, sensory impairments, and birth weight less than or equal to 1,000 grams. Biological risks included medically complex/technology dependent, illness or trauma associated with delays, drug exposure, chronically ill mother associated with delays, neonatal intensive care, birth weight 1,000–1,500 grams, birth weight 1,501–2,500 grams with complications, and factors impinging on developmental progress. Environmental risks included teen mother with less than a high school completion, history of abuse or neglect, no legal guardian established, in shelter or foster care, parent unable to consistently perform essential parenting functions, history of abuse or violence in the home, migrant or homeless, and family exposure to poisons or toxins.

A prevalence survey involving about 800 children and their families in Palm Beach County was conducted in July 1990. Based on a draft eligibility definition developed by FICCIT, the survey questionnaire covered established conditions and delays, risk factors, family stressors, and other demographic information. Family stressors included family immigrated in the past year; death in the home in the past year; family member retarded, seriously ill, or incapacitated; family moved more than twice in the past year; parents separated or divorced in the past year; family member under 18 pregnant in the past 3 years; family member has been a victim of a serious crime in the past year; and children often left without supervision.

The sample drew children from privately paid health care services, publicly paid health care services, and children identified on the active case rolls of four programs that provide services to young children and their families. Using synthetic estimation for demographic analysis, rates determined for the three groups of children in Palm Beach County were applied to the same age segments for the state of Florida for the years 1990, 1992, 1995, and 1999. This method of projection took into account racial variations of the population segments and prevalence rates. From the survey, prevalence rates by group were determined for each of the four state programs. These rates were applied to their total case rolls to estimate the rate of early intervention service participation in Palm Beach County as of July 1990 by eligibility group. The ratio of participation to prevalence provided the utilization by group. To provide detailed information on these children and their families, case studies were conducted on 55 of the survey respondents. Purposeful, maximum-variation sampling ensured a wide range of relevant conditions and circumstances (Therapeutic Concepts, Inc., 1991). Of the 55 case studies, 9 were conducted in languages other than English. The case studies were used to verify the prevalence survey data, examine the needs of children within the context of the family, identify services needed and received, and illuminate what life is like for these children and their families.

Virginia

The state of Virginia combined state-level vital statistics data and local survey data to develop prevalence estimates. Three policy option groups were identified for study: children who are Part H eligible; children who are Part H eligible plus children who have three or more risk factors; and children who are Part H eligible, children who have three or more risk factors, plus children who have one or two risk factors. The eligible service population consisted of children born with developmental delays, atypical behavior or development, and/or who have a diagnosed handicapping condition. Developmental delay is defined as functioning below 25% of their chronological age in one or more of the following skills: cognitive, physical, speech and language, psychosocial, and self-help. Atypical behavior or development was defined as abnormal muscle tone, reflexes, or posture; poor quality of movement; oral motor problems such as feeding difficulties; failure to respond to social interaction; or excessive fear or distress that does not respond to comforting. Diagnosed physical or mental condition with a high probability of resulting in a delay included seizures, infection at birth, effects of substance abuse, hearing or vision difficulties, and chromosomal abnormalities such as Down syndrome. The risk factors included: maternal age 15 or less, birth weight less than 1,500 grams, cleft palate or ear deformities, positive maternal HIV, meningitis, no well-child care by 6 months, diagnosed genetic disorders, chronic ear infections, child abuse/neglect, lead poisoning, lack of adequate shelter, parent's mental or developmental disability, and parent's substance abuse.

Five areas of the state were surveyed in 1990, with a second, more targeted survey conducted in 1991 (G. Barker, personal communication, June 5, 1992). Survey participation included local hospitals, physicians' groups, health departments, social service agencies, mental health service providers, and private entities. Participants were asked to provide information about every new child in their caseloads during the 5-month study period who might have any one of the above conditions or risk factors. A unique child identification code was developed for each child on the basis of name and birthdate. This code was used to eliminate duplication of forms submitted by multiple participants. To estimate the accuracy of the counts, collections were compared to birth certificate information concerning birth weights under 1,500 grams, teenage mothers, and low Apgar scores.

Estimated rates determined for the three groups of children were projected for Virginia for fiscal year 1997 (Virginia Department of Mental Health, Mental Retardation and Substance Abuse Services, 1992). The number of children served for fiscal year 1991 was based on December 1, 1990 child-count information submitted by local interagency councils and local education agencies. For Established Conditions, it was projected that the growth rate would be higher in fiscal years 1992 through 1994 than for fiscal years 1995 through 1997, due to an initial increase in awareness and a subsequent leveling off. For the other two groups combined, the estimated change between fiscal years 1991 and 1997 was divided evenly, assuming straight line growth in participation over that time period.

The study derived the estimated prevalence rates for Virginia. Of the children born each year, estimates were 2.6% born with developmental delays, atypical behavior or development, and/or with a diagnosed handicapping condition; 12.7% born with one or two risk factors; and 0.3% born with three or more risk factors. This resulted in a rate of 15.6% of children from birth to age 3 that could benefit from early intervention services (Virginia Department of Mental Health, Mental Retardation and Substance Abuse Services, 1992).

Maryland

Maryland was one of the few states that had made the policy decision to proceed with fifth-year Part H participation at the time this chapter was written. When asked for information about prevalence estimates, service utilization information was provided (Governor's Office for Children, Youth, and Families, 1992). A follow-up inquiry found that Maryland had entitled early intervention services to the group of children having an established handicapping condition and/or developmental delay (C. A. Bagland, personal communication, June 7, 1992). Although at-risk children were not included in the entitlement group, they were tracked on a database when services were requested and received.

The reason that service utilization information was sent in lieu of prevalence information was that Maryland relied on service utilization and other service-based information for planning future services. After more than 10 years of experience with prevalence, which was estimated at 4%, prevalence became a moot point. Every time prevalence information was published, government officials expressed concern that there would be a large surge in service delivery requirements. The state found that the best predictor of service delivery requirements had not been prevalence estimates, but trends in service utilization. In the beginning, the utilization rate was only 0.5%. The state increased this rate to 1.8 or 1.9% through careful service planning such as attending to the location of service provision, affecting parent's perceptions of the needs for services, and improving access to services. Thus, Maryland relies on service utilization rates for planning and budgeting incremental changes in the capacity of its service system.

Summary

States have used a variety of ways to estimate prevalence of their Part H eligible children. A state should use a method that provides the best fit with its definition of the target group of interest and its associated determination factors. Available to states are nationally derived estimates, as well as estimates described in the literature. States can use existing databases, or conduct surveys to gather new information. In most cases, states have relied upon a combination of methods and data sources in order to obtain estimates of prevalence. Estimating prevalence is an important piece of the people puzzle. The other two pieces are program participation and service utilization.

PROGRAM PARTICIPATION AND SERVICE UTILIZATION

This section discusses the concepts of program participation and service utilization and how they may be measured and applied. Illustrations of how these measures have been used by a state with programs and services for infant and toddler populations are provided.

Program Participation

Program participation, as used here, refers to the portion of children in a defined target population who are identified and served in a given program. A rate is determined by dividing the number of persons participating in a program by the expected prevalence in the service area at that point in time. For example, if the prevalence rate for children in need of early intervention services were 6% of the infant and toddler population, if a county had 1,000 eligible infants and toddlers, and if 300 of the eligible children were served through the local early intervention program, then the rate of participation by children in the target group would be 30% for that county at that time. Participation is an important measure for advocates, policy makers, and program managers because it reveals the size of the estimated unidentified, and presumably unserved, portion of the target group. This is the group at greater risk of poor developmental outcomes due to the lack of intervention to mitigate those factors associated with poor outcomes. By not finding and serving this remainder of the target group immediately, greater developmental problems and their consequences will have to be addressed later at greater cost. Thus, in the example given, some 70% of the target group remain unidentified and at increased risk of potentially preventable adverse outcomes.

An exploration of program participation was undertaken in the studies sponsored through Florida's Part H interagency council as part of its planning activities. One study activity explored program participation by infants and toddlers in a variety of programs associated with early intervention services (Therapeutic Concepts, Inc., 1991). As described earlier, the study team used Palm Beach County, Florida, as a study site, because that county contained the demographic characteristics necessary to represent the state as a whole when using synthetic estimation techniques to develop state projections. The study team used survey sampling techniques to estimate prevalence and used existing data from local and state agency databases to measure participation and service use. For purposes of presentation of findings, the study team formed three groups of infants and toddlers for consideration of entitlement by policy makers. The first group consisted of infants and toddlers with developmental delays and/or an established handicapping condition; a prevalence rate of 6.9% was found. The second group consisted of infants and toddlers having three or more predisposing risk factors but no current indication of developmental delay nor an established risk condition; a prevalence rate of 4.2% was found. The third group consisted of infants and toddlers having one or two predisposing risk factors but no current indication of developmental delay nor an established risk condition; a prevalence rate of 17.0% was found. These prevalence estimates reflected a draft definition that the state interagency council was using at the time the study began.

Once prevalence estimates for the three groups of children were developed, the study team analyzed survey data to determine the extent to which children in these three groups were present within various programs of interest. Determining the incidence of the three groups within the active caseloads found in programs of interest was a first step in describing program participation. Because this was an exploratory activity, a single-point-in-time count was used for all programs reviewed. The point in time selected was concurrent with the prevalence surveys conducted. Programs in two areas of interest were examined: (1) traditional child development programs for children with disabling conditions and at elevated biological risk due to prematurity or other birth complications and (2) programs provided for abused or neglected children. The first set of programs were Florida's developmental disabilities early intervention program, regional perinatal intensive-care program, public school child-find registry, and special education (birth to age 3) programs for sensory-impaired children. These represented the state's traditional child development programs providing early intervention services. Prevalence survey results were applied to caseload information from each program's database count to determine the incidence of the three groups in each program area. The same process was repeated for selected child welfare programs provided by the state for children admitted for confirmed abuse or neglect. Programs included in this area were child protective services, foster care, adoptions, and family support services. The incidence rates within these two areas were determined as follows, using results of the prevalence survey.

Group of interest	Child developmental programs	Child welfare programs
Established conditions/ developmental delay	78.8%	13.7%
3+ predisposing risks	9.5%	45.2%
1–2 predisposing risks	8.4%	31.4%

These findings indicate that a significant majority (78.8%) of infants and toddlers in the traditional developmental programs have developmental delays and/or established handicapping conditions. These were children admitted to services under eligibility definitions already in use by the state but not exactly the same as the proposed Part H definition provided by the state interagency council to the study team.

Approximately 13.7% of the infants and toddlers in the child welfare programs were found to have developmental delays or disabling conditions. This is almost twice the estimated prevalence rate for this group in the general population of 6.9%. Based on a computerized comparison of children in the traditional developmental program caseloads, most of the children with established conditions identified in the child welfare programs were not currently enrolled in nor receiving developmentally oriented early intervention services. Most (58.9%) of the infants and toddlers in the child welfare caseloads were determined to be members of either the established conditions group or the 3+ predisposing risks group, placing these children at very high risk of poor developmental outcomes including developmental delay, disability, or later social dysfunction (e.g., school failure, school dropout, teen pregnancy, delinquency, unemployment, or adult dependency). Few were currently receiving developmentally oriented early intervention services of an appropriate, substantial, and enduring nature.

Because person-specific information on the use of particular services (e.g., physical therapy, respite care, infant stimulation, etc.) by infants and toddlers participating in the programs was not available, the study team used program participation as an alternative to service utilization. An unduplicated estimate of the number of children currently participating in one or more of the programs providing developmental or child welfare related services was made using an ad hoc analysis of local database information. The unduplicated counts produced for each group then were divided by the state's demographic projections for the county's infant and toddler population for the point in time that synchronized with child counts for the prevalence studies and ad hoc caseload analysis. This resulted in an estimate of the proportion of the infant and toddler population that currently was participating in the programs of interest (see Column 1 in the table below). The numbers of children identified as participants in three groups were then divided by Column 2, the estimated prevalence of children in each group as determined through the prevalence survey work. This produced a single-point-in-time program participation measure (Column 3) for each potential eligibility group of interest to the state's interagency coordinating council.

Group of interest	(1) General population served	(2) Estimated prevalence rate	(3) Participation rate
A: Established conditions/ developmental delay	1.7%	6.9%	24.6%
B: 3+ predisposing risks	2.2%	4.2%	52.4%
C: 1–2 predisposing risks	1.5%	17.0%	8.8%
Groups A + B	3.9%	11.1%	33.3%
Groups A + B + C	5.2%	28.1%	18.5%

As indicated above, Group A children, who were found to be receiving services from one or more programs providing special child development or child welfare services, comprised 1.7% of the general population of infants and toddlers in Palm Beach County. Group A children, through the prevalence survey, had been estimated to comprise 6.9% of the infants and toddlers in the county. Using this information, it can be deduced that about a quarter (24.6%) of the infants and toddlers in Group A were participants in a program that provided some type of intervention service, either developmental or protective. Thus, the program participation rate for members of Group A was 24.6%. Participation rates for Groups B and C and for group combinations are indicated in Column 3 above. This approach is helpful in understanding participation by infants and toddlers in available programs that provide various types of early intervention services. But, to understand the utilization of particular services, a different method is necessary.

Service Utilization

What is service utilization, how is it measured, and how is service utilization information actually used? Service utilization usually refers to the number of persons in a program using a specific service, such as physical therapy. As states move to a service unit approach for planning and payment purposes, service utilization is expanding to include not only the number and percent of participants using individual services within a given service array, but it includes the number of units of services being used. People involved in the planning, budgeting, funding, and management of service delivery are the principal users of service utilization information. Thus, the concept of service utilization, its methods of measurement, and its use in planning and budgeting are continuing to evolve. As with any concept and method in an evolutionary state, there are problems associated with the definition of service utilization and its application to early intervention services.

Problems associated with measuring the utilization of prevention/early intervention services usually arise from three sources. The first problem is defining what is meant by early intervention and then identifying the associated programs and services that are encompassed within that definition. Are only those programs and services historically associated with child development interventions for infants and toddlers having developmental delay and/or established handicapping conditions included, such as those traditionally provided through developmental disability services and prekindergarten special education? Should child protective interventions associated with abuse and neglect be included as early intervention services? Should generic family support services be considered early intervention? What about preventive health care strategies and routine primary health care? Or nutritional interventions for impoverished infants and their mothers? Clearly, decisions must be made about the programs and services that will be defined and counted as early intervention services before service utilization can be measured. States using a narrow eligibility definition of the service population and a narrow set of child developmental focused services will have a much easier time defining and measuring service utilization than will states that include a broader range of intervention strategies and related services. A significant contributing problem for states taking the broad approach is the multitude of noncompatible databases that must be reconciled and used to count participants and track their services.

The second problem in measuring service utilization is deciding whether to count persons who are participating at any level in selected programs that provide early intervention services or to measure only utilization of the specific services offered within particular programs. State-sponsored programs that may be considered to provide early intervention services, such as special education, public health, child welfare, or developmental disabilities services, provide a range of services to their participants. Some of the services provided are unique to particular programs. For example, typically only health programs provide immunization services and only child welfare programs provide protective supervision services. Other more generic services may be provided by several programs. For example, family support services may be provided by child welfare, economic assistance, mental health services, and developmental disabilities services. Because the same child/family may participate in several different programs simultaneously and receive both unique and generic services, a decision must be made about whether to simply count program participation or to focus measurement efforts on use of specific units of discretely defined services across all programs providing those services. To measure participation and service utilization by persons across programs requires the ability to merge databases to produce an unduplicated count of program participants. To measure units of services used by an unduplicated count of individuals within and across programs requires even more complex database design and file-merge capabilities. Clearly, this level of analysis represents the state of the art of information management in human services and special education.

The third problem in measuring service utilization is one of time reference. Should the measurement of service utilization be based on a single-point-in-time count or should it count all persons served and the services they used over a fixed time period, such as a year? The answer depends on two considerations. The first consideration involves the flow characteristics of persons moving through the early intervention service system. If the target population consists largely of persons with established handicapping conditions who are participating in traditional programs for infants and toddlers with disabilities, the persons who enter are likely to remain in the programs over the course of several years. The number of persons moving through the system over a year will be close to the number served on any day of a year, plus new admissions during the course of the year. Conversely, children moving through a child welfare program may enter the program and remain only a few months. In such a program, the flow of children over the course of a year could be two or three times the number of children being served by the program on any given day. Thus, the flow characteristics of children moving through whatever a state defines as its early intervention program is a major consideration in designing measures of participation and utilization. The second consideration involves determining the purpose of measuring of service utilization. Is the purpose to count people using services or to count units of services used by a group of participants? The answer to this question will influence the choice of a single-point-in-time measure or a cumulative measure over a given time period.

Maryland, which has identified roughly the equivalent of Florida's established conditions group as its eligible population, uses services recommended on Individual and Family Service Plans for children participating in the state's early intervention program as a measure of service utilization (Governor's Office for Children, Youth, and Families, 1992). This data system enables state planners to count the number of children using each specific service (e.g., audiology, speech therapy, respite care, etc.) offered through the program. By dividing the number of users by the total number of program participants, a utilization rate is established. For example, the 1992 state report indicated that in 1991, 343 infants and toddlers in Maryland used audiology services. The number of users (343) divided by the identified eligible population currently served (2,315) yielded a service utilization rate of 14.8% for audiology services. This method of measuring service utilization is helpful in planning future services based on knowledge of current usage patterns.

The value of this type of information could be enhanced with the use of further information indicating how the 14.5% current rate of service utilization compared with the actual need for this service among program participants. If 29% of current participants needed this service, then only half of the known demand was being addressed by the program. Thus, service utilization rates and assessed need rates for services should be evaluated together for program planning and budgeting purposes.

Because prevention/early intervention services usually are provided though a multiplicity of public and private agencies often having noncompatible databases, producing an accurate, unduplicated measure of program participation may be a challenging undertaking in many states, especially those that broadly define early intervention services across a variety of programs. To go beyond counting program participants to measuring utilization of service units by certain groups of children participating across numerous state and local programs will be a continuing challenge for planners and managers of early intervention services.

FACTORS INFLUENCING PROGRAM PARTICIPATION AND SERVICE UTILIZATION

There are a variety of circumstances and events that influence program participation and service utilization. Provided below is an array of factors that were identified through case studies conducted as part of an early intervention prevalence and service utilization study conducted in Florida (Therapeutic Concepts, Inc., 1991). The following factors were found to promote or inhibit program participation and service utilization:

- Definition of the target population (affects group size, composition, range of needs).
- Parent and professional awareness and acceptance of early intervention concepts.
- Frequency of screening children likely to meet the eligibility definition.
- Reliability of tools and procedures used to determine eligibility and service needs.
- Quality of case management: role, competence, personal style, and availability.
- Actual needs of children for particular services at given points in time.
- Availability of the major services required by the entitled group.
- Choices of providers, locations, and schedules of services available to parents.
- Ease of accessing a service by parents (location, time of day, transportation support).
- Parent's perceived value of the services and benefits received compared to the inconvenience and family intrusion endured to achieve those benefits.
- Desire of parents to request or to use particular services.

Thus, a variety of factors are likely to influence participation of eligible children and their families in early intervention programs as well as their use of particular services that are recommended. Planners and policy makers should be mindful of these factors. Usually, several of these factors addressed together are more likely to increase service utilization than any one factor taken alone. For example, expanding an eligibility definition alone will not increase participation and utilization without simultaneously increasing public awareness, screening, case management, and service availability. However, when all of these factors are addressed together, the combined efforts should result in an increase in service utilization over time.

THE IMPORTANCE OF PREVALENCE, PARTICIPATION, AND UTILIZATION INFORMATION

Information about prevalence, program participation, and service utilization can illuminate many important issues for advocates, planners, and policy makers. First, if prevention is the goal, then knowing the size of the population at risk and the proportion of the at-risk population receiving services is necessary for sound program planning. The unidentified portion of the population at risk remains to be found and served. If an undesired condition with serious adverse effects can be prevented or its effects minimized for a relatively small cost now, and later costs for more extensive and expensive services can be avoided, then intensified efforts to find and serve the unidentified population as quickly as possible should be undertaken. Knowledge of target group size and the portion of that group participating in prevention and early intervention programs is essential in planning future policy and budget initiatives.

Second, if a government program is planning to entitle a new group of persons to services and a high program participation and service utilization rate is expected to occur in a relatively short amount of time, then knowing the size of the target group is essential for cost projections to make sure that policy commitments will not "break the bank." Legislators and budget planners are especially aware of this issue. Estimated service utilization rates for successive years of operation will be necessary for program planning and budgeting.

Third, if an entitlement to a target group is made to address certain critical needs through entitled services, then service utilization should be commensurate with service needs. Measures of service utilization should be coupled with measures of service needs to identify gaps that could result in inadequate services, which in turn could lead to avoidable and undesired developmental outcomes for infants and toddlers. Parents, child advocates, program managers, and service providers are especially focused on this issue. The importance of these issues in sound planning and management is obvious and central to the delivery of adequate services to a group of children in need of early intervention services.

CONCLUSION

Addressing prevalence and service utilization should be an ongoing process for planners, policy makers, and funders of early intervention services. Prevalence rates for developmental delay and disability may vary through time as a result of ever-changing socioeconomic conditions and through the changes in population characteristics produced by prevention strategies. Any changes in the size and composition of the population of infants and toddlers in need of early intervention services require that programs respond to those changing needs and to adapt their focus and structure accordingly. As new risk factors emerge, eligibility definitions will require modification to target and mitigate those risks. As new forms of intervention are developed and new technologies introduced, service arrays by necessity will be modified, thus altering utilization patterns. Shifting public interests may result in increased efforts to prevent developmental delay among children at elevated risk due to environmental circumstances. Shifting political interests could result in a freeze or roll back in the use of entitlements to target support for particular groups in need of government-funded services. To guide the direction of future prevention/early intervention programs, planners will have to answer four perennial questions: Whom shall we serve? How many persons in the target group could qualify for services if all were screened? How many persons are participating in programs and using services? Which services are needed and being used? These questions will have to be answered to focus and fund the programs that will address the needs of those to be served.

REFERENCES

Benn, R. (1990, February). *Defining eligibility criteria for a state-wide definition under P.L. 99–457: Part H.* Research report submitted to the State Board of Education, Michigan Department of Education. Detroit, MI: Merrill Palmer Institute.

Gortmaker, S. L., & Sappenfield, W. (1984). Chronic childhood disorders: Prevalence and impact. *Pediatric Clinics of North America, 31*(1), 3–18.

Governor's Office for Children, Youth, and Families. (1992). *Maryland Infants and Toddlers Program, 1991 Part H data collection overview.* Baltimore, MD: Author.

Human Services Research Institute. (1989, May 10). *Estimates of the incidence of conditions that can lead to developmental disabilities as defined by the state and of the prevalence of developmental disabilities as defined by the state and federal governments, by county and statewide: California 1990.* Report prepared for the California State Council on Developmental Disabilities, and Berkeley Planning Association.

National Center for Health Statistics. (1962). *Vital and Health Statistics Series, Data from the National Health Survey.* Washington, DC: U.S. Department of Health and Human Services.

Newacheck, P. W. (1991, June). *State estimates of the prevalence of chronic conditions among children and youth.* San Francisco: Institute for Health Policy Studies, University of California, San Francisco.

Therapeutic Concepts, Inc. [now Improvement Concepts, Inc.]. (1991, July). *Florida's cost/implementation study for Public Law 99-457, infants and toddlers phase II findings: Prevalence/utilization study summary of activities, findings and policy implications.* Report prepared for the Florida Department of Education by the Florida State University, Policy Studies Clinic, College of Law, and The Center for Prevention and Early Intervention Institute of Science and Public Affairs.

Virginia Department of Mental Health, Mental Retardation and Substance Abuse Services. (1992, January 7). *Early intervention services.* Presentation to the Joint Legislative Subcommittee Studying Early Intervention Services for Infants and Toddlers with Disabilities.

CHAPTER 5

Creating Family-Centered Programs and Policies

SUSAN M. DUWA

CONNI WELLS

PAULA LALINDE

Families of children with special needs, policy makers, and individuals providing services are all finding themselves in the midst of a service delivery overhaul as a result of Part H of Public Law 99-457, now referred to as the Individuals with Disabilities Education Act (IDEA), and the reorientation of early intervention systems and services that this legislation mandates. The heart and soul of this dramatic change is the reconceptualization from a child-centered to a family-centered service delivery system and approach to working with young children and their families. Recent research supports what most families, practitioners, and bureaucrats struggle with every day at many different levels—that these are major changes accompanied by a multitude of known and unknown challenges (Bailey, Buysse, Edmondson, & Smith, 1992; Bailey, Palsha, & Simeonsson, 1991; Dunst, Johanson, Trivette, & Hamby, 1991).

The concept of a family-centered service delivery system and approach to service delivery is neither a new idea nor an exclusive Part H conceptualization of best practice. Part H has provided the impetus and a new lens through which current approaches to building systems and working with families can be examined.

Historically, service delivery systems and approaches have shown little ability to perceive the needs of children in relation to their larger unique environment of family and community. This old paradigm further perceives the family as being an isolated group, not individualized, with no interrelationships to community or other educational, social, or health systems. Many of our systems and programs for meeting the needs of families and their children were developed by professionals and outside consultants (Turnbull,

1991). Few of these persons understand the impact of regulations or program rules on families living in today's society. Families, primary stakeholders because they are the prime recipients, have been traditionally and systematically excluded from the decision-making process. The new lens through which we view early intervention services creates a focused vision for working with children and families that recognizes the family as the consumer, respects a family's priorities and decisions, and provides service and support options to assist families in achieving their identified goals.

This chapter is an attempt to define the concept of family-centered within the philosophical and best-practice framework of Public Law 99-457, Part H. A family-centered approach is considered best practice for creating systems and working directly with young children and their families, regardless of the context for services (Vincent & Beckett, 1993). The service delivery system that is discrete and categorical, whether health, education, or social services, is being replaced with a community-based service delivery system that provides services in the context of family supports and resources individualized for each family (Weissbourd & Patrick, 1988).

In this chapter the principles and elements that provide the framework of effective, meaningful, family-centered early intervention systems and services are described. These include family-centered parent involvement; definition of family-centered programs and policies; community-based resources; family and professional relationships; respect for family diversity; effective interagency coordination; family involvement in system design; determination of effective system design; family-centered concerns, priorities, and resources; family-centered child evaluations; family-centered individual family service plans; and family-centered service coordination. Putting these principles and essential elements into practice is illustrated by sharing best practices and strategies for implementation. Finally, strategies are presented for successful family-centered systems and approaches for all programs and families.

FAMILY-CENTERED SYSTEMS AND SERVICES

I called the social worker to let her know I could not make it to the parent meeting that morning. I started crying. I didn't mean to. . . . I was just worried they would think I didn't care about Maria if I couldn't make it to every meeting.

Family-Centered Parent Involvement

From the perspective of families an emerging critical concern is the definition and application of family-centeredness (Frederick & McGonigel, 1992).

There is growing consensus and alarm that the interpretation of "family-centered" is running amuck, leaving families at risk of being left in the status quo of current policy and practice.

Many authors and researchers have contributed concepts, principles, and components to our current knowledge about family-centered early intervention systems (Dunst, Trivette, & Deal, 1988; McGonigel, Kaufmann, & Johnson, 1991; Vincent & Beckett, 1993). As a result, many different terms have been used synonymously and interchangeably with family-centered. These terms include family-focused, family involvement, family participation, family-responsive, family-allied, family-friendly, family-inclusive and family-driven. This list is probably not exhaustive but representative of common as well as new Part H-generated terms. This new terminology has added to the confusion in attempts to define family-centered. Confusion has also resulted from the fact that the degree to which a system is family-centered depends on the program's and the individual's perception of the definition.

Terms we often hear used interchangeably are family-centered and family or parent involvement. Providers and others have come to believe that their program is family-centered if it involves parents. However, family involvement through inclusion opportunities is only one component of a system or program that is family-centered in design. A program professing to be family-centered may in reality have a prescribed, system-driven parent involvement program. Vincent and Beckett (1993) believe that family participation occurs when families are equal members, that is, partners with staff, and take part in all aspects of the early intervention system, including all aspects of their child's care and all levels of decision making.

Traditionally, family involvement in child-centered programs prescribed extensive mother-focused activities that included parent training, parent support, parent education, and parent advocacy (Robinson, Rosenberg, & Beckman, 1990). Bringing cookies to Valentine parties, fund raising, and other traditional parent involvement activities have been replaced by a vision of assisting parents to gain the skills, knowledge, and confidence to become equal partners in making decisions for their child (Healy, Keesee, & Smith, 1989). In the past, the parent involvement opportunities were neither individualized nor appropriate for every family. Table 5.1 provides a comparison between the "old way of doing business" and a family-centered approach to family involvement.

Historically, program goals for parent involvement were written by professionals, essentially prescribing the parent services to be offered. Today, a program striving to be family-centered will include families as program designers in creating a family-centered program with family involvement activities as one component of service options. Family involvement activities in turn will be delivered with a family-centered approach.

TABLE 5.1. Comparison between Traditional and Family-Centered
Parent Involvement

Traditional	Family-centered
Parent involvement is an array of supports given to parents	Families are included as decision makers, policy makers, and program designers, as well as receiving supports
Parents are involved so their children can get "fixed" quicker and to make the professional's job easier (i.e., follow-through with therapists and intervention at home)	Families are included so that the professionals working with the child and family can know that they are serving the child and the family in the most appropriate meaningful manner
Parents are judged based on their "willingness" to comply with prescribed parent involvement activities or treatments to their child	Families choose their own level of involvement and are not judged, penalized, or displayed as shining examples

Current research has found that early intervention policies and practice are most often described as being family-focused when defined as a collaboration model between families and professionals to determine what families need with the emphasis on professionally delivered traditional services (Dunst et al., 1991). Given this reality, special care must be taken to ensure families fully realize the potential of family-centered practices and are able to make distinctions between a family-centered program and programs that are merely renaming parent involvement activities as being family-centered. To complete the family-centered circle, policies and services need to be evaluated by families.

Defining Family-Centered Programs and Policies

Some professionals sound like car salesmen with all of their promises of what they are going to "do" for us. I don't want promises, I don't want them to "DO" for me, I want to learn how to get my family back to where we are in control again.

As the parent quote above illustrates, there is a persistent need for institutionalized system reform in the way we serve children and families in early intervention. The ability to assimilate best practice and create new structures for supporting families with infants and toddlers requires a careful reconfiguration and reorientation of our policies and programs. To do so is to adopt a family-centered approach toward working with families that supports and builds on family strengths and resources and deals with family issues and concerns in a holistic, culturally appropriate manner.

Family-centered services are a primary component of quality programs (Turbiville, Turnbull, Garland, & Lee, 1993; Vincent & Beckett, 1993). Research has shown that to ignore the family and focus narrowly on the child reduces the effects of early intervention (Bronfenbrenner, 1977; Healy et al., 1985). Programs that adopt a joint focus on both the child and family are the most effective in achieving their goals. By strengthening and supporting the entire family, not just the child, the probability of achieving positive outcomes is greatly enhanced. Families have identified a positive outcome as one that results in the ability to recruit help from others and utilize social supports (Summers et al., 1990). A family-centered environment that will enhance the competency of families, based on a belief that families are competent or are capable of becoming competent, promotes families' ability to be interdependent with their environment (Dunst et al., 1988).

Specifically, families have stated that meeting the need for information is an expected outcome from early intervention programs (Coulter, Johnson, & Innis, 1991; Summers et al., 1990). Families who are provided with the information, skills, and tools necessary to become informed decision makers will be able to access the service delivery system and develop their knowledge and confidence so as to become advocates. Families also identified (1) meeting needs for the whole family and (2) individual well-being as the next most important expected outcomes (Summers et al., 1990). Thus, the definition of family-centered should include that an environment must be developed that promotes the growth, development, and health of the family as well as the child. This would be an environment that focuses its energy on strengths, resources, and solutions, not weaknesses, deficits, and problems.

Outcomes related to enhancing family–professional relationships and parent–child relationships are also desired by families (Summers et al., 1990). Families stated they expected early intervention programs to assist them in developing skills to work with professionals and the service delivery system. Thus, being family-centered requires offering opportunities for growth, change, and control without families being forced to compromise their values and integrity to participate.

CORE INGREDIENTS OF FAMILY-CENTERED PLANNING

Nolan wasn't eligible for their program, but definitely needed some help. They gave me a stack of books and papers to use as guides to work with him myself until his next evaluation. After she left, I took the papers home and put it on top of the stuff the other places had given me; the stack was already 3 feet high and he isn't even 2 years old yet.

Family-centered programming includes many core ingredients that help support families and assist them in reaching their goals and dreams for their child (Turnbull & Turnbull, 1990). The challenge facing professionals today stems from the theory that the family-centered components must be individualized from family to family as well as from one individual to another (Bailey et al., 1992). Basic components of a family-centered program must then be broken down into practical applications to meet individual needs. These components encompass community-based resources, family–professional relationships, respect for family diversity, and interagency coordination.

Community-Based Resources

I don't want to go someplace else for services for Cedrick. I don't know those people. They don't know us. They will never have to look us in the eye if they make a mistake. I don't like maps. What if the car breaks down? What if we can't find the place? How will I know if they are doing the right things?

Communities play an increasingly prominent role in the lives of families today. They influence the lifestyle and values of families and protect the cultural roots of community members (McKnight, 1992). Because of an increased focus on the community, many families measure the success of their lives through their own level of participation and acceptance in their community. Communities form and bond together through work environments, celebrations, holidays, schools, agencies, landmarks, and friendships, so it is natural for a family to desire to remain within the boundaries of that community for services. It is here that families have developed relationships that they use as a support system during difficult times.

Services based within the normal environment promote the family's sense of belonging (McKnight, 1992). Self-image and family security will be enhanced by inclusion in a service delivery system that is similar to that of other families living in their community. For example, in research using focus groups, families of children with special health care needs tended to feel more secure and accepted when they were receiving community-based services that acknowledged that their child is a child first, with many needs not unlike those of others the same age (Diehl, Moffitt, & Wade, 1991).

Most communities, and the families that live within them, have built a network that supplies services and supports in a locally accepted manner. It is essential that we build upon existing networks in the early intervention process. Many communities are suspicious of outside influences that threaten familiar services already in place. Families are at risk of becoming outsiders within their own community if forced to use services and supports not within their community network.

Thus, programs that are community-based can also enhance family-centeredness. Administrators must ensure that mechanisms are in place that will allow programs to meet family needs in a community-based fashion. The need to ensure consistency and equity in service delivery must be balanced with the flexibility to adapt to existing, local resources (Dunst et al., 1991).

Family and Professional Relationships

> *The professionals begin to get uneasy when we start to get emotional. They want us to focus on Katrina's future. Can't they understand that we are talking about what is left of our dreams and the impact it will have on our family forever? Forever is a long time. . . . Who can see beyond forever?*

The relationship between the family and the professionals working with them is considered a key to successful early intervention (Dunst et al., 1991). The collaborative efforts that result in relationships are the building blocks for a family foundation of independence (Dunst et al., 1988). Collaboration is working together, with mutual respect and acceptance, in an effort to reach a commonly recognized goal. Although collaboration fosters a relationship, it is obvious that some serious changes in attitudes and roles will be required.

Because most families are receiving services from several sources (Diehl et al., 1991), a collaborative team approach is necessary. Collaboration will be dependent upon several significant factors. The first factor is delineation of the roles each individual will be playing. Traditionally, those with the most education assumed the dominant role in decision making and services for families (Harry, 1992). Because parents seldom had the most education, professionals have been the driving force behind services. Unfortunately, these professionals changed frequently, as did family direction. When society recognized that the family was often the only constant in a child's life (Shelton, Jeppson, & Johnson, 1987), a new perspective developed. To develop and deliver family-centered systems, professionals must learn new behaviors (Bailey et al., 1992) and develop new attitudes toward families' role in early intervention. This will be an ongoing process for both families and professionals.

The second factor in a collaborative effort is respect. Collaboration requires that everyone respect each other's talents and special skills. Families and professionals alike must work within their own parameters to reach a common goal and be recognized for their ability to contribute to a successful ending. Families who are serious about enhancing the success of their child will seek the services and the respect of those professionals who support them.

The final factor in the collaborative process is communication. Lack of effective communication can be blamed for the failure of most collaborative efforts (Veninga, 1985). Each person has a unique and individualized communication style that becomes developed and finely tuned over years of influence from family, culture, education, environment, and personal temperament. With so many influencing factors, it is essential for communication efforts to focus upon a variety of techniques that will enhance a successful outcome. Professionals and parents will often present themselves with very narrow communication abilities (Bailey et al., 1991). Enhancement of communication skills is a major challenge in today's society. Professionals develop communication skills by participating in seminars, workshops, and trainings, and by working with a variety of people with different communication styles. Families will learn their main communication skills from those persons surrounding them, including the professionals and other role models in their lives (Kuenning, 1987).

Respect for Family Diversity

You can't even begin to imagine what it is like in our home. We have to deal with a lot more than Courtney's problems. If we can't get the other things done, we can't take care of her.

Everyone has a set of unique strengths and coping mechanisms based upon generations of family values (Roberts, 1990). Community lifestyle, economics, culture, religion, and personal values play a significant role in how a person will react to situations. This is a commonality shared by everyone, professionals and families alike (Adams, 1990). A common barrier to family-centered service delivery is that professional diversity and resulting values influence the ability to relate to a family. Professionals can fail to recognize their own prejudices, resulting in inappropriate judgmental interactions with families (Harry, 1992). Divesting professional relationships of personal opinions and values can be a difficult task. A family-centered philosophy requires professionals to respect family beliefs.

Family sensitivity is part of assuring respect for the families. It is impossible for professionals to understand all the influences that govern families' behavior and decisions concerning their child (Kaufmann & McGonigel, 1991). We have learned through our work that it is unfair to families to ask or allow professionals to make assumptions about families based upon small pieces of information. If we are to support the philosophy of allowing a family to make their own decisions, then our role also will include assisting them in recognizing their right to do so. History has led families to misunderstand their evolving role of full participation. Old attitudes in both the family and professional sectors must be changed to create a new atmosphere that recognizes the vital contributions that both families and professionals make to enhance the lives of children.

Effective Interagency Coordination

> *By the time Janell was 2 years old we had weekly contact with 14 doctors, 11 nurses, 2 home health agencies, 4 case managers, 4 state agencies, 3 therapists, 2 insurance companies, 2 pharmacies, 3 tertiary care centers, 2 durable medical equipment companies, and special education teachers.*

Few children and their families are served exclusively by one agency or program (Diehl et al., 1991). Through our work in developing family-centered programs we have found that many families may become involved with as many as 40 professionals at one time to meet the needs of their child. Early intervention often requires a concentrated effort by an entire team to develop the most appropriate program and supports for the family (Able-Boone, Sandall, Loughry, & Frederick, 1990). The reason many families are dealing with multiple sources of assistance stems from an attempt to individualize services; however, when each program or service operates segregated from the others serving that family, it minimizes effectiveness. Without coordination, families often become confused and frustrated and have difficulty identifying improvements in their child (Saunders, Miller, & Cates, 1989). To serve a family fully, there must be a coordinated understanding of all players involved with the family and of the roles they play. Coordination dictates consistent shared information between each program, agency, service, and the family.

Besides the obligations to coordinate services in a way that will best meet family needs, there remain issues of financial responsibility. As programs face budget restraints, coordination becomes a survival tactic to minimize duplication, enhance child outcomes, and decrease family dependence upon systems and services. Duplication of services and competition between agencies have been replaced with a forced interdependence among agencies to negotiate the rising volume of services and scarce resources.

The recognition and acceptance of coordinating services for families has become widespread. One such effort exists in St. Joseph County, Michigan, where the coordination of services for families within the early intervention system has become the rule, rather than the exception. Multi-agency team meetings occur regularly to review Individualized Family Service Plans

(IFSPs), coordinate payment for necessary services, and assign fiscal responsibility to the appropriate source. Those attending are expected to have authority to commit agency money for eligible services at the meeting. The results of these efforts have shown that families receive services in a more timely manner and agencies are confident in their role and responsibility in relation to the services outlined in the IFSP.

OPERATIONALIZING FAMILY-CENTEREDNESS

Family Involvement in System Design

> *I didn't agree with some of the ways that our family was treated so I asked to talk to someone at the main office. I found out that they were really interested in helping, but they were so far away that they didn't always know what we needed.*

Many of today's programs and systems designed to meet the needs of families and their children were developed without input from the families/consumers to be served (Turnbull, 1991). Families often express frustration that the programs do not connect with the reality of their lives (Diehl et al., 1991). Realistically, we cannot expect people without a child with special needs to understand the impact of regulations or program rules on family living (Harbin, 1992). Systems are beginning to recognize their limitations in being able to appreciate how components will affect families (Dunst et al., 1991). Families who have successfully worked toward meeting their child's needs must be involved in the formulation of the guidelines that will direct their lives for the years ahead. Their insight and understanding of program structure from a family perspective will enhance programs' abilities to direct energy where families feel the most need or frustration.

One state's response to the increased need for parent involvement in early intervention initiatives is Florida's Parent Resource Organization (PRO). Fifteen parents of children with special needs work together to review policies, procedures, programs, and rules that will affect the special needs population, birth through age 5. Major statewide committees, agencies, and programs that focus on early intervention have PRO representation to ensure that all state efforts are sensitive to family needs. The group develops best practice guidelines in relation to family-centered philosophies to provide technical assistance to programs across the state. PRO has been instrumental in designing a foundation for a family-centered future.

Families are being asked to give input and redirect professional practice into practical ideas that will help systems be sensitive to the real needs of families as illustrated in Table 5.2. By hiring family members as consultants,

TABLE 5.2. Family-Centered System Design

Traditional approach	Family-centered approach	Strategies for change	Expected outcomes
Systems developed by professionals and outside consultants	All components of system development and planning include families and professionals, as well as necessary support consultants	Make parents and family members integral members of *all* system-planning teams and internal work groups	System will know real needs of populations served; planning will be directed at needs of diverse groups as represented
Professional philosophy drives system planning and services	Families direct philosophies toward realistic needs and issues	Family members are participants on all levels of system development	Dollars are maximized as focus stays on family-prioritized issues; solutions to needs will be more successful as they reflect family concerns and priorities
Planning issues are developed before allowing family input	Families are involved from the beginning on all system issues and planning	Families are assigned to workgroups at the beginning of projects; family roles in workgroups are delineated by collaboration and coordination among all members of the group; families are paid for their time and expertise	It will never be "too late" to get family input; all products will reflect family-centeredness; each program will be family-centered, with sensitivity toward family needs; families will recognize and support programs, services, and issues because of their knowledge and participation

programs are consistently considering how a program will work, what effect it will have, how sensitive it is, and how successful it will be in relation to family-centered philosophies (Whitmore, 1991). Family consultants for early intervention programs can encourage input from consumer groups previously overlooked and ensure consideration of cultural, economic, ethnic, and environmental issues (Adams, 1990). Programs utilizing families in planning and development are richer in their missions toward families and have services that can encompass the diverse populations they serve.

Effective System Design

Many programs serving families and children undergo intensive evaluations and frequent monitoring to ensure compliance with state and federal regulations. This effort is usually attached to laws and rules that require certain standards to be met to continue to receive funding (Whitmore, 1991). Most programs and agencies have built-in procedures that recognize evaluation and monitoring as a component of their regulatory structure. The program/ agency's main interest is to comply while protecting its funding status. Most monitoring/evaluation teams also look at the level of services provided as part of quality assurance (Dunst, 1986).

Today, family-centered programs are beginning to involve families and consumers as a part of the evaluation/monitoring team (Murphy & Lee, 1992). The more appropriate term seems to be program "screening" because the teams and the program work collaboratively in identifying strengths and weaknesses, as well as the participants' concerns and priorities and the program's resources. Families and consumers are in an excellent position to provide a close look at the family-centered principles within each program and to identify the program's weaknesses and strengths. Tools to assist teams in utilizing family members and consumers in the process already exist (Greene, 1991) and may be modified for program-specific needs. Program enhancements can involve a collaborative effort between the families, screening team, and staff. Success of this method of ensuring family-centeredness lies in administrative ability to hold programs accountable for the resolution of deficits uncovered during the screening process.

Family participation in the screening process can assure that the needs of the families in relation to their child are addressed (Selener, 1991) and that programs are family-centered. Children's Medical Services in Florida employs a State Parent Consultant to develop an assessment tool in conjunction with the monitoring and evaluation teams. As part of the outreach to maintain family-centered standards throughout the state, the consultant travels with the teams to evaluate and monitor offices, programs, and clinics. The goal of the consultant position is to ensure that the state programs are fulfilling the federal mandates in the Omnibus Budget Reconciliation Act 1989 regulations requiring all Title V programs to deliver services in a family-centered manner. Screening of program strengths and needs is accomplished through parent/consumer interviews, record reviews, random phone interviews, and the utilization of a checklist of family-centered components necessary in the clinics. Results of the screening are presented at the exit conference, and a full report with recommendations is passed on to the district administrator, medical director, nursing supervisor, and the state program office. Offices and programs are commended for family-centered strengths and given technical

TABLE 5.3.   Family-Centered Program Screening

Traditional approach	Family-centered approach	Strategies for change	Expected outcomes
Professional team assesses programs	Families and consumers play a role in screening programs	Programs are screened with team members consisting of professionals and consumers	Programs will be assured of recognizing family needs; families will become more familiar with program operations; collaborative efforts will enhance programs
Programs are assessed for compliance and quality	Programs are screened to identify strengths and weaknesses	Program strengths are identified and are basis for improvements	Programs are less defensive and more willing to change due to an attitude of assistance rather than policing
Program assessments pertain to compliance and regulation only	Family-centered components are an ongoing part of program screenings	A screening tool to identify program strengths and weaknesses in family-centeredness is developed	Family-centeredness becomes an integral part of screening programs
After assessments, programs are accountable only for noncompliance with law and regulation	Programs focus accountability on family-centered components as well as regulation and law	All gaps identified in screenings will be addressed and programs are held accountable	Programs adopt family-centered philosophy; families feel more control over services

assistance to improve weak areas. Table 5.3 summarizes the strategies for change and expected outcomes in family-centered program screening.

Family-Centered Focus on Concerns, Priorities, and Resources

All of us parents sat around talking about what all of this early intervention was doing to our "normal" children. Would they remember that we didn't have the time or the energy to deal with their little problems? We wondered if they would hate us when they grew up because we didn't give them what they deserved.

The heart of any family-centered process is the recognition that families can identify their own concerns, priorities, and resources (Kaufmann & McGonigel, 1991). Because families "own" the outcomes of all efforts related to their child (Turnbull, 1991), they must have ownership of the plans to create those outcomes. A program that assumes this role itself or attempts to provide services regardless of family input will produce a frustrated family unit that is still unable to meet its child's needs.

Family concerns are those issues and problems that will impact the family's ability to meet the child's needs (Kaufmann & McGonigel, 1991) as well as concerns that extend beyond the immediate needs of the child. There is little separation between a problem that affects the family and one that affects just their child. A family-centered approach knows no boundaries between the family's needs and those of the child (Harbin, 1992). Professionals often consider it a part of their service to direct families' attention to concerns the professionals feel are "appropriate." Many concerns that professionals identify are shared by the family, but these concerns often are narrow in the context of everything that the family must deal with. In addition, professionals are careful to address only those concerns that relate directly to their own field of training, which neglects some family needs. From a family-centered approach, however, families will learn that they are the most important factor in the success of their child (Harbin, 1992). With the recognition that they determine the needs of their family, they can embrace their family concerns as a unit, not in a fragmented form.

Before we had the baby, a priority was staying on our budget and eating healthy meals. I'm not sure what a priority is anymore. The old ones don't seem to have anything to do with us anymore.

Many forms of assistance and support offered to the family may not be interpreted as useful because the family did not see them as a priority in the first place. Family priorities will determine the agenda of early intervention involvement with the family (Kaufmann & McGonigel, 1991). As families' environments and needs change, so will their agendas. For example, with one family we have collaboratively developed a family-centered plan to meet the needs of their child. When the father unexpectedly lost his job, the entire plan became moot because their priorities and resources had changed. A family will have difficulty following priorities that are not congruent with what most concerns them at that particular moment (Kaufmann & McGonigel, 1991). A family often continues to work toward what *they* feel is important with the same amount of energy as before intervention, and use what is left over to accomplish professionally driven priorities. Collaboration requires the understanding of the investment of each party involved. Collaborative efforts will support a family to identify and select priorities by putting their concerns into perspective. This will also give the family a sense of ownership that may translate into increased investment in the outcomes.

> *I had to start looking at everything a new way. Things that I never thought were a big deal, like having our own car or a washing machine, are suddenly resources. I learned that what we had was what would get us through the months ahead.*

The strengths, abilities, and supports that can be mobilized to meet the family's concerns and priorities will become their resources (Kaufmann & McGonigel, 1991). Professionals often refer families to those resources with which the professionals are most familiar, giving little consideration to the family's strengths and inner resources. They also shy away from resources over which they have little control or are uncertain about. For example, doctors refer to medical resources and state agencies refer families to other state agencies. Early intervention programs founded upon a family-centered approach will build upon all resources available to a family, formal and informal. These programs will give families the opportunity to formulate their own resource lists and select what they feel would be acceptable within the parameters of their family structure and needs. It is recommended to begin with those resources closest to the family in an effort to build from the family upward (Pizzo, 1990). A family-centered method will allow families to start with what is familiar to them and encourage simple solutions to be identified. Families will begin to coordinate resources with real needs as they learn their roles in the process. Also, when the resources are selected by the family themselves, there is assurance that the culture, values, and diversity of the family will be fully protected (Roberts, 1990).

> *This is a very important, but difficult job I am doing. I am human and possess all of the wonderful and not so wonderful emotions that go with it. There will be times when I will cry, when I will laugh, when I will be angry, sad, or when I just won't care. Please don't overreact or read too much into my human emotions. I have as much right to them as you do.*

The Identification Process

Professionals must temper their ambition to help families identify their needs and set priorities in the issues that they are facing (Kramer, McGonigel, & Kaufmann, 1991). Multiple family assessment tools have evolved to assist in the process. Many of these tools have family-centered intentions of supporting the family and guiding them to make their own choices based upon their input. The concentration must be maintained upon an outcome generated by the family, not by professionals who have used family information to develop their own judgments. Those tools that allow the family to assess themselves in relation to their own strengths and needs are the most effective in protecting family values and diversity (Whitehead, Deiner, & Toccafondi, 1990). Families should be offered a wide array of assessments in several different modes to ensure that the process itself is not contrary to the family-centered efforts intended. Flexibility in the use of tools and how they are presented to the family will ensure that the identification of concerns, priorities, and resources enables professionals to support families in determining their own strengths and needs.

We prefer a description of the activity, such as identifying concerns, priorities, and resources, to "assessment of the family." Many professionals use the term "assessment" to relate an action that uses the information to formulate an opinion of ability. Tools that generate a label that reflects functions or need are based upon the assumption that most families are alike and that there should be an accepted median (Turnbull, 1991). A celebration of individuality and family diversity is slowly shifting focus from one of deficit orientation to that of self-generated identification of concerns, priorities, and resources. A family-centered approach to identifying concerns, priorities, and resources will allow families to become a part of the solution process and not simply provide a label of functioning ability that still lacks the capacity for changing weaknesses. Labels do not change people; people must ignite change from within themselves.

When families begin to work from within, looking at their own needs and strengths, they will become better able to recognize their options to develop solutions in relation to their needs. Professional support will enhance the success of families by giving them an inside look at factors that influence their own efforts within their family (Adams, 1990). Often families will share information through the identification of concerns, priorities, and resources that can give insight to professionals, which enables them to address previous barriers to providing services.

Previous assessments traditionally have not addressed the emotional issues that accompany the difficulties that modern families experience (Harbin, 1992). Today we recognize that the emotional issues of families must be included and accepted as part of a family process to produce necessary changes. Because emotions carry a powerful influence on family needs, decisions, and direction, recognition of the importance of emotions must be incorporated into any process that involves change within the family. When families are identifying the concerns, priorities, and resources involved in their lives, we can be assured that the emotions impacting them will play a dominant role in the resulting process of change. Table 5.4 summarizes the strategies for change and expected outcomes when identification of concerns and priorities is family-centered.

TABLE 5.4. Family Identification of Concerns, Priorities, and Resources

Traditional approach	Family-centered approach	Strategies for change	Expected outcomes
Concerns are based upon those determined by professionals	All concerns evolve from the family based upon their culture, values, and lifestyle	Allow the family to discuss and form opinion on what concerns them	Families will know that they are the important factor in their child's life; families will be ready to accept more responsibility; families will learn to recognize needs
Professional concerns are formulated according to the field of the professional	Concerns encompass the entire family unit and their lifestyle, culture, values, etc.	Families are not presented with boundaries on their concerns about their child and resulting effects on the family	Everything that can improve families' abilities to meet their child's needs will be recognized and addressed; all components of the family will be considered to affect the child
Priorities are chosen according to professional evaluation of necessity	Priorities are based upon what the family wishes to focus their energy on	Priorities are born from effective collaboration with the family	Families will develop the ability to recognize their needs and put them into perspective; families will have a sense of ownership of outcomes; family energy will be maximized
Professionals select resources they are familiar with	Formal and/or informal resources will be utilized as selected by the family	Resources should begin with those closest to the family	Families will build upon familiar resources; overlooked and simple solutions will be identified
Professionals decide where and when the family will access resources	Families identify what resources are acceptable from a complete list of what is available	Families are offered what is available with all options to choose from	Families will learn to coordinate resources with needs; family values and culture will be respected; families will be more responsive as what is offered will be derived from themselves

(continued)

TABLE 5.4. (*continued*)

Traditional approach	Family-centered approach	Strategies for change	Expected outcomes
Professionals assess needs by giving assessments to judge the level of family functioning	Families are encouraged to visualize needs and assess family strengths and weaknesses themselves	Self-assessment tools in a variety of modes are offered to the family along with nonjudgmental support	Families will recognize their own strengths and weaknesses based upon their own values; professionals will serve families in a more sensitive manner; families will feel part of the process instead of part of the problem
Families are kept on the outside of the decision making to control emotional input	Families use their emotions to sort out their strengths, weaknesses, concerns, priorities, and resources	Encourage families to express their emotions and feelings	Families will be addressing the issues most pressing to them; professionals will learn what factors may be interfering with communication with families

Assessments: How Family-Centered Are They?

Programs that are using assessments as a part of understanding and identifying family needs should look carefully at the tools they are using. The questions in Table 5.5 should receive a positive answer as a reflection of sensitivity to the family.

Family-Centered Child Evaluations

> *She stops breathing several times a night, her heart rate drops to 40 or soars into the 300s, she shakes all the time, and throws up most of what I feed her. I am sorry I don't remember how old she was when she rolled over for the first time.*

Evaluation is a term used for the procedure to determine eligibility for services or to describe the child's current status in a variety of developmental areas. Assessment is defined as the use of ongoing procedures to identify a

TABLE 5.5.   Checklist for Evaluating the Family-Centeredness of Assessments

1. Will the completion of the tool result in a family-generated identification of concerns, priorities, and resources, *not* a label or diagnosis of family functioning?
2. Does the family have a choice about participating in the assessment?
3. Is the tool free of acronyms and program jargon?
4. Is the answer to *every* question going to play a role in planning and serving the family according to their own identified needs?
5. Are the answers based upon the family's perception of themselves and their needs?
6. Can the family answer the questions in privacy if they wish?
7. Will/could the process involve the entire family unit, including the spouse and siblings?
8. Do family members have the opportunity to discuss the questions with the interviewer or each other?
9. Is the tool culturally sensitive and available in another language, if necessary?
10. Can the resulting information be used by other agencies and programs with family permission?
11. Were families involved in the creation and development of the tool to be used?

---

child's unique needs. Assessment begins after a decision has been made to initiate early intervention and is conducted throughout the period during which services are provided. Evaluation for eligibility is one step in the assessment process. Because of the overlap in use of the terms "evaluation" and "assessment," they are often used interchangeably (Graham, 1990). For the purpose of this discussion we will refer only to evaluation as described above.

In entering an early intervention system, families, as consumers, often encounter evaluation as a beginning step to determine eligibility. Traditionally, these first contacts have been to gather information about the child and family to make an eligibility determination. In a family-centered system the goal for first contacts is to assist the family in beginning to identify the family's agenda for themselves and their children. It is then determined if and how an early intervention program will become involved in their life. These first encounters with the system may influence, positively or negatively, the tone for future collaborations and relationships to come.

As best practice moves from a child-centered evaluation system to a family-centered system, parents are being significantly recognized and utilized as the experts on their children. Professionals are creating opportunities for meaningful family participation in the evaluation process, although the shift to family-centered evaluations is evolving slowly. A review of research on parent involvement in selecting educational goals for their children showed that over 90% of goals were chosen by professionals (Brinkerhoff & Vincent, 1986). In a more recent national study of 180 professionals, a substantial discrepancy remains between the extent to which families currently participate and their ideal level of involvement in the following areas: parent involvement in decisions about child assessment, parent participation in assessment, parent participation in the team meeting and decision making, and the provision of family goals and services (Bailey et al., 1992).

Table 5.6 suggests that the evaluation process begins with assisting the family in preparing for their role in the process. For many families this will be a new experience that will require support and information as well as options for involvement. It is important to remember that family members' responses to the opportunity for participation will be likely to change over time as they become knowledgeable and comfortable with professionals and the process. A family-centered approach will provide families with the opportunity to participate in all evaluation decisions. Some families will choose to be intensely involved and others will choose a less active role. The key is to respect individual family preferences for participation in the process and to provide opportunities for the level of involvement that feel right for each family. Child evaluations should be based upon a respect for the knowledge and experience the family has with the child. Parents are the experts on their child and they know their child best. They also know the interventions that could work in their lives and therefore be successful, and those that could not.

To obtain the best picture of the child's abilities and to elicit information from the family regarding their concerns, evaluations and observations should be conducted in environments that are familiar to the child. These may include child care sites, extended-family homes, or playgrounds. This will require flexibility and creativity in planning, scheduling, and providing supports to accommodate not only system requirements but family schedules and need for support.

Too often, evaluation reports become an endless list of the child's deficits and fail to mention the abilities present. The family perspective on their child's strengths and needs is a vital component of evaluation and one that early interventionists often do not know how to elicit. Parent report has been found to be as reliable as some screening instruments, such as the widely used Denver Developmental Screen (Squires, Nickel, & Bricker, 1990). Tools are available to help parents structure their observations of their child in categories necessary for evaluation. Families should be encouraged to discuss their child's activities, strengths, and likes/dislikes that are exhibited at home. It is appropriate to ask what types of behaviors the child demonstrates under certain conditions, and to ask families about information that has been gathered from other sources, such as the baby-sitter or child care site. For a truly comprehensive view of the child, family–child interactions should be observed and family reports of child behavior obtained.

Any individual designated as a family member is part of the team. Find-

TABLE 5.6. Family-Centered Child Evaluations

Traditional approach	Family-centered approach	Strategies for change	Expected outcomes
Professionals decide which children are to be evaluated and in which developmental areas	Family concerns and decisions about evaluations drive evaluation planning	A designated person (service coordinator, resource parent, etc.) provides information and options to families	Evaluations address family concerns as well as professional concerns
Single source of information: professionally administered tests	Multiple sources of information used, including parent report, observations, and tests	Procedures changed to routinely elicit parent report and include time for observation	More reliable evaluation of child increases appropriateness of interventions
Single-discipline evaluations with much duplication	Integrated, comprehensive, multidisciplinary evaluations with collateral information shared	Create efficient systems through policy and funding changes	Less time, less expense for professionals, fewer appointments for families
One-time evaluation and labeling of child in isolation from the family	Continuing and evolving process based on changing needs of child and family	Develop a mechanism for ongoing, informal (observation) and formal multidisciplinary process	Child's developmental needs are routinely addressed within the context of the family
Evaluations are scheduled around the professional's time and located at his/her convenience	Families involved in choosing time, location, team, tools, dissemination of results	Collaborative decision making, providing family with supports (child care, transportation) and options	Families are able to participate in process to elicit child's best performance and share information
Discipline-specific jargon used throughout process	Clear, understandable, jargon-free language used during process	Communication style and language of families used	Information understood by family; families ask questions, make corrections, give input
Professionals decide how, when, and what information is shared with the family—often limited, overwhelming, and confusing	Complete, unbiased sharing of results with family questions answered; support offered as needed in a timely fashion	Use language of families, schedule enough time for sharing, answering questions, repeat as necessary	Families' understanding of child's abilities and needs increased; informed decisions made
Focus on child's deficits and weaknesses	Includes strengths and functional abilities	Develop skills and tools to elicit parent report, observational skills, and language control	Families not overwhelmed with negatives, allowed to "brag" about child and hear positives

(continued)

TABLE 5.6. (*continued*)

Traditional approach	Family-centered approach	Strategies for change	Expected outcomes
Evaluation process not explained to families, yet families expected to comply with process	Process explained to families, families involved in every aspect	Develop mechanism to ensure time, staff availability, and skills are in place	Families have increased understanding of importance of process and there is respect for family values and decision-making style

ings are discussed as a team with the family's input and decisions respected and acknowledged. Professionals and family will then jointly integrate their concerns and resources into a single intervention plan for the child and family. Table 5.6 summarizes strategies for change and expected outcomes when child evaluations are family-centered.

Family-Centered Individualized Family Service Plans

> *When they wrote the program it never occurred to them that it just doesn't work that way in a home. The phone rings, brothers and sisters get hurt and need bandages, there are Cub Scout meetings, the never-ending advice of grandparents, and of course, someone has to feed the family. The plan never considered someone has to cook.*

To refer to a family-centered Individualized Family Service Plan (IFSP) may sound redundant to some, but we cannot assume that an IFSP is going to be family-centered. The IFSP has the monumental responsibility of embodying a process that is the essence of a changing delivery system. This "leap of faith" for families into uncharted territory hinges on the process by which the IFSP is developed and implemented. Without emphasis and accountability focused on the process, we may do nothing more than change the name of a form, or worse yet, the IFSP could become "one more" document used by professionals to continue to direct the child and family. Constant vigilance is required to prevent this from occurring. Barriers to implementation spring not from the components of the plan, but rather from the requirement that professionals must make concessions in the way they work with each other and with families in order to comply with the principle and philosophy of family-centeredness.

Turbiville et al. (1993) identified principles upon which best-practice indicators for the IFSP and Individualized Education Plan (IEP) are based.

The primary guiding principle identified is that the family is the decision maker in the process of generating the IFSP or IEP. The second guiding principle in the development of the IFSP and IEP is the plan's importance to the family outcome. In order for the IFSP to be an umbrella plan, it is critical that it reflect all of the services and supports the family has identified as priorities and emphasizes the need for collaboration and partnership between professionals and agencies.

In training over 1,800 professionals in interagency IFSP workshops in Florida, the obstacle to creating an IFSP most often expressed was the inability of professionals to write collaborative plans with each other (Duwa, 1993). Time constraints, unresolved policy conflicts, funding, and turf-guarding were the issues raised that seemed the most overwhelming to participants. The notion of families as the final decision maker on the IFSP drew the most resistance from therapists. As participants perceived that family-centeredness was a practice that went far beyond just encouraging parent participation, their ability to assimilate this fact, plus the requirement to jointly plan with one other, was hindered by a narrow view of their discipline and perceived systemic barriers. Their ability to conceptualize family-centeredness as a positive approach to planning appeared to diminish as they felt their authority to make decisions threatened.

Being family-centered is an ongoing process that does not end with the completion of an IFSP. The IFSP process encompasses all of the best-practice family-centered strategies found in this chapter. Table 5.7 illustrates the change from our traditional planning practices to family-centered strategies for achieving viable, successful outcomes.

Family-Centered Service Coordination

> *I knew we needed some help so I started to call around. Each person I spoke with had the name and number of another person for me to call. Ten phone calls later I still didn't have the information I needed.*

With the reauthorization of Public Law 99-457 (Part H of IDEA) in 1991, the term "service coordination" formally replaced the term "case management services." This change was a result of families and professionals expressing their objections to the implications that families are "cases" to be "managed" (Hobbs, 1975). This new terminology more accurately reflects a shift in paradigms than it does a creation of just two more new words. This shift in paradigms (Edelman, 1991) reflects a whole new way of doing business with families.

To many, the term "service coordination" in and of itself has come to represent a family-centered approach. This is true to such a degree that to say family-centered service coordination seems to be redundant. Meanwhile,

TABLE 5.7. Family-Centered Family Support Plans

Traditional approach	Family-centered approach	Strategies for change	Expected outcomes
Reflects only child's developmental needs as determined by professionals	Outcomes reflect family concerns, priorities, and resources as related to the development of the child	Identify family's concerns, priorities, and resources	Child's *and* family's strengths and resources drive service delivery
Plan reassessed semi-annually with annual review	Plan modified and updated to respond to changing family situations	Identified primary service coordinator who is responsible for implementation of plan	Plan is dynamic and responds to changing needs of family and child
Each provider writes a separate plan	One umbrella plan for each child and family	Restructuring of planning systems	Coordinated and integrated supports and services for child and family
Information about the family (i.e., psychosocial) is part of the plan with or without parental consent	Only information regarding family's concerns, priorities, and resources that the family chooses to share is reflected on the IFSP	Family has final decision regarding shared information	Family is final decision maker in the process; reduces inappropriate or irrelevant judgments about families
Family signs completed plan	Family develops plan as part of the team	Family's strengths, needs, and resources drive planning process	Family "owns" plan that reflects their priorities and are invested in outcome
Expected outcomes of early intervention are all child related	Expected outcomes reflect both child and family needs	Identify family strengths, needs, and resources during planning process	Support services and interventions are designed for needs of all family members
Family is involved to meet legal requirements	Family is involved to increase positive outcomes for child and family	Define professional's role to include meeting family's desired outcomes	Increase positive outcomes for child and family

the term "case management" has been shunted to the side by many family advocates and others as it has come to represent the old school of managing and controlling families.

In this section, distinctions are drawn between service coordination and case management, the belief systems behind service coordination are identified, and strategies for moving from a case management approach to a service coordination approach are shared.

Service Coordination

Service coordination can be seen as a way of working that moves from the known to the unknown. The service coordinator, for example, knows concrete information about the child and family (e.g., income level, ethnicity, child's special needs, number of children in the family). However, what is best for the child and the family is not set when the relationship between the service coordinator and family begins. What is best for the child and family is perceived as an empty canvas upon which the family will paint its own picture with assistance from the service coordinator.

In this regard, the service coordinator's role can be seen as the orchestration of meaningful interactions that can lead to problem solving, decision making, goal setting, and accomplishments. To achieve these objectives, the service coordinator needs to create a nurturing environment for families to do whatever they are comfortable achieving, in an undetermined timeframe. The canvas is the family's to paint on and it is understood that they will take however long they need to complete it.

With a service coordination approach, the family measures the success of the service being provided rather than the "beauty or timeliness" of the painting itself. Questions about whether the family felt their concerns and priorities were heard or comprehended become essential. This shift in approach would explain the need for and the recent development of parent/consumer program evaluation tools (Summers, Turnbull, Murphy, Lee, & Turbiville, 1991).

Case Management

Case management, on the other hand, can be seen as moving from the known to the known. The case manager knows both the concrete information about the family and has a set of preconceived notions about what is best for the family with timeframes attached. This may result in the case manager selecting from the available options (programs and services within his/her agency or, less typically, community-wide) and presenting the narrowed list to the family. The family would then choose from this narrowed list with the understanding that some of the choices are actually "better" than others.

With a case management approach, success is measured by whether the case manager was able to "convince" the family to take the necessary steps to arrive at the preconceived notion about what would be best for them. Thus, the beauty and timeliness of the painting is the yardstick that determines whether case management services were effective. The following is a typical scenario of this approach. Upon receipt of a referral, the case manager determines that the child should be enrolled in a full-time early intervention program. The case manager establishes the goal of enrolling the child in program X. The case manager then sets out with her array of strategies to convince the family of this need. Regardless of whether that goal is shared by the family, the case manager still adheres to that goal. Furthermore, she may believe that it was her technique that worked to convince the family of the need for a full-time early intervention program, even if the goal was desired by the family. The dilemma that this creates is that the family never is seen as owning the goal, and thus is never allowed the success for achieving the goal. The success and achievements are attributed to the case manager. In this approach, the process is not as important as the outcome and it is the outcome that measures effectiveness. Family/consumer evaluations are thus not important in determining successes.

Distinctions

In essence, service coordination involves facilitating a family's decision-making process while case management helps a family "pick the right plan or goal from a predetermined list." Success in the former is measured by the family's evaluation of the service, whereas success in the latter is determined by the case manager's perceptions of his/her ability to achieve the goals that he/she has in mind for the family.

In part, this shift from case management to service coordination can be seen as the result of a shift in beliefs about families. The years of work by the Turnbulls, and families and researchers like them, has been a tremendous contribution and impetus to this shift in beliefs and perceptions (Behr, 1990; Summers, Brotherson, & Turnbull, 1989). By addressing the strengths and resources of families with members with special needs, as well as celebrating the contributions of persons with disabilities, the field has come a long way in dispelling the old myths of overwrought, perpetually grieving, helpless families and individuals. Viewing families in a new way has become a prerequisite to effective family-centered service coordination. To be successful in this new role, case managers must go beyond acquiring new skills and learning new strategies to adopting a new belief system about families.

Beliefs about Families

A service coordination approach is based on the belief that families have the ability to find their own directions and solutions and that families are very diverse with each family unique in its structure, roles, values, beliefs, and coping style (Johnson, McGonigel, & Kaufmann, 1989). Believing that families are the best judges as to what will or will not work for them, service coordinators perceive their role as interacting with families in such a way that the family maintains or acquires a sense of control over their family life and are able to attribute positive changes that result from early intervention to their own strengths, abilities, and actions (Dunst et al., 1988).

Service coordinators also should have no preconceived notions about what a family should or should not do. Such notions should be released so as to allow the relationship with the family to be the vehicle through which the family will discover what works for them. The service coordinator gives up the need to be right, to heal, and to "fix" the family.

Strategies for Becoming Family-Centered

The two beliefs about families mentioned above underscore many of the service coordinator's decisions and will determine the skills and practices the service coordinator will need to acquire. The acquisition of these necessary skills, practices, and beliefs is a process of evolution and internalization. Table 5.8 presents a matrix describing both the traditional approach and a family-centered approach, as well as strategies to achieve a more family-focused, family-driven process.

ARE WE FAMILY-CENTERED?

On most days I am an occupational therapist, physical therapist, nurse, teacher, case manager, taxi driver, social worker, and dietitian. Some days I just want to be her mom; nothing else, just her mom. Please don't make me feel wrong for that.

Family-centered development, delivery, and evaluation of service to young children and their families is causing a fundamental shift in how families and professionals perceive their own and each other's roles in early intervention. A result of this shift is a substantial amount of uncertainty, resistance, and frustration. Research suggests that although professionals understand the concept of being family-centered, there is great difficulty in putting theory into practice (Bailey et al., 1991, 1992; Dunst et al., 1991).

TABLE 5.8.   Family-Centered Service Coordination

Traditional approach	Family-centered approach	Strategies for change	Expected outcomes
Case management client-focused	Service coordination is family-focused and family-driven	View child in context of family and address needs of all family members	Needs of all family members are met, enhancing child outcomes
Several programmatic case managers	One family-identified service coordinator	Family chooses one primary service coordinator; family choice is respected	Coordinated, integrated, family-driven service coordination
Case management focus on child and family dysfunction	Service coordination focus on child and family strengths and resources	Protocols and training specify process focused on strengths; tools are specified to help identify strengths	Family confidence increased; strengths are built upon increasing likelihood of success
Case manager offers only options their agency provides	Service coordinator provides options across agencies	Improve information sharing and cooperative agreements across agencies	Needs of whole family are met
Case manager views family in the context of the child's disability	Service coordinator views the child in the context of the family	Professionals are trained and skilled in meeting family concerns	Child outcomes are enhanced as family needs are met
Case manager provides family with information using professional jargon and shares only what they feel family can handle	Service coordinator provides unbiased, uncensored information in the family's language (both level and native)	Training is supplied so professionals skillfully provide information on family level	Family understands and has same information as professionals
Case managers make assumptions/decisions about what child needs	Service coordinator assists families in identifying their concerns, priorities, and resources	Establish trusting relationship with family; identify most appropriate way to assist families in identifying their concerns, priorities, and resources	Family makes decisions resulting in increased control of their lives
Case manager must be trained professional	Service coordinator may be the patient(s), another family member, another family, or paraprofessional	Provide opportunity, ongoing skill building/ training	Family choices are expanded

According to a recent survey of professionals in early intervention programs in four states, perceptions of family involvement differ between current and ideal practices in four areas: parent involvement in decisions about child assessment; parent participation in assessment; parent participation in the team meeting and decision making; and the provision of family goals and services (Bailey et al., 1992). When asked to identify the barriers to practicing a family-centered approach, professionals in this study listed family barriers first, followed by system barriers, and finally professional barriers, specifically related to lack of skill.

In contrast to the professionals' view of barriers, research shows that families perceive professionals' attitudes and behavior as the major barriers to receiving the respect, dignity, and compassion they deserve (Coulter et al., 1991). The importance of sensitivity to families, including offering critical emotional support, is seen as a primary responsibility of providers in addition to their important clinical expertise (Able-Boone et al., 1990; Coulter et al., 1991; Summers et al., 1990). Families of children receiving early intervention services voiced the importance of professionals recognizing family priorities, concerns, and resources; respecting parental observations; providing emotional support; coordinating services and providing referrals; and not making unrealistic demands on families (Coulter et al., 1991).

Head Start is one model that has institutionalized family-centered policy and practice. The principles of family-centeredness were inherent in Head Start programs from the inception of the 25-year-old antipoverty, prevention program. Head Start policy brings parents into the decision-making process, beginning in the classroom and continuing to the national level. On a national scale, Head Start exhibits all of the attributes of successful family-centered programs described by Schorr (1988), which include comprehensive and intensive services for the child and family; basic premise of the child as part of the family and the family as part of a community; commitment to meet local needs where their programs are located; parent involvement policies that establish and accept parents as key players; and staff provided with the time, training, skills, and other necessary resources to build trusting, respectful relationships with children and families (Mallory & Goldsmith 1990; Zigler, 1989).

SUMMARY

As policies and programs respond to the requirement of developing and delivering family-centered systems and services, professionals will be increasingly forced to learn new behaviors (Bailey et al., 1992). Family-centeredness is an attitude, one that challenges the way we think about services, families, and ourselves, and is manifested in the way policy is developed, programs are designed, and services are delivered. The distant, almost inaudible murmur of change in early intervention has become a full-blown movement fueled by Public Law 99-457 and kept alive by the commitment of families and professionals to the evolving concept of family-centeredness. Are we family-centered? If you answer yes, think again. Family-centeredness requires a constant vigilance to resist the habitual and explore the possibilities of change and creativity.

REFERENCES

Able-Boone, H., Sandall, S. R., Loughry, A., & Frederick, L. L. (1990). An informed, family-centered approach to Public Law 99-457: Parental views. *Topics in Early Childhood Special Education, 10*(1), 100–111.

Adams, E. M. (1990). *Policy planning for culturally comprehensive special health services.* Washington, DC: U.S. Department of Health and Human Services.

Bailey, D. B., Buysse, V., Edmondson, R., & Smith T. M. (1992). Creating family-centered services in early intervention: Perceptions of professionals in four states. *Exceptional Children, 58,* 298–308.

Bailey, D. B., Palsha, S. A., & Simeonsson, R. J. (1991). Professional skills, concerns, and perceived importance of work with families in early intervention. *Exceptional Children, 58,* 156–165.

Behr, S. (1990). *Positive contributions of person with disabilities to their families.* Lawrence, KS: Beach Center on Families and Disabilities.

Brinkerhoff, J. L., & Vincent, L. J. (1986). Increasing parental decision-making at their child's individualized educational program meeting. *Journal of the Division for Early Childhood, 11,* 46–58.

Bronfenbrenner, U. (1977). Toward an experimental ecology of human development. *American Psychologist, 32,* 513–531.

Coulter, M., Johnson, J., & Innis, V. (1991). *Selected Florida Counties Early Intervention Project: The family perspective.* Tallahassee, FL: College of Public Health, University of South Florida; Florida Department of Education, Office of Early Intervention and School Readiness.

Diehl, S., Moffitt, K., & Wade, S. (1991). Focus group interview with parents of children with medically complex needs: An intimate look at their perceptions and feelings. *Children's Health Care, 20*(3), 170–179.

Dunst, C. J. (1986). Overview of the efficacy of early intervention programs. In L. Brickman & D. L. Wetherford (Eds.), *Evaluating early intervention programs for severely handicapped children and their families* (pp. 51–63). Austin: Pro-Ed.

Dunst, C., Johanson, C., Trivette, C., & Hamby, D. (1991). Family-oriented early intervention policies and practices: Family-centered or not? *Exceptional Children, 58*(2), 115-126.

Dunst C. J., Trivette C. M., & Deal, A. G. (1988). *Enabling and empowering families: Principles and guidelines for practice.* Cambridge, MA: Brookline Books.

Duwa, S. (1993). *Florida's family support plan process: Training professionals.* Tallahassee, FL: Florida State University Center for Prevention and Early Intervention Policy. Unpublished manuscript.

Edelman, L. (1991). *Getting on board: Training activities to promote the practice of family-centered care*. Baltimore, MD: Project Copernicus; The Kennedy Institute National Center for Family-Centered Care.

Frederick, L., & McGonigel, M. (1992, August). *Conversations about family involvement versus family-centered in relation to services integration*. Workshop presented at Partnerships for Progress V: National Early Childhood Technical Assistance System, Washington, DC.

Graham, M. (1990). *Evaluation, assessment, and IFSP development*. Tallahassee, FL: Florida State University Center for Policy Studies in Education.

Greene, J. (1991). On the practice of normative evaluation. *Networking Bulletin, 2*(2), 17–20.

Harbin, G. L. (1992). Family issues of children with disabilities: How research and theory have modified practices in intervention. In N. J. Anastasiow & S. Harel (Eds.), *At-risk infants: Interventions, families and research* (pp. 101–109). Baltimore: Paul H. Brookes.

Harry, B. (1992). Restructuring the participation of Afro-American parents in special education. *Exceptional Children, 59*(2), 123–131.

Healy, A., Keesee, P. D., & Smith, B. S. (1989). *Early services for children with special needs: Transactions for family support*. Baltimore: Paul H. Brookes.

Hobbs, N. (1975). *The futures of children*. San Francisco: Jossey-Bass.

Johnson, B. H., McGonigel, M. J., & Kaufmann, R. K. (Eds.). (1989). *Guidelines and recommended practices for the Individualized Family Service Plan* (1st ed.). Chapel Hill, NC, and Bethesda, MD: National Early Childhood Technical Assistance System and Association for the Care of Children's Health.

Kaufmann, R. K., & McGonigel, M. J. (1991). Identifying family concerns, priorities, and resources. In M. J. McGonigel, R. K. Kaufmann, & B. H. Johnson (Eds.), *Guidelines and recommended practices for the Individualized Family Service Plan* (2nd ed., pp 47–55). Bethesda, MD: Association for the Care of Children's Health.

Kuenning, D. (1987). *Helping people through grief*. Bloomington, MN: Bethany House.

Kramer, S., McGonigel, M., & Kaufmann, R. K. (1991). Developing the IFSP: Outcomes, strategies, activities, and services. In M. J. McGonigel, R. K. Kaufmann, & B. H. Johnson (Eds.), *Guidelines and recommended practices for the Individual Family Service Plan* (2nd ed., pp. 57–66). Bethesda, MD: Association for the Care of Children's Health.

Mallory, N., & Goldsmith, N. (1990). Head Start works! Two Head Start veterans share their views. *Young Children, 45*(6), 36–39.

McGonigel, M. J., Kaufmann, R. K., & Johnson, B. H. (Eds.). (1991). *Guidelines and recommended practices for the Individualized Family Service Plan* (2nd ed.). Bethesda, MD: Association for the Care of Children's Health.

McKnight, J. (1992, July & August). Are social service agencies the enemy of the community? *Utne Reader*, pp. 88–90.

Murphy, D. L., & Lee, I. M. (1992). *Family-Centered Program Rating Scale. User's Guide*. Lawrence, KS: Beach Center on Families and Disabilities.

Pizzo, P. (1990). Family centered Head Start for infants and toddlers: A renewed direction for Project Head Start. *Young Children, 45*(6), 30–35.

Roberts, R. N. (1990). *Developing culturally competent programs for families of chil-*

dren with special needs. Washington, DC: Georgetown University Development Center.

Robinson, C. C., Rosenberg, S. A., & Beckman, P. J. (1990). Parent involvement in early childhood special education. In J. B. Jordon, J. J. Gallagher, P. L. Huttinger, & M. B. Karnes (Eds.), *Early childhood special education: Birth to three* (pp. 109–127). Reston, VA: Council for Exceptional Children.

Saunders, R., Miller, B., & Cates, K. (1989). Pediatric family care: An interdisciplinary approach. *Children's Health Care, 18*(1), 53–58.

Schorr, L. R. (1988). *Within our reach, breaking the cycle of disadvantage.* New York: Anchor Press/Doubleday.

Selener, D. (1991). Participatory evaluation: People's knowledge as a source of power. *Networking Bulletin, 2*(2), 25–27.

Shelton, T. L., Jeppson, E. S., & Johnson, B. H. (1987). *Family-centered care for children with special health care needs.* Washington, DC: U.S. Government Printing Office.

Squires, J. K., Nickel, R., & Bricker, D. (1990). Use of parent-completed developmental questionnaires for child-find and screening. *Infants and Young Children, 3*(2), 46–57.

Summers, J., Brotherson, M., & Turnbull, A. (1989). *The impact of handicapped children on families.* Lawrence, KS: Beach Center on Families and Disabilities.

Summers, J. A., Dell'Oliver, C., Turnbull, A. P., Benson, H. A., Santelli, E., Campbell, M., & Siegel-Causey, E. (1990). Examining the Individualized Family Service Plan process: What are family and practitioner preferences? *Topics in Early Childhood Special Education, 10*(1), 78–99.

Summers, J., Turnbull, A., Murphy, D., Lee, I., & Turbiville, V. (1991). *Family-Centered Program Rating Scale.* Lawrence, KS: Beach Center on Families and Disabilities.

Turbiville, V., Turnbull, A., Garland, C., & Lee, I. (1993). IFSPs and IEPs. In *DEC Task Force on Recommended Practices: Indicators of quality in programs for infants and young children with special needs and their families* (pp. 30–36). Reston, VA: Council for Exceptional Children.

Turnbull, A. P., & Turnbull, H. R. (1990). *Families, professionals and exceptionality* (2nd ed.). Columbus, OH: Merrill.

Turnbull, A. P. (1991). Identifying children's strengths and needs. In M. J. McGonigel, R. K. Kaufmann, & B. H. Johnson (Eds.), *Guidelines and recommended practices for the Individual Family Service Plan* (2nd. ed., pp. 39–46). Bethesda, MD: Association for the Care of Children's Health.

Veninga, R. (1985). *A gift of hope.* New York: Ballantine Books.

Vincent, L. J., & Beckett, J. A. (1993). Family participation. In *DEC Task Force on Recommended Practices: Indicators of quality programs for infants and young children with special needs and their families* (pp. 19–25). Reston, VA: Council for Exceptional Children.

Weissbourd, B., & Patrick, M. (1988). In the best interest of the family: The emergence of family resource programs. *Infants and Young Children, 1*(2), 46–54.

Whitehead, L. C., Deiner, P. L., & Toccafondi, S. (1990). Family assessment: Parent and professional evaluation. *Topics in Early Childhood Education, 10*(1), 63–77.

Whitmore, E. (1991). Evaluation and empowerment: It's the process that counts. *Networking Bulletin, 2*(2), 1–7.

CHAPTER 6

Traditions in Family Assessment
Toward an Inquiry-Oriented, Reflective Model

DONALD B. BAILEY, JR.
LAURA W. HENDERSON

Family assessment and family assessment procedures have their roots in three distinct, although overlapping, traditions. These traditions have had a powerful influence on the purposes and methodologies that have come to characterize family assessment and have important implications for teachers, therapists, health care professionals, and others who work in the early intervention arena. In this chapter we distinguish among these traditions and argue for an inquiry-oriented, reflective model based heavily on the professional's ongoing attempts to view events from the family's perspective. In the process of describing this model, we discuss guidelines and considerations when engaging in family assessment and provide examples of family assessment activities framed around this overarching goal.

TRADITIONS IN FAMILY ASSESSMENT

In its most general form, family assessment may be defined as the process by which information is gathered about families. In individual assessment, the focus is on a child, youth, or adult, with an emphasis on gathering information about the individual's development, abilities, feelings, or behavior. Although individual assessment may include a documentation of social relationships, the primary focus is on a single person. In contrast, family assessment typically includes more than one individual; furthermore, the information gathered almost invariably addresses some aspect of the relationship between two or more family members. In theory, family assessment should be able to accommodate the wide variation in the definition and construction of families, so long as two or more people are involved who define themselves as a family and are engaged in a meaningful and enduring relationship (Hanson & Lynch, 1992).

Family assessment strategies have used diverse methodologies for gathering information, including direct observation, rating scales, and self-reports. Although these methodologies vary considerably from each other, it is the historical traditions associated with various family assessment strategies that most clearly differentiate the procedures. Three such traditions are evident in the literature: research, clinical, and support. An understanding of the assumptions and purposes underlying each tradition is helpful in evaluating the usefulness of family assessment procedures for early intervention.

Research Traditions

The research tradition of family assessment has been driven by the desire to develop an understanding of the general nature of families and how they function (Massey, 1986). This goal led to the development of hundreds of measures to assess various aspects of family functioning. Simeonsson (1988) groups these measures into three broad categories. *Structural measures* assess the composition of the family, interactions and relations among family members, and the systemic properties of families. *Developmental measures* are based on the assumption that a family is a developing unit and are used to assess the extent to which families grow and change over time. *Functional measures* assess various needs, tasks, or functions experienced by families in their efforts to adapt to demands, events, or other stressors.

The goals of the research tradition have been to describe those characteristics of families and family functioning that are universal and identify factors that contribute to variability across families. Although individual families are certainly of interest and, indeed, constitute the basic unit of measurement in the research tradition, the primary focus has been on gathering quantitative data with large samples to determine patterns or styles of functioning (LaRossa & Wolf, 1985). In the research tradition, there is rarely a meaningful relationship between the professional gathering the data and the family member providing the information. In fact, the researcher may never even meet an individual family if the study relies on paper and pencil measures for data collection. The family exists as an object for study; although the researcher may be quite interested in the families under study, the relationship is almost certainly one way. Rarely does the family benefit directly from the information gathered because the measures were not designed for clinical assessment purposes, nor is the information used in any kind of clinical or supportive context.

The research tradition has led to a large number of theories and models of family functioning (e.g., Beavers & Voeller, 1983; Bentovim, 1986; Combrinck-

Graham, 1985; McCubbin & McCubbin, 1987; Tseng & McDermott, 1979; Turnbull, Summers, & Brotherson, 1984). Although it is generally recognized that the field is far from any kind of theoretical consensus about the fundamental nature of families (Cowan, 1987; Grotevant & Carlson, 1989), systems theory is generally regarded as the best framework for understanding the complex interrelationships and influences that characterize families (Campbell & Draper, 1985). As Steinglass (1984) suggests, systems theory is a broad-based model built on three basic assumptions. The first assumption is that although families consist of individual members, they function as organizational units in which each member influences and is influenced by the other. The second assumption is that families, like other living systems, continually strive to achieve balance or stability in functioning. Finally, the concept of systemic growth assumes that family systems become increasingly complex over time. The implication of systems theory for therapists and interventionists is a recognition of the complexity of the family context and how integral the child with a disability is to each family's ecology.

Clinical Traditions

The clinical tradition of family assessment has focused on the need to provide therapeutic support for families who, for one reason or another, are experiencing significant difficulties in some aspect of family relationships (e.g., marital dissatisfaction, infidelity, child abuse, ineffective or unfulfilling interactional styles). Assessment procedures developed in the context of this tradition typically have been designed to pinpoint problems that then become the focus of therapy. The assessment techniques range from specific paper and pencil measures to lengthy and more diffuse assessment in the context of multiple interview sessions with family members. Families may be classified into typologies derived from research or clinical practice (e.g., McCubbin & Thompson, 1987), specific dysfunctional styles may be described, or individual feelings or behaviors may be identified. Although the clinical tradition also seeks to document family resources and strengths, its primary goal is to identify problems for the purpose of therapeutic remediation.

In contrast with the research tradition, where the professional may not even know the families from whom data are collected, professionals in the clinical tradition are likely to have detailed knowledge of each individual family. Through multiple sessions, therapists often become privy to intimate details about family functioning and individual styles. Although the relationship is rarely reciprocal because therapists generally do not share details about their own lives with clients, it is two-way, as therapists "give opinions, share judgments, make suggestions, and assume overt relational positions vis-à-vis family members for the purpose of trying to influence family relationships"

(Aponte, 1985, p. 323). With the exception of court-mandated circumstances, families voluntarily seek out therapists, usually with the explicit goal of gaining assistance to improve some aspect of the family relationship.

Support Traditions

Family support constitutes the third tradition underlying family assessment strategies. This tradition lies in a broader social movement in the United States designed to help families cope with the challenges faced by circumstances such as unemployment, homelessness, poverty, chronic illness, or having a child with a disability. According to Zigler and Black (1989), the ultimate goal of family support programs is to "enable families to be independent by developing their own informal support networks" (p. 11).

Family assessment strategies for early intervention have emerged primarily out of the support tradition. Several terms and models have been used to characterize the family support movement in early intervention, including family-focused intervention (Bailey et al., 1986), parent empowerment (Dunst, 1985; Dunst, Trivette, & Deal, 1988), and family-centered care (Shelton, Jeppson, & Johnson, 1987). Two features common to each of these models are the assumption that family support is a primary goal of early intervention and the belief that families should be able to choose both the services they want and their level of involvement in the decision-making process.

Public Law 99-457, passed in 1986, and subsequent amendments to the law passed in 1991 (Public Law 102-199), provide a legal context for family assessment. In the process of requiring an Individualized Family Service Plan (IFSP) for infants and toddlers with disabilities, the law also establishes the expectation that early intervention programs will offer "family-directed assessments." According to the regulations, the purpose of family assessment is to assist each family to determine their resources, priorities, and concerns related to enhancing their child's development. Family assessment must be voluntary on the part of families, conducted by personnel trained to use appropriate methods and procedures, based on information provided by the family through a personal interview, and should incorporate the family's own description of its resources, priorities, and concerns.

Family assessment strategies evolving out of the support tradition typically seek to determine the resources and supports available to families and the needs or concerns that families might have. In the research tradition, family assessment is designed to gather information in order to make general statements about family functioning and development; in the clinical tradition, family assessment is designed to identify overt or underlying problems. In the support tradition, however, the goal of family assessment is to gather information needed to determine family priorities for goals and services, as well as resources available to meet those priorities (Bailey, 1991). The relationship between parent and professional is fundamentally different from the relationship between therapist and patient. In the clinical tradition, families approach therapists because of specific problems in family functioning. In the support tradition, in the context of early intervention, families interact with professionals because they have a child with a disability. Although families desire assistance in both cases, the support tradition makes no assumptions about the nature of the problem residing within the family or the task of the interventionist being to "fix" families. Rather, the role of the professional is to serve as a resource and support for families, working with families to help them achieve goals they have for themselves and their children. Thus assessment activities are driven by the need to develop a greater understanding of individual family circumstances and perspectives.

In summary, it is evident that the research, clinical, and support traditions differ with respect to the functions and goals of family assessment, the assessment strategies used, and the nature of the relationship between professionals and family members. Recognizing that early intervention has its roots in the family support tradition is an important step in developing an effective and appropriate approach to family assessment. Because the nature of the relationship between family and professional differs fundamentally across the three traditions, the assessment strategies developed and used in the research or clinical traditions may not be applicable within the context of early intervention.

CONSIDERATIONS IN DEVELOPING
A FAMILY ASSESSMENT MODEL

Given this framework, what factors should be considered in constructing an approach to family assessment that is consistent with the goals and traditions of early intervention? Among the many variables likely to be important, we discuss four. We assume that effective family assessment (1) recognizes the importance of individual perceptions of events and the likelihood that different individuals will have different perspectives; (2) is an ongoing process taking many forms; (3) requires reflective thinking centered around an inquiry-oriented approach; and (4) may function as an intervention, with potentially negative and positive implications.

Individual Perspectives

If all individuals or families viewed life in the same way, there would be no need for family assessment strategies. Professionals could simply learn general or specific truths about families and provide a single set of services that would meet the needs of all. Fortunately, we all have different beliefs, values, styles, and skills. Although this variability makes life much richer and more interesting, it creates special challenges for early intervention professionals. Because we cannot make assumptions about family needs or priorities, some form of assessment (information gathering) is needed.

Research by McCubbin and Patterson (1983) led to the development of a theoretical model that demonstrates the importance of perception or appraisal of an event. They argued that any event could take on positive or negative attributes depending upon one's perspective. Furthermore, how one defines a stressful event is likely to have a direct bearing on how successfully one copes with that event. Consider, for example, two families whose daughters, both of whom have spina bifida and cannot walk, attend a mainstreamed child care program. Both families observe an outdoor play scene in which their child at one minute is surrounded by playmates and the next minute is left alone as the other children run off to another section of the playground. The parents of one child question the wisdom of placing their daughter in a situation in which circumstances serve as constant reminders of her disability, and subsequently decide to keep her at home. The parents of the other child say they are truly glad their daughter is experiencing these situations as a youngster in a supervised environment so that she will learn how to cope with them. Both families saw the same event, but interpreted it from different perspectives and drew different conclusions about the desirability of a placement option.

Aponte (1985) suggests that individual assessment is essential because every family has a different set of values that must be taken into account if intervention is to be at all successful:

> A therapist can understand an individual and his family only in the value framework of their ecostructural context. This means understanding *what* they are doing (function) and *how* (structure) in reference to the values that are guiding them, which, for example, include their cultural standards. (p. 328)

Bernheimer, Gallimore, and Weisner (1990) make a similar point in describing the concept of ecocultural niche, the assumption that every family develops a definition of its place and function, a definition that fits their culture and circumstances. They argue that this niche can only be understood if professionals assess both the objective components of the family's ecology and how the family members actually perceive those components.

The stories told by families of children with disabilities often carry a consistent theme of frustration with professionals who have not listened or given credence to the family's point of view. We argue that the fundamental intent of family assessment is to ascertain that point of view. Thus family assessment comes to be defined as the process by which the early intervention professional actively seeks to understand the family's perceptions of their resources, priorities, and concerns within the context of the family's value system.

An Ongoing Process Taking Many Forms

Given the goals and definitions of family directed assessment, how does the early intervention professional go about providing family assessments? A variety of strategies are available, ranging from structured to unstructured, written to verbal, and brief to extensive. However, at the outset we maintain that every interaction a professional has with a family or family member constitutes an assessment. This is so because it is likely that any interaction, whether a phone call, a home visit, arrival at a child care center, or a handwritten note, contains important information that, if attended to, would provide the professional with greater insight into family resources, priorities, or concerns. Some research suggests that parents actually prefer these informal, naturally occurring contexts as the mechanism by which information is shared (Summers et al., 1990; Winton & Turnbull, 1981). Thus the first guideline for conducting family assessments is to take the opportunity to learn from every interaction with families.

In the context of interacting with families, professionals have several strategies available to them for providing a structure or framework for gathering information. Three such strategies are person-to-person communication, paper and pencil measures, and direct observation procedures.

Person-to-Person Communication

The most frequently used and probably most useful general family assessment strategy is the process of communicating directly with one or more family members. These interactions, which can be informal (e.g., arrival and departure times) or formal (e.g., structured interviews), provide repeated opportunities for gathering information about family resources, priorities, and concerns. Although they provide the context in which critical information is likely to be obtained, it is clear that not all professionals have the skills needed to make optimal use of these opportunities (Winton & Bailey, 1990). Two key skills are those of effective listening and effective questioning.

Effective listening requires that the professional attend to the verbal and nonverbal statements made by family members, reflect on them, and try to understand the messages and feelings that underlie those statements (Winton,

1988). Effective listening is an active process in which the listener lets the communicator know that the message has been heard, acknowledged, and accepted as valid. One way to do this is by reflecting back to the speaker the feelings or content that you perceive to underlie the statements made. This lets the speaker know that you have been listening and provides an opportunity to verify, correct, or expand the message.

Effective questioning requires that the professional ask questions that are not threatening to the family member, that show a genuine interest and concern (rather than collecting information for legal or programmatic purposes), and that promote rather than inhibit the conversation. Reviews of the literature on question asking suggest three broad recommendations (Tomm, 1987; Winton, 1988; Winton & Bailey, 1993). First, ask questions that are open-ended (e.g., "What are bedtimes like at your house?") rather than closed-ended (e.g., "Does Alecia have a regular bedtime?"). Open-ended questions open the door to a variety of answers and allow the family member to communicate aspects of the experience that are most important to them. Second, do not ask questions that may appear to be investigative and judgemental in nature (e.g., "Why didn't you do Kyle's therapy activities this week?"). Such questions may put a family member on the defensive and reduce the likelihood of meaningful exchange. A more effective strategy would be to reflect on the family's circumstances (e.g., "Sounds like you had a pretty busy week.") and ask questions that help you understand the reasons why therapy was not possible for this family at this time (e.g., "How do you manage to get all the things done that you do with all of this going on?"). Third, refrain from making too many suggestions in the context of questioning (e.g., "Why don't you hire a babysitter so that you can get Kyle's therapy done?"). This approach puts the professional in the position of solving the problem rather than the family member and often may constitute suggestions that are unreasonable or inconsistent with family priorities. A more effective strategy may be to ask questions that encourage the family member to think of options themselves (e.g., "Can you think of any ways that you can get in his therapy and meet all your other responsibilities as well?").

Paper and Pencil Measures

A second category of assessment strategies is the use of paper and pencil measures completed by one or more family members. The content and format of these measures varies widely, as does the usefulness of the information gathered. In the context of early intervention, probably the most frequently used versions of paper and pencil measures are surveys of family needs, resources, or concerns. Examples include the Family Needs Scale (Dunst, Cooper, Weeldreyer, Snyder, & Chase, 1988), the Parent Needs Survey (Seligman & Darling, 1989), How Can We Help (Child Development Resources, 1989), and the Family Needs Survey (Bailey & Simeonsson, 1988). All of these surveys include a list of items (e.g., "I would like more information about my child's disability"; "We have a strong network of supportive friends and extended family members") that the family member rates as to the extent the item is applicable to their family situation. This provides important information about the family that could then be used as the context for further discussions and perhaps the establishment of certain goals or the provision of specialized services.

Professionals considering the use of needs surveys, however, should be aware of several recent research findings (Bailey & Blasco, 1990; Bailey & Simeonsson, 1988; Bailey et al., 1988). First, although most families appreciate the opportunity to share information such as that contained on the surveys described, they strongly prefer it being presented as a choice rather than a program requirement. Second, the wording of items is particularly important. Families do not like items that appear judgmental, of a personal nature, or that seem to be an admission of weakness or lack of competence. Third, open-ended formats are essential if adequate information is to be gathered. This should take the form of open-ended questions on the survey itself as well as follow-up discussions with family members. Fourth, some family members prefer sharing information in a written format, whereas others prefer a conversational format. Providing choices such as these can help build a more trusting and collaborative relationship with families. Finally, families have expressed considerable concern about being asked questions for which there has been no follow-up. The message behind these concerns is that family members are willing to share information if they feel it will help them or their child receive more appropriate services. They strongly resent, however, being asked an array of questions about family life for no apparent purpose.

Direct Observation

A final broad category of assessment procedures involves the use of direct observational measures. Typically, direct observation in early intervention takes place through the use of various measures of parent–child interaction (Comfort, 1988). The purpose of these measures, which can take the form of rating scales or behavior counts, is to document the amount, quality, or appropriateness of the parent's behavior with the child. Another commonly used procedure is documentation of the home environment, which could include the physical structure and social dimensions of home life that can influence parent–child interactions and development.

Direct observation provides extremely useful information that usually cannot be obtained through discussions or paper and pencil measures. However, professionals should recognize that many such procedures may be threatening to family members, in part because they may feel that they are being evaluated by an outsider or that their behavior will be compared with that of a norm group to determine whether or not they are "good parents." This possibility suggests that direct observation is best used after professionals have gotten to know a family and in response to concerns expressed directly by family members. For example, a parent–child interaction measure might be used as a way to help respond to a parent who expresses frustration in not being able to teach her child effectively.

Reflective Thinking and Inquiry

A recognition of the individuality of each family's perspectives and a knowledge of strategies for assessing families is critical to the work of early intervention professionals. How does one use this information, however, in developing a broader framework for family assessment? Selvini, Boscolo, Cecchin, and Prata (1980) argued that the successful family therapist creates a set of questions about a family, develops hypotheses regarding the answers to those questions, engages in active information gathering to confirm or disconfirm those hypotheses, and maintains an open and nonjudgmental stance in the attempt to seek answers. Likewise, in the educational literature, the importance of reflective teaching has been emphasized. Effective teachers are those who continually ask questions about student performance, reflect on performance with respect to the activities provided, and modify instruction to teach children in a more effective fashion.

Although family assessment instruments exist, it is not likely that early intervention professionals will be engaged in frequent and formal family assessment activities in the same way that child performance is regularly documented to plan intervention programs. Thus professionals are left with the task of constructing their own assessment strategies that are informal, yet systematic and ongoing. Reflective questioning may be defined as the process of continually asking a set of basic questions about a particular family, seeking to gather information with respect to those questions, reflecting on the information that is available, generating hypotheses about that information vis-à-vis the questions posed, and attempting to validate potential hypotheses. Through such a process, professionals are likely to learn considerably more about a family in ways that are more likely to be functional for both the professional and the family members.

Family Assessment as Family Intervention

A final general point that must be made about family assessment is that the assessment process itself is likely to serve as an intervention. Tomm (1987) describes a family therapy session in which it became clear that the questions he asked the family, simply for the purpose of information gathering, had a direct influence on their behavior. This discovery let him to conclude the following:

> It is impossible for a therapist to interact with a client without intervening in the client's autonomous activity. The therapist assumes that everything she or he says and does is potentially significant with respect to the eventual therapeutic outcome. For instance, every question and every comment may be evaluated with respect to whether it constitutes an affirmation or a challenge to one or more behavior patterns of the client or family. . . . Within this perspective, no statement or nonverbal behavior is assumed, a priori, to be inconsequential. Nor is the absence of certain actions considered trivial. By not responding to particular events the therapist may knowingly or unknowingly disappoint or fulfill certain expectations of one or more family members. . . . *Thus interventive interviewing refers to an orientation in which everything an interviewer does and says, and does not do and does not say, is thought of as an intervention that could be therapeutic, nontherapeutic, or countertherapeutic.* (p. 4, italics in original)

Although early intervention professionals are not engaged in family therapy, they may play similar roles for families, especially with respect to their perceived knowledge about disabilities and their role as advisors about intervention services. At the least, actions by early intervention professionals communicate messages to families about their competence, the accuracy or veracity of their statements, and their status vis-à-vis professionals in the context of decision making. For example, conducting an observation of parent–child interactions may send a message that the professional is concerned about the mother's ability to parent. In general, the assessment process communicates the message that the one conducting the assessment is in a better position than the one being assessed to make judgments about the proper course of action.

Assessments can also have a direct influence on behavior. For example, asking both parents to complete a survey of family needs could result in a conflict between mother and father over family priorities, a conflict that might not have emerged without the assessment. On the other hand, completing a survey may help a parent begin to think about needs and services that he or she had not previously recognized or considered.

The point of this discussion is that family assessments are rarely neutral events. They often bear emotional consequences for families and certainly communicate messages to families. As Tomm (1987) suggests, however, the actual effect of the assessment is always determined by the family, not by the professional. The key is recognizing the potential for the assessment itself to fundamentally influence a family or to alter the relationship between family members and early intervention professionals.

DOMAINS FOR FAMILY ASSESSMENT

Given the above considerations, what are the appropriate domains for family-directed assessment in early intervention? In many respects this is a difficult question to answer. Although we can readily agree on the basic domains for child assessment (e.g., cognitive, communication, adaptive, social, motor), core family-related domains are not so apparent. Any number of domains could be identified from the literature, such as parent–child interaction, family needs, support systems and resources, stages of grief, coping and adaptation, critical events, or locus of control. Consistent with our earlier discussion about reflective thinking and inquiry, however, we argue that the legitimate questions that may be asked in the context of family assessment are those that, if answered, would help the professional provide services that are consistent with each family's values, priorities, and resources. In order to illustrate the implications of such an approach, we describe three questions likely to be of importance to every professional who interacts with a child or family: (1) How does this family want to participate in decision making and service provision? (2) What does this family want from the service system? and (3) How do family members perceive the child with a disability? We suggest that these questions be combined with other important questions (e.g., How do these parents feel about their competence as parents? How does this family perceive the supports that are available to them? Is this family experiencing or about to experience a particularly stressful event?) to form the basic content of family assessment processes.

How Does This Family Want to Participate in Decision Making and Service Provision?

One fundamental tenet of Public Law 99-457 and of the family-centered movement in early intervention is an explicit acknowledgment of the rights and responsibilities of parents to serve as primary decision makers with respect to the services provided for them and their child. Also, it has been argued that supporting parents in making choices about their children can enable and empower families in ways that could not be achieved if professionals made all of the decisions (Dunst, Trivette, & Deal, 1988). It would be erroneous, however, to assume that every family wants to be fully involved in every aspect of this process. Thus, one of the first questions of importance in the context of family assessment is the extent to which family members want to participate in the process of making decisions, coordinating services, and providing interventions. As Simeonsson and Bailey (1990) suggest, families may vary considerably in their choices regarding these roles. Some will elect not to be involved at all, some will elect to participate in selected roles, and others will want to be fully involved in every facet of early intervention. Because this information is unlikely to be known initially to early interventionists, strategies for assessing preferences and responding accordingly are needed.

The roles that families can play in decision making and service delivery are many. For example, Bailey, McWilliam, Winton, and Simeonsson (1992) describe a range of roles that parents could fulfill in the child assessment process; these include receiving information from professionals, observing professional assessments, informing professionals about their child's behavior and development, interpreting their child's behavior, or conducting the actual child assessments. In the context of team meetings, parents may choose to listen quietly to what professionals have to say, to participate as active and equal team members, or to lead the team meeting. With respect to service coordination, some parents may prefer to have a professional take responsibility for identifying, accessing, and coordinating services, whereas others may elect to coordinate services themselves. Finally, in terms of service provision, some families may want to provide extensive educational and therapeutic activities for their child at home, whereas others will prefer that professionals fill those roles.

Explicit acknowledgment of the decision-making roles of parents bears several important implications for professionals and families. From the professional's perspective, it means giving up some of the power or authority traditionally reserved for those with specialized expertise. This change does not diminish the professional's role or level of responsibility. In actuality, the professional's job now requires more competence and flexibility in order to accommodate roles as both facilitator and consultant. This shift in roles calls for a more diversified base of expertise and experience in that the professional is still expected to share knowledge and opinions, as well as recommend assessment and intervention plans. The main difference is that families are now full partners throughout the process and are recognized as the final decision makers.

From the parents' perspective, the movement toward family-centered services may inadvertently result in some families feeling guilty if they choose not to participate as actively as professionals may like. With the push toward more family-centered assessment and intervention, the deliberate choice for a more passive parental role may be mistaken by professionals as noncompliance or neglect for their child's development. This situation suggests that professionals need to be especially careful in maintaining a balance between providing choices and providing leadership. Offering parents the choice to be involved or uninvolved in decision making and service provision is the first step in acknowledging the value and worth of families. Respecting their decisions in these areas provides concrete evidence that the professional is committed to a meaningful partnership with families. Thus the first "family assessment" domain can serve not only as an important information-gathering framework, but also as an intervention in that it may enable some families to strengthen their views of themselves.

What Does This Family Want from the Service System?

Given that families want to be involved in some aspect of the decision-making process and desire some form of early intervention services, the next step in the context of family assessment is determining their specific goals and their preferences for the role the service system will play in helping them achieve their goals. Asking this question assumes, of course, that the early intervention program is willing to provide an individualized program of services in accordance with family needs, priorities, and concerns. Services likely to emerge in this process include direct interventions or therapy for children, provisions for satisfying informational needs, family support services, respite care, parent training, service coordination, assistance with finances, or community support services.

The research literature provides some basis for professional awareness of the preferences typically expressed by parents in early intervention programs. For example, Summers et al. (1990) questioned focus groups of professionals and families about their preferences for early intervention services, including what outcomes they might expect from each type of service. Four areas emerged as high-priority needs: meeting the informational needs of the family, promoting the well-being of the family unit and individual family members, enhancing the parent–child relationship, and enhancing the parent–professional relationship. In a study of more than 400 parents of young children with disabilities, Bailey, Blasco, and Simeonsson (1992) found the need for information to be the most consistently expressed need.

Studies such as these provide helpful insights about the kinds of services that families may be expected to request, if asked. In reality, however, each family constitutes a unique set of resources, priorities, and concerns. Bailey, Blasco, and Simeonsson (1992), for example, found that the expression of needs generally could not be predicted on the basis of birth order, age, race, socioeconomic status, or the child's disability type. The only reliable finding was that mothers expressed more needs than fathers, especially in areas related to family and social support, explaining their child's condition to others, and child care. These results reinforce the individuality of each family and provide evidence for the importance of ascertaining each family's desires for services so that services can be matched to perceived needs.

In addition to respecting family preferences for services, there are other reasons to determine the match between services and the family's perceived needs. For one, because resources are scarce, it is critical that professional time and agency resources are maximized. A second reason for matching services to needs derives from the consumer-based nature of early intervention; because it is not mandated that parents participate in early intervention, responsive and individualized services will likely be more acceptable and more heavily used than a single "take it or leave it" program. A final reason for matching services to perceived needs is suggested in research by Affleck, Tennen, Rowe, Roscher, and Walker (1989). This study examined the effects of a weekly home visit program provided for parents of children who had been in the neonatal intensive care unit. An evaluation of the program found that the intervention was beneficial for parents who, prior to discharge from the hospital, indicated a need for such support. However, for the parents who indicated that they did not need the help, but got it anyway, the program appeared to have a negative effect. At the end of the 15-week program, those mothers felt less competent, had a lowered sense of control, and were less responsive to their infants than they were before the program started. This study suggests that failure to individualize services may have negative ramifications, even when the program provided is well-intentioned and well-designed.

In the phase of family assessment involving decisions about resource allocation, the professional's primary responsibility is to assist families in identifying desired outcomes and services likely to achieve those outcomes. This information can be obtained through informal discussions with families or through the use of surveys or checklists that describe frequently mentioned needs or services. A combination of approaches is likely to be best, with options provided for how parents want to share this information. One dilemma frequently faced by professionals in this context is how much to offer with respect to services. On the one hand, we want to be open and responsive to any needs the family might express, yet we all know that resources are limited and that some needs could never be addressed through the early intervention network.

The use of open-ended approaches to information gathering makes it especially likely that a wide range of needs will be expressed. Therefore, it is important that families realize that the service system exists to provide *support* for families as they seek to meet their own needs. Sometimes this support is provided through direct service provision and in other cases through referral to other service systems. An equally important goal of the assessment process, however, is providing support for families as they seek to identify solutions to needs or problems themselves. Once again we see the family assessment process having the potential to serve as an intervention. Through inquiring about resources, priorities, needs, and concerns, professionals may open the door for more extended discussions with some families. In many cases the assessment process will simply involve listening, responding in a sensitive fashion, and helping families generate and evaluate alternative solutions. Although interactions among parents and professionals provide the context for discussing options, the "service" may actually turn out to be something that the parents seek or do themselves.

How Do Family Members Perceive the Child with a Disability?

A third question described in this chapter regards the family's perception of the child with a disability. Historically, this question has been aimed at the parents' knowledge about their child's ability or the extent to which parents have "accepted" their child's disability. However, other dimensions of perception are likely to be important as well. For example, how do the parents and siblings view the child in the context of full family membership? How do parents perceive their child's personality? What existential interpretations or meanings have families used to explain why they have a child with a disability? Weisner, Beizer, and Stolze (1991), for example, found that religious parents described the purpose of their children in ways that conveyed strong emotions and substantial meaning. A large proportion of religious families used their religious beliefs to explain why they had a child with a disability. Asking questions about family perceptions of their child (yet taking care not to offer explanations or imply that families should have thought this topic through) demonstrates to families that professionals are interested in the significance of their child in the context of their family rather than their child's attainments in reference to a set of external standards or norms. Answers to questions such as these will help professionals understand how families have come to construct a view of their child that is meaningful for them in the context of their culture, values, beliefs, and life experiences.

When we usually talk about parental perceptions of the young child with a disability, particularly from an assessment perspective, we tend to think of parental estimates of specific skill achievement and global cognitive competence. Much research has been done in this area, especially comparing parental estimates of development either to the child's actual performance on standardized test items or to professional estimates of the child's developmental abilities (Beckman, 1984; Blacher-Dixon & Simeonsson, 1981; Gradel, Thompson, & Sheehan, 1981; Handen, Feldman, & Honigman, 1987; Schafer, Bell, & Spalding, 1987; Sexton, Hall, & Thomas, 1984; Sexton, Kelley, & Scott, 1982; Sexton, Miller, & Murdock, 1984; Totta & Crase, 1982). And, although some studies have found evidence of parental, usually maternal, overestimation, others have not. Although the former finding has been discussed in terms of parental overestimation and/or professional underestimation (Gradel et al., 1981), we need to question the true value of such studies before fully reorganizing the structure of child and family assessment based on these and other interpretations. Given certain limitations of standardized testing (sterile environment, unfamiliar adult, limited number of test items) and the advantage of parental observations (viewing the child in a variety of situations over an extended period of time), does it even make sense to compare the two types of assessments? Ultimately, we must recognize that both parents and professionals have legitimate views of the child's abilities. So, rather than trying to achieve congruence in ratings of behavior, professionals may want to use disagreements as opportunities for learning about how parents view their child and how they interpret their child's abilities in the context of the environment in which the child and family live. Any assessment of the child's development must include assessing that child's needs within the context of the entire family's needs and current level of functioning.

A related topic is the extent to which professionals perceive parents to be "accepting" or "denying" their child's disability. This preoccupation with parent denial is, in our view, not likely to lead to productive interactions between families and service providers. What goals are achieved by having a parent accept the fact that their child has a disability of some magnitude? Many parents have expressed frustration of this goal and have interpreted it as a pessimistic view of their child's potential. In reality, what is perceived as denial by professionals may very well be an effective coping strategy for families (Winton, 1988).

Huntington (1988) describes three child characteristics that have an impact on the family's perceptions of the child, including the child's temperament, readability, and behavior. Parental perceptions of the child's temperament, whether the child has an easy or difficult behavioral style, have been linked with overall family functioning, particularly the relationship between the parent and child (Sprunger, Boyce, & Gaines, 1985). These perceptions of temperament are likely to be influenced by the child's readability, or how easy or difficult it is for the parents to identify and meet the child's needs. A child who clearly and consistently communicates his or her needs is easier to console than a child who does not or cannot communicate needs as distinctly. This latter child is likely to incite feelings of frustration and incompetence in the parents who try unsuccessfully to comfort their child. Specific child behaviors also play a large part in regulating family stress in that certain aspects of children's behaviors may have more impact than others. Beckman (1982) found that families of children who require more caregiving attention and families with children who fail to display behaviors that fit in with society's expectations tend to experience higher levels of parental stress.

This does not mean that every child exhibiting behaviors associated with higher levels of parental stress or more negative outcomes for family functioning will actually have a negative impact on his or her family unit. Some studies suggest that the child's and family's characteristics interact through the family's coping skills, their capacity to meet the child's needs, and their expectations for the child with a disability, to determine whether an adaptive and positive relationship will exist to promote the healthy development of the family unit (Chess & Thomas, 1986; Nihira, Meyers, & Mink, 1983).

The extent to which the family adapts to the child's disability will determine how well the family continues to function as a unit promoting family and child well-being. Adaptability and cohesion, or the extent to which families are committed to each other yet manage to maintain their individual roles and responsibilities, are two characteristics of a family that will affect family goals and the outcomes for intervention (Turnbull & Turnbull, 1986). The professional must determine where the family is operating in terms of adaptability and cohesion in order to determine realistic expectations for successful family participation. Only then can goals and strategies be mutually agreed upon that will provide a transition from everyday life that is more amenable to that family's style.

The family's perceptions of the child with a disability are not only affected by family characteristics such as cohesion and adaptability, but also by the family's cultural style and socioeconomic status, both of which can affect levels of cohesion and adaptability. Recognizing and respecting family values, which may or may not be founded in the family's cultural heritage, is a crucial yet often difficult responsibility for the early interventionist. Because our own values tend to govern our perceptions of the way we believe things should be done, we must make a conscious effort to consider the family's preferences for handling situations.

Families from diverse ethnic backgrounds may view the child with a disability differently, including the cause of the disability and proposed treatment or intervention plans (Hanson, Lynch, & Wayman, 1990). The early interventionist must realize that intervention efforts may not be interpreted as beneficial by all family members. For example, an attempt at family assessment may seem intrusive and impractical to families who value their privacy or see the responsibility of the child's early development belonging solely within the child's family unit. Although some ethnic groups may be characterized by certain values and behaviors (e.g., Italian-Americans as close-knit families who are supportive of each other yet reluctant to let others in their family circle), we cannot generalize to other families with similar ethnic backgrounds. Because each family is unique, stereotyping is not the answer to dealing effectively with families. However, recognizing that cultural influences exist and can play a large part in what a family values and practices is a step in the right direction.

In addition to the family's ethnic background, cultural style may also refer to other aspects of the family, such as socioeconomic status. Several studies have investigated the association between socioeconomic status and the family's reactions to the birth of a child with disabilities (Dunlap & Hollingsworth, 1977; Farber, 1960). These studies uncovered an interesting trend in that middle-class families seemed more concerned with the child's future, including anticipated emotional demands, whereas lower socioeconomic families expressed more concern with the immediate financial constraints and excessive caregiving demands.

In all aspects of family assessment, the professional must recognize and respect the family's values and associate these with the family's preferences for intervention plans. If goals and values do not match, intervention services will not be successful. This is difficult for professionals to do because families may agree with and seem in favor of identified goals, yet also may be passively noncompliant. If a conflict exists between established goals and values, intervention efforts may never have a chance.

Professionals must focus on getting to know families and obtaining information from all family members, including parents, siblings, and extended family members. The early interventionist must discover who is influential in decision making and include this person or these people in order to promote the success of the program. Some professionals may question how to do this without offending parents or seemingly doubting their control over their child. However, if the early interventionist provides the family with the necessary information and options, then the family can determine priorities for assessment procedures and services, make knowledgeable choices for intervention plans, and follow through on their roles and responsibilities with the assistance and support of the early interventionist.

EVALUATING THE USEFULNESS
OF FAMILY ASSESSMENTS

How does one evaluate the ultimate usefulness of family assessments? This question is important for families, professionals, and researchers alike because it is a process in which early interventionists will likely make considerable investment over the next few years. It is also important because of the potential pitfalls associated with the process. Although the family assessment movement is well-intentioned and has the potential for creating more positive and productive relationships between families and professionals, it also bears the possibility of creating negative or adversarial relationships, especially if families view the process as intrusive. Slentz and Bricker (1992) frame this problem in the context of possible messages that we may be sending families if we approach them with a battery of family assessment tools:

> First, we may lead families to assume that early intervention services will include efforts to impact general family functioning, when in fact many

community-based services do not and cannot. . . . Second, some parents may assume that the early interventionist plans to address the needs of all family members in all the areas assessed. . . . Third, and most seriously, the process of family assessment can carry the hidden message that because a child has special needs, the family must have problems. . . . Finally, early interventionists who attempt to conduct comprehensive family assessments assume the expertise of other professionals and may unwittingly contribute to difficulties in interagency and interdisciplinary coordination. (pp. 14–15)

Our own experiences with parents and professionals validate these concerns and point to the importance of continuing research regarding the usefulness and appropriateness of various family assessment strategies.

A variety of strategies should be used to evaluate the usefulness of family assessment procedures. McGrew, Gilman, and Johnson (1992), for example, reviewed 15 scales developed or suggested for use in assessing family needs in the context of early intervention. The instruments were evaluated in terms of administration format, content validity, and psychometric characteristics. The authors concluded that the measures generally were limited in scope, lacked reliability data, and offered little evidence for the validity of their content. They suggested caution in using the scales for psychometric purposes such as evaluating program effectiveness or assessing change in individual families.

Such reviews are helpful and provide important information about the usefulness of various instruments. Henderson, Aydlett, and Bailey (in press), however, suggest that two fundamental questions should be asked of all family assessment procedures. First, does the instrument or procedure provide information that is helpful for families in identifying and communicating their resources, priorities, and concerns? Second, is the instrument or procedure one that is acceptable to the family members with whom it is used? Although psychometric information about measures is useful, it is safe to conclude that if an instrument does not provide useful information and is not acceptable to families, then any other evaluation of that measure is not likely to contribute substantially to our understanding of its relevance in early intervention.

This statement draws us back to our initial point in this chapter. Family-directed assessment in the context of early intervention evolves out of the support tradition and thus should be evaluated from that perspective. The ultimate goal of family assessment is to facilitate the process by which professionals provide support for families of young children with disabilities. It is within this supportive relationship that families are encouraged to build upon and maintain their independence, therefore promoting the healthy development of the family unit, including the child with a disability.

REFERENCES

Affleck, G., Tennen, H., Rowe, J., Roscher, B., & Walker, L. (1989). Effects of formal support on mothers' adaptation to the hospital-to-home transition of high-risk infants: The benefits and costs of helping. *Child Development, 60,* 488–501.

Aponte, H. J. (1985). The negotiation of values in therapy. *Family Process, 24,* 323–338.

Bailey, D. B. (1991). Issues and perspectives on family assessment. *Infants and Young Children, 4*(1), 26–34.

Bailey, D. B., & Blasco, P. M. (1990). Parents' perspectives on a written survey of family needs. *Journal of Early Intervention, 14,* 196–203.

Bailey, D. B., Blasco, P. M., & Simeonsson, R. J. (1992). Needs expressed by mothers and fathers of young children with disabilities. *American Journal on Mental Retardation, 97,* 1–10.

Bailey, D. B., McWilliam, P. J., Winton, P. J., & Simeonsson, R. J. (1992). *Implementing family-centered services in early intervention: A team-based model for change.* Cambridge, MA: Brookline Books.

Bailey, D. B., & Simeonsson, R. J. (1988). Assessing needs of families with handicapped infants. *Journal of Special Education, 22,* 117–127.

Bailey, D. B., Simeonsson, R. J., Isbell, P., Huntington, G. S., Winton, P. J., Comfort, M., & Helm, J. (1988). Inservice training in family assessment and goal-setting for early interventionists: Outcomes and issues. *Journal of the Division for Early Childhood, 12,* 126–136.

Bailey, D. B., Simeonsson, R. J., Winton, P. J., Huntington, G. S., Comfort, M., Isbell, P., O'Donnell, K. J., & Helm, J. M. (1986). Family-focused intervention: A functional model for planning, implementing, and evaluating individualized family services in early intervention. *Journal of the Division for Early Childhood, 10,* 156–171.

Beavers, W. R., & Voeller, M. N. (1983). Family models: Comparing and contrasting the Olson model with the Beavers systems model. *Family Process, 22,* 85–98.

Beckman, P. J. (1982). Influence of selected child characteristics on stress in families of handicapped infants. *American Journal of Mental Deficiency, 88,* 150–156.

Beckman, P. J. (1984). Perceptions of young children with handicaps: A comparison of mothers and program staff. *Mental Retardation, 22,* 176–181.

Bentovim, A. (1986). Family therapy when the child is the referred patient. In S. Block (Ed.), *An introduction to the psychotherapies* (pp. 198–221). Oxford: Oxford University Press.

Bernheimer, L. P., Gallimore, R., & Weisner, T. S. (1990). Ecocultural theory as a context for the Individual Family Service Plan. *Journal of Early Intervention, 14,* 219–233.

Blacher-Dixon, J., & Simeonsson, R. J. (1981). Consistency and correspondence of mothers' and teachers' assessments of young handicapped children. *Journal of the Division for Early Childhood, 3,* 64–71.

Campbell, D., & Draper, R. (1985). *Applications of systematic family therapy.* London: Grune & Stratton.

Chess, S., & Thomas, A. (1986). *Temperament in clinical practice.* New York: Guilford Press.

Child Development Resources. (1989). How can we help? In B. H. Johnson, M. J. McGonigel, & R. K. Kaufmann (Eds.), *Guidelines and recommended practices for the Individualized Family Service Plan* (pp. D9–D11). Washington, DC: Association for the Care of Children's Health.

Combrinck-Graham, L. (1985). A developmental model for family systems. *Family Process, 24,* 139–150.

Comfort, M. (1988). Assessing parent–child interaction. In D. Bailey & R. Simeonsson (Eds.), *Family assessment in early intervention* (pp. 65–94). Columbus, OH: Merrill.

Cowan, P. A. (1987). The need for theoretical and methodological integrations in family research. *Journal of Family Psychology, 1*(1), 48–50.

Dunlap, W. R., & Hollingsworth, J. S. (1977). How does a handicapped child affect the family? Implications for practitioners. *Family Coordinator, 26*(3), 286–293.

Dunst, C. J. (1985). Rethinking early intervention. *Analysis and Intervention in Developmental Disabilities, 5,* 165–201.

Dunst, C. J., Cooper, C. S., Weeldreyer, J. C., Snyder, K. D., & Chase, J. H. (1988). Family needs scale. In C. J. Dunst, C. M. Trivette, & A. G. Deal, *Enabling and empowering families: Principles and guidelines for practice.* Cambridge, MA: Brookline Books.

Dunst, C. J., Trivette, C. M., & Deal, A. G. (1988). *Enabling and empowering families: Principles and guidelines for practice.* Cambridge, MA: Brookline Books.

Farber, B. (1960). Family organization and crisis: Maintenance of the integration in families with a severely retarded child. *Monographs of the Society for Research in Child Development, 25*(1).

Gradel, K., Thompson, M. S., & Sheehan, R. (1981). Parental and professional agreement in early childhood assessment. *Topics in Early Childhood Special Education, 1,* 31–39.

Grotevant, H. D., & Carlson, C. I. (1989). *Family assessment: A guide to methods and measures.* New York: Guilford Press.

Handen, B. L., Feldman, R. S., & Honigman, A. (1987). Comparison of parent and teacher assessments of developmentally delayed children's behavior. *Exceptional Children, 54,* 137–144.

Hanson, M. J., & Lynch, E. W. (1992). Family diversity: Implications for policy and practice. *Topics in Early Childhood Special Education, 12*(3), 283–306.

Hanson, M. J., Lynch, E. W., & Wayman, K. F. (1990). Honoring the cultural diversity of families when gathering data. *Topics in Early Childhood Special Education, 10,* 112–131.

Henderson, L. W., Aydlett, L. A., & Bailey, D. B. (in press). Evaluating family needs surveys: Do classical methods tell us what we want to know? *Journal of Psychoeducational Assessment.*

Huntington, G. S. (1988). Assessing child characteristics that influence family functioning. In D. B. Bailey & R. J. Simeonsson (Eds.), *Family assessment in early intervention* (pp. 45–64). Columbus, OH: Merrill.

LaRossa, R., & Wolf, J. H. (1985). On qualitative family research. *Journal of Marriage and the Family, 47,* 531–541.

Massey, R. F. (1986). What/who is the family system? *American Journal of Family Therapy, 14*(1), 23–39.

McCubbin, H. I., & Patterson, J. M. (1983). Family transitions: Adaptation to stress. In H. McCubbin & C. Figley (Eds.), *Stress and the family: Vol. 1. Coping with normative transitions* (pp. 5–25). New York: Brunner/Mazel.

McCubbin, H. I., & Thompson, A. I. (1987). Family typologies and family assessment. In H. I. McCubbin & A. I. Thompson (Eds.), *Family assessment inventories for research and practice* (pp. 35–62). Madison, WI: University of Wisconsin.

McCubbin, M. A., & McCubbin, H. I. (1987). The T-Double ABCX model of family adjustment and adaptation. In H. I. McCubbin & A. I. Thompson (Eds.), *Family assessment inventories for research and practice* (pp. 3–32). Madison, WI: University of Wisconsin.

McGrew, K. S., Gilman, C. J., & Johnson, S. (1992). A review of scales to assess family needs. *Journal of Psychoeducational Assessment, 10,* 4–25.

Nihira, K., Meyers, C. E., & Mink, I. (1983). Reciprocal relationships between home environment and development of TMR adolescents. *American Journal of Mental Deficiency, 88,* 139–149.

Schafer, P. S., Bell, A. P., & Spalding, J. B. (1987). Parental versus professional assessment of developmentally delayed children after periods of parent training. *Journal of the Division for Early Childhood, 12,* 47–55.

Seligman, M., & Darling, R. (1989). *Ordinary families, special children: A systems approach to childhood disability.* New York: Guilford Press.

Selvini, M. P., Boscolo, L., Cecchin, G., & Prata, G. (1980). Hypothesizing–circularity–neutrality: Three guidelines for the conductor of the session. *Family Process, 19,* 3–12.

Sexton, D., Hall, J., & Thomas, P. J. (1984). Multisource assessment of young handicapped children: A comparison. *Exceptional Children, 50,* 556–558.

Sexton, D., Kelley, M. F., & Scott, R. (1982). Comparison of maternal estimates and performance-based assessment scores for young handicapped children. *Diagnostique, 7,* 168–173.

Sexton, D., Miller, J. H., & Murdock, J. Y. (1984). Correlates of parental–professional congruency scores in the assessment of young handicapped children. *Journal of the Division for Early Childhood, 8,* 99–106.

Shelton, T. L., Jeppson, E. S., & Johnson, B. H. (1987). *Family-centered care for children with special health care needs.* Washington, DC: Association for the Care of Children's Health.

Simeonsson, R. J. (1988). Unique characteristics of families with young handicapped children. In D. B. Bailey & R. J. Simeonsson (Eds.), *Family assessment in early intervention* (pp. 27–43). Columbus, OH: Merrill.

Simeonsson, R. J., & Bailey, D. B. (1990). Family dimensions in early intervention. In S. J. Meisels & J. P. Shonkoff (Eds.), *Handbook of early childhood intervention* (pp. 428–444). Cambridge, England: Cambridge University Press.

Slentz, K. L., & Bricker, D. (1992). Family-guided assessment for IFSP development: Jumping off the family assessment bandwagon. *Journal of Early Intervention, 16,* 11–19.

Sprunger, L. W., Boyce, W. T., & Gaines, J. A. (1985). Family–infant congruence: Routines and rhythmicity in family adaptations to a young infant. *Child Development, 56,* 564–572.

Steinglass, P. (1984). Family systems theory and therapy: A clinical application of general systems theory. *Psychiatric Annals, 14*(8), 582–586.

Summers, J. A., Dell'Oliver, C., Turnbull, A. P., Benson, H. A., Santelli, E., Campbell, M., & Siegal-Causey, E. (1990). Examining the Individualized Family Service Plan process: What are family and practitioner preferences? *Topics in Early Childhood Special Education, 10*(1), 78–99.

Tomm, K. (1987). Interventive interviewing: Part 1. Strategizing as a fourth guideline for the therapist. *Family Process, 26,* 3–13.

Totta, A. R., & Crase, S. J. (1982). Parents' and day-care teachers' perceptions of young children's skills. *Perceptual and Motor Skills, 54,* 955–961.

Tseng, W. S., & McDermott, J. F. (1979). Triaxial family classifications: A proposal. *Journal of the American Academy of Child Psychiatry, 18,* 22–43.

Turnbull, A. P., Summers, J. A., & Brotherson, M. J. (1984). *Working with families with disabled members: A family systems approach.* Lawrence, KS: Kansas University Affiliated Facility.

Turnbull, A. P., & Turnbull, H. R. (1986). *Families, professionals, and exceptionality: A special partnership.* Columbus, OH: Merrill.

Weisner, T. S., Beizer, L., & Stolze, L. (1991). Religion and families of children with developmental delays. *American Journal on Mental Retardation, 95,* 647–662.

Winton, P. (1988). Effective communication between parents and professionals. In D. Bailey & R. Simeonsson (Eds.), *Family assessment in early intervention* (pp. 207–228). Columbus, OH: Merrill.

Winton, P. J., & Bailey, D. B. (1993). Communicating with families: Examining practices and facilitating change. In J. Paul & R. J. Simeonsson (Eds.), *Children with special needs: Family, culture, and society* (2nd ed., pp. 210–230). New York: Holt, Rinehart & Winston.

Winton, P. J., & Bailey, D. B. (1990). Early intervention training related to family interviewing. *Topics in Early Childhood Special Education, 10*(1), 50–62.

Winton, P. J., & Turnbull, A. P. (1981). Parent involvement viewed by parents of preschool handicapped children. *Topics in Early Childhood Special Education, 1,* 11–19.

Zigler, E., & Black, K. (1989). America's family support movement: Strengths and limitations. *American Journal of Orthopsychiatry, 59,* 6–19.

CHAPTER 7

Sensible Strategies for Assessment in Early Intervention

STEPHEN J. BAGNATO
JOHN T. NEISWORTH
SUSAN M. MUNSON

Young children with neurodevelopmental delays and their families have special needs that demand unique professional perspectives and practices. One of the most important practices is how professionals assess and plan for effective early intervention programs for infants and preschool children. Traditional psychoeducational methods are ineffective, antithetical to the missions of early intervention, and, arguably, illegal with infants and preschoolers who have developmental disabilities.

The passage of federal and state mandates in the form of Public Law 99-457 and the Individuals with Disabilities Education Act (IDEA) amendments have institutionalized both the requisite purposes and practices for early intervention. In response, many professional organizations have published formal policy statements regarding early childhood assessment, intervention, and professional training (see Table 7.1), including the National Association of School Psychologists (NASP) (Bracken, Bagnato, & Barnett, 1991; Schakel, 1987), the Council for Exceptional Children—Division for Early Childhood (DEC) (Neisworth & Bagnato, in press; Odom, in press), and the American Speech and Hearing Association (ASHA) (1990).

Similarly, several professional resources and inservice training manuals have been published recently that guide early educators, psychologists, and other interdisciplinary team members in applying these "best practices" for early intervention, particularly assessment (Bagnato & Neisworth, 1991; Bagnato, Neisworth, & Munson, 1989; Bailey & Wolery, 1989; Barnett & Carey, 1992; Bracken, 1991; Gibbs & Teti, 1990; Meisels & Shonkoff, 1991; Nuttal, Romero, & Kalesnik, 1992; Odom & Karnes, 1988; Wachs & Sheehan, 1988).

TABLE 7.1. Themes of the NASP and DEC Early Intervention Service and Early Childhood Assessment Position Statements and Public Law 99-457

Unique developmental needs of young children
"Whole-child" intervention plans
Valid screening procedures
Flexible team assessment approaches
Family's primary influence on development
Noncategorical diagnosis and service delivery
Broad intervention options for developmental and family support services
Inclusion and mainstreaming
Inadequacy of standardized assessment procedures
Collaborative parent–professional team decision making
Multidimensional and ecological assessment approaches
Documentation of response to intervention
Functional, curriculum-based developmental assessment
Assessment–intervention linkages
Specialized training and credentialing

Through creatively designed and federally funded interdisciplinary pre-service/inservice training programs, many professionals are beginning to acquire the skills necessary to work effectively and sensitively with infants and preschoolers with special needs and their families. Unfortunately, many uninformed administrators and traditionally trained professionals persist in following outdated methods and regulations that subvert the missions and hinder the delivery of early intervention services.

This brief chapter synthesizes professional best-practice guidelines from many sources and offers commentary to translate these principles into action. Wider knowledge of early intervention principles among all team members will help to provide a common foundation for increasing the quality and breadth of early childhood services.

EARLY INTERVENTION PRINCIPLES AND PRACTICES

With the passage of Public Law 99-457 (Parts H and 619) and the IDEA, several field-validated principles of early intervention have become mandated in state special education and/or public welfare standards and regulations. The cornerstones of these principles are *noncategorical diagnosis* and *noncategorical service delivery.* "Developmental delay" is recognized as an appropriate "nonclassification" to declare a young child's eligibility to receive developmental and family support services (i.e., variable state criteria). Other major principles and themes include multidisciplinary team assessments, family-centered practices, Individualized Family Service Plans (IFSPs), full inclusion in regular education settings, longitudinal progress monitoring, accountability for program efficacy, and transition services.

The following principles or qualities of assessment in early intervention are culled from numerous sources, but are adapted and summarized largely from two major resources by the authors (Bagnato & Neisworth, 1991; Bagnato, Neisworth, & Munson, 1989). Each principle underscores the uniqueness and complexity of assessment in infancy and early childhood that make it fundamentally different from traditional school-age psychoeducational testing. The discussion of each principle offers guidelines for direct application by interdisciplinary professionals.

Collaborative and Convergent

One of the most unique attributes of assessment for early intervention is that it fosters teamwork, family–professional collaboration, and consensus decision making about child status and needs. This collaboration occurs through the use of a "check-and-balance" system of "converging" information culled from multidimensional information (i.e., multidomain, multisource, multimeasure, multioccasion, multisetting, and multipurpose) and distilled into a consensus through a process of group dynamics and problem solving. Seasoned early childhood professionals recognize that "tests don't make decisions, people make decisions." A broader and more flexible definition of assessment for early intervention has been offered that celebrates this collaborative and convergent process:

> Assessment for early intervention is not a test-based process, primarily; early childhood assessment is a flexible, collaborative decision-making process in which teams of parents and professionals repeatedly revise their collective judgments and reach consensus about the changing developmental, educational, medical, and mental health service needs of young children and their families. (Bagnato & Neisworth, 1991, p. xi)

Guidelines for Application

1. Select the mode of teaming that fits the child's and family's needs the best (e.g., modified multi-, inter-, or transdisciplinary models).
2. Use a curriculum-based developmental assessment system to unify the assessments of all members of the team including the family (e.g., Carolina Curriculum for Infants and Preschoolers with Special Needs, Johnson-Martin, 1991).
3. Employ a team decision-making format to promote group dynamics

and problem solving about service delivery decisions (e.g., Nominal Group Technique, Delbecq & Van de Ven, 1971; System to Plan Early Childhood Services [SPECS], Bagnato & Neisworth, 1990).

Developmental and Responsive

A developmental perspective and approach underlies early childhood assessment. The traditional psychometric approach emphasizes rigid adherence to standardized procedures, testing aimed at interindividual comparisons for diagnostic classification, and an overemphasis on single dimensional trait measurement (e.g., intelligence).

In contrast, a developmental approach presumes a more "whole-child" view in which multiple functional domains are sampled and intraindividual differences are highlighted so that the child's previous performance serves as the referent to monitor progress. A flexible, rather than lockstep, approach is used in which professionals choose toys that are motivating for the child (i.e., often the child's own toys!) and are responsive to the fact that young children rarely sit still at tables or respond on command to typical structured tasks. Assessment measures whose floors sample only picture identification skills and require no object and social play skills are clearly inappropriate with infants and preschoolers. Simply, a developmental approach acknowledges that professionals must adjust their own language, behavior, and expectations to the young child's level of developmental maturity. Thus, a more natural, play-based approach is used that is more familiar to the child and does not force conformance to standardized testing procedures that are at odds with typical behavioral styles in normal early child development.

A developmental perspective presumes known sequences of developmental skills or processes that emerge at various ages or stages in longitudinal order. Professionals first must acquire an internalized knowledge of both typical and atypical development. This knowledge enables them to sample these skills guided by various developmental assessment instruments. Such an approach emphasizes the observation and analysis of purposeful and teachable behaviors rather than reliance on testing for statistically derived traits.

Guidelines for Application

1. Learn an approach to play-based assessment such as Transdisciplinary Play-Based Assessment (Linder, 1991).

2. Gain an understanding of typical and atypical child development expectancies for various disabilities and be sensitive to the ways in which functional impairments distort development in interrelated skill areas (e.g., language–social–behavioral).

3. Learn the clinical sampling approach to preschool assessment (LeVan, 1990) and how multisensory and response-contingent toys are important to elicit developmental skills at various ages.

Intervention-Based and Valid

Assessment for early intervention has treatment validity—it prescribes and gauges the impact of developmental and family support services. Assessment approaches are dead ends unless they demonstrate a direct link to programming. For this reason, 90% of infant and preschool programs rely upon some form of criterion- or curriculum-referenced assessment (Johnson & Beauchamp, 1987).

Early intervention teams rely on curriculum-based developmental assessment procedures so that the functional behaviors tested and taught are similar. The developmental task analysis of sequential and prerequisite competencies forms the basis for identifying ranges of fully acquired, emerging, and absent skills and for monitoring child progress and treatment outcome.

The technical adequacy of early intervention assessment procedures resides in such issues as social validity and treatment validity—do the measures target skills that can be taught and are these skills important to team members and parents? It is critical that assessment measures in early intervention be field-tested and validated on various disability groups because reliability and validity are characteristics that do not reside in the instruments themselves, but rather vary with the type of child assessed (Neisworth & Bagnato, 1992).

Guidelines for Application

1. Consider the use of a hybrid measure such as the Battelle Developmental Inventory (Newborg, Stock, Wnek, Guidubaldi, & Svinicki, 1984) to accomplish the purposes of eligibility determination and initial linkage to curriculum goal planning.

2. Choose a central developmental curriculum system for your program based on several child, program, and family considerations.

Family-Directed and Ecological

Early childhood assessment procedures focus beyond the child and help the family to conduct a self-appraisal of their needs to help their child to develop and learn. Families are viewed as active partners in the assessment process, eliciting optimal behavior and performance, interacting with their child, and contributing with an equal voice during team collaboration and decision making about service needs and options.

Early childhood professionals recognize that assessments must be conducted in natural environments (e.g., home and preschool) with peers, everyday activities, and typical toys in order to gain a representative view of skill acquisition. An ecological assessment analyzes the environmental supports that a child needs to show such important functional skills as self-initiation, social competence, responsiveness, self-regulation, and independent learning.

Guidelines for Application

1. Conduct initial assessments of most infants and preschoolers in the home.
2. Broaden the assessment by observing trial-inclusion in the preschool program.
3. Use a combination of methods acceptable to the family to foster family self-appraisals (i.e., interviews, rating scales, service menus).
4. Analyze the match between environmental features of the program and the child's developmental and behavioral needs using such scales as the Infant/Toddler Environment Rating Scale (Harms, Clifford, & Cryer, 1989) and the Early Childhood Environment Rating Scale (Harms & Clifford, 1980).

Functional and Adaptive

Developmental assessment activities in early intervention target competencies that are truly functional and foster the goals of normalization, inclusion, and increasing independence. Traits such as intelligence and perceptual–motor integration are eschewed in favor of competencies that integrate skills across several different developmental domains: initiating social interactions with peers, discrimination, classification, attention and task orientation, and forms of communication.

Assessment activities accommodate the child's clear sensory and response capabilities through various field-tested modifications contained in many curriculum task sequences for visual, hearing, neuromotor, language, and behavioral deficits.

Guidelines for Application

1. Incorporate response-contingent toys with microswitches, windup toys, computers, and augmentative communication devices into the assessment of the child.

2. Use only instruments that allow flexible adaptations for alternate sensory and response modes for all young children.

Sensitive and Longitudinal

Appraisals of child progress and treatment outcome are two of the most important, but often neglected, purposes of assessment for early intervention. A central principle of early intervention is that prediction of developmental outcome is impossible (and unethical!) unless one monitors the child's response to individualized intervention. For this reason, programs rely on the use of curriculum-based instruments that contain dense, finely graded sequences of developmental skills that enable teams to monitor the gradual acquisition of functional capabilities under different instructional conditions (manual prompts, verbal prompts, independence).

Only curriculum-based measures have the sensitivity necessary to enable teams to sample a wide range of primitive to advanced skills that can document current levels, set individualized goals, and monitor incremental accomplishments longitudinally. Different metrics such as number of curricular goals achieved during a period of intervention and local norms provide the more sensitive statistics and learning curves required to make informed predictions and, later, diagnoses, after a reasonable period of early intervention services. Note that federal regulations require that early intervention programs be able to document the frequency, intensity, and duration of services provided to children and families so that they can be accountable for the efficacy of their treatment.

Guidelines for Application

1. Choose curricula that have continuity across the birth to 72-month age range and sample graded sequences of developmental skills.
2. Identify various metrics that sensitively chart child progress.
3. Consider the use of System to Plan Early Childhood Services (SPECS) (Bagnato & Neisworth, 1990), which creatively documents child progress and program impact through team ratings of the inverse functional relationship between increases in developmental competencies and decreases in program intensities (e.g., type, amount, and degree of service options selected).

SUMMARY

Assessment for early intervention is a team-based process of family–professional collaboration and decision making. The philosophy, styles, approaches, and missions of infant and early childhood assessment are fundamentally different from the psychoeducational methods associated with school-age prac- tices. These basic differences require specialized preservice and inservice prepa- ration and specialty credentialing for professionals who work with young children who have neurodevelopmental disabilities. The new legal mandates regarding early intervention services and parallel best practice statements from professional organizations will underscore the unique needs of young chil- dren and families and will fuel the thrust for special interdisciplinary training.

ACKNOWLEDGMENT

This chapter originally appeared in *Child Assessment News*, 1992, *2*(4), 1–4. Copyright 1992 by The Guilford Press.

REFERENCES

American Speech and Hearing Association. (1990). *Guidelines for practices in early intervention.* Rockville, MD: Author.

Bagnato, S. J., & Neisworth, J. T. (1990). *System to Plan Early Childhood Services (SPECS).* Circle Pines, MN: American Guidance Service.

Bagnato, S. J., & Neisworth, J. T. (1991). *Assessment for early intervention: Best prac- tices for professionals.* New York: Guilford Press.

Bagnato, S. J., Neisworth, J. T., & Munson, S. M. (1989). *Linking developmental assess- ment and early intervention: Curriculum-based prescriptions* (2nd ed.). Rockville, MD: Aspen.

Bailey, D., & Wolery, M. (1989). *Assessing infants and preschoolers with handicaps.* Columbus, OH: Merrill.

Barnett, D., & Carey, K. T. (1992). *Designing interventions for preschool learning and behavior problems.* San Francisco, CA: Jossey-Bass.

Bracken, B. (1991). *The psychoeducational assessment of preschool children.* Boston, MA: Allyn & Bacon.

Bracken, B., Bagnato, S. J., & Barnett, D. (1991). *Early childhood assessment: Position statement.* Silver Spring, MD: National Association of School Psychologists.

Delbecq, A. L., & Van de Ven, J. T. (1971). A group process model for problem iden- tification and program planning. *Journal of Applied Behavioral Science, 1,* 466– 492.

Gibbs, E. D., & Teti, D. M. (1990). *Interdisciplinary assessment of infants: A guide for early intervention professionals.* Baltimore, MD: Paul H. Brookes.

Harms, T., & Clifford, R. (1980). *Early Childhood Environment Rating Scale.* New York: Teachers College Press.

Harms, T., Clifford, R., & Cryer, D. (1989). *Infant/Toddler Environment Rating Scale.* New York: Teachers College Press.

Johnson, L. J., & Beauchamp, K. D. (1987). Preschool assessment measures: What are teachers using? *Journal of the Division for Early Childhood, 12*(1), 70–76.

Johnson-Martin, N. (1991). *Carolina Curriculum for Infants and Preschoolers with Special Needs.* Baltimore, MD: Paul H. Brookes.

LeVan, R. (1990). Clinical sampling in the assessment of young handicapped children: Shopping for skills. *Topics in Early Childhood Special Education, 10*(3), 65–79.

Linder, T. (1991). *Transdisciplinary play-based assessment: A functional approach to working with young children.* Baltimore, MD: Paul H. Brookes.

Meisels, S. J., & Shonkoff, J. P. (Eds.). (1991). *Handbook of early childhood intervention.* New York: Cambridge University Press.

Neisworth, J. T., & Bagnato, S. J. (1992). The case against intelligence testing in early intervention. *Topics in Early Childhood Special Education, 12*(1), 1–20.

Neisworth, J. T., & Bagnato, S. J. (in press). Best practice recommendations for early intervention assessment. In S. Odom (Ed.), *Best practices in early intervention.* Allen, TX: Pro-Ed.

Newborg, J., Stock, J., Wnek, J., Guidubaldi, J., & Svinicki, S. (1984). *Battelle Developmental Inventory.* Chicago: Riverside.

Nuttal, E. V., Romero, I. R., & Kalesnik, J. (1992). *Assessing and screening preschoolers.* Boston, MA: Allyn & Bacon.

Odom, S. (Ed.). (in press). *Best practices in early intervention.* Allen, TX: Pro-Ed..

Odom, S., & Karnes, M. B. (1988). *Early intervention for infants and children with handicaps: An empirical base.* Baltimore, MD: Paul H. Brookes.

Schakel, J. (1987). *Early intervention services in the school: Position statement.* Silver Spring, MD: National Association of School Psychologists.

Wachs, T. D., & Sheehan, R. (1988). *Assessment of young developmentally disabled children.* New York: Plenum Press.

CHAPTER 8

Instruments for the Screening, Evaluation, and Assessment of Infants and Toddlers

RONALD L. TAYLOR

Accurate and appropriate assessment is a vital part of the educational process and can be used for a variety of purposes. In fact, Part H of Public Law 99-457 makes a specific distinction between screening, evaluation, and assessment. Specifically, *screening* refers to any activity that is used to identify children who are in need of further evaluation or assessment. *Evaluation* refers to the determination of the child's initial and continuing eligibility including the determination of the status of the child in each of the developmental areas. *Assessment* refers to the ongoing procedures used by qualified personnel to identify (1) the child's unique needs, (2) the family's concerns and priorities related to the child's development, and (3) the nature and extent of early intervention services that are required by the child and the child's family to meet those needs. In other words, evaluation refers to procedures that are used to determine eligibility, whereas assessment refers to the gathering of information that will be used in the development of specific interventions for the child. Five developmental areas are traditionally addressed (and required in Part H) throughout the assessment process: cognition, physical/motor, speech and language, psychosocial, and self-help. In reality, many instruments designed for the infant and toddler population measure more than one of these areas; in some cases developmental tests might measure all of these areas. In this chapter, instruments will be discussed in the context of screening, evaluation, and assessment; further, they will be cross-referenced to the five developmental areas. It should also be noted that many tests used in early childhood extend the entire preschool age range (usually birth to age 6 or 7).

GENERAL BEST PRACTICES

Recommendations have been made regarding several best practices that should be incorporated into the assessment of infants and toddlers (Division for Early Childhood [DEC], 1993). For example, a team approach should be used and information should be gathered from a variety of sources. In addition, it is important to recognize that the testing instruments and testing environment itself might need to be adapted. These practices are discussed in the following sections.

Team Approach

Widespread consensus exists regarding the need for a team approach for evaluating young children (e.g., Bagnato & Neisworth, 1991; Taylor, 1993). It is important that professionals, in conjunction with the family, work together to gather and coordinate assessment information that results in the best educational decisions. One way to accomplish this is through the use of the *System to Plan Early Childhood Services* (SPECS) (Bagnato & Neisworth, 1990). SPECS was developed to provide a way in which professionals can communicate results from testing and other sources of information. SPECS consists of three sections or components. *Developmental SPECS* provides the opportunity for various professionals to convert assessment information into mutually understood ratings regarding the child's development in 19 areas. *Team SPECS* allows the team to compare those ratings and arrive at a consensus regarding the child's level of functioning across the developmental areas. Finally, *Program SPECS* includes a set of service options that are available. The amount or intensity required for specific services is also indicated. By completing all three components of SPECS, a team should have some consensus on the child's developmental status, and an idea of the type, extent, and intensity of needed services.

Ecological Evaluation/Multiple Sources of Information

An ecological evaluation requires that information be collected from a child's total environment. Lerner, Mardell-Czudnowski, and Goldenberg (1987) noted that this approach involves the assessment of the child, the environment, and the interaction of the two. Bagnato (1992) made several recommendations regarding the application of the ecological model. These included conducting the initial assessment in the home and using a combination of methods. Clearly, a young child's performance in a test situation may not provide a true picture of the child's abilities. Information about performance in the home environment should be collected through interviews, observation, checklists, and/or histories. In fact, information other than formal test information should always be gathered, particularly when results are used for evaluation (i.e., identification) purposes. The Division for Early Childhood (DEC) of the Council for Exceptional Children made several recommendations regarding appropriate assessment procedures that are consistent with these suggestions. Among those were to (1) gather information from multiple sources, (2) gather information on multiple occasions, and (3) make sure that the measures are sensitive to child and family change (DEC, 1993).

Adaptation of Testing Instruments and Environment

The assessment of young children requires that the evaluator have different skills and more flexibility than those testing older children, adolescents, or adults. This frequently will require that materials and/or procedures be adapted to accommodate the child's sensory (input) and response (output) capacities (DEC, 1993). The examiner must be aware of a few guidelines that will facilitate the testing. Paget (1983) noted several of these general guidelines.

- Reduce the complexity, the level, and the length of instructions.
- Make the evaluation more playlike; be more physically active and interact with the child.
- Be aware of the issue of separation from parent(s); understand the child's reaction to new and different situations.
- Be flexible and use different procedures and techniques.
- Be adaptive, confident, encouraging, enjoyable, and interesting and provide numerous praise statements.
- Make sure that behavioral observations during the testing session are carefully noted; these can help put the test results into proper perspective.
- Provide frequent breaks during the testing session.

Although these general guidelines provide suggestions for the examiner when testing one on one, they often are not sufficient to allow for the most meaningful assessment. As noted previously, some type of team approach is helpful. Wolery and Dyk (1984) described three models that involve progressively more communication among the team members. The *multidisciplinary approach* involves a number of professionals who work together with a minimum of interaction, usually to share the results of their evaluation with each other. The *interdisciplinary approach* emphasizes more interaction among the team members and usually involves regular consultation to share information, which results in the coordinated evaluation of a child in all the developmental areas. In the *transdisciplinary approach* the assessment is conducted within disciplines but the treatment plan is implemented by one or two team members across the various disciplines. An extension of the transdisciplinary approach is *arena assessment,* a very useful technique for working with young children. In this approach, one or two team members assess the child while the other team members (and parents) observe, take notes, and even "score" portions of their tests. For example, the evaluator might work with the child with blocks, allowing the psychologist to score certain items on an intelligence test and the physical therapist to score items on a motor test.

Another effective approach that is very useful with young children is *play assessment.* By observing play behavior, social and developmental skills can be observed in a more naturalistic setting. Linder (1989) described a six-phase process that allows for the observation of the child in a variety of situations. Those are:

1. Unstructured facilitation: The child chooses own activity (20–25 minutes).
2. Structured facilitation: The evaluator chooses the tasks and elicits behaviors not seen in the unstructured phase (10–15 minutes).
3. Child–child interaction: Two children are observed in an unstructured setting (5–10 minutes).
4. Parent–child interaction: This phase allows the parent and child to interact in both unstructured and structured settings; the child's reaction when the parent leaves is also noted (10–15 minutes).
5. Motor play: Motor skills are elicited in both structured and unstructured settings (10–20 minutes).
6. Snack: The child is observed eating a snack (5–10 minutes).

Regardless of the approach that is used, it is important that the results are interpreted carefully, put into proper perspective and translated into appropriate educational decisions. In fact, professionals should report the results in such a way that it is useful for educational program planning for teachers and parents (DEC, 1993).

TYPES OF INSTRUMENTS AVAILABLE

The two major types of instruments are norm-referenced and criterion-referenced. In general, norm-referenced tests are used to determine eligibility and general goals (evaluation) whereas criterion-referenced tests are used to determine specific strengths, weaknesses, and intervention objectives (assessment). Both norm-referenced and criterion-referenced instruments are used for screening.

Norm-referenced tests compare an individual's score with a reference group called the normative sample or standardization sample. Usually, raw scores (number of items passed) are converted to one of a variety of derived scores based on the individual's performance compared to that of the normative sample. Common derived scores yielded by tests for young children are age equivalents, percentiles, and standard scores. An age equivalent is expressed in years and months. Suppose that a girl aged 3 years 4 months received a raw score of 16 on a developmental motor test. If the raw score of 16 was converted to an age equivalent of 2-6, it would indicate that the average performance (raw score) of the children aged 2 years 6 months from the standardization sample was 16. In other words, norm-referenced tests compare the child's performance to children of various ages in the standardization sample. Percentile ranks range from 1 to 99. A percentile rank of 23 would indicate that the child performed better than 23% of the children in the standardization sample. The description of a standard score is beyond the scope of this discussion. However, most developmental tests yield standard scores with an average of 100 and a standard deviation of 15. On these tests, approximately 68% of the standardization sample score between 85 and 115 and 96% between 70 and 130. Obviously the lower or higher the standard score, the more the child's performance can be considered a significant weakness or strength relative to the standardization sample.

The other major type of assessment instrument, a *criterion-referenced test*, does not allow direct comparison of a person's performance with that of other individuals. Rather, it is more directed at what an individual can and cannot do. For younger children, this would mean that the examiner would determine which specific developmental skills the child does and does not exhibit.

TECHNICAL CHARACTERISTICS OF INSTRUMENTS

Two important qualities that must be considered when choosing a test are its reliability and validity. Data that establish these characteristics are routinely provided for norm-referenced tests although the nature of criterion-referenced tests makes it more difficult to determine these characteristics. For example, many criterion-referenced tests are extremely comprehensive and only portions are administered to a given child. Consequently, determining the reliability and validity of the total test would be very difficult. Both reliability and certain types of validity are usually stated in terms of correlation coefficients that range from −1.0 (perfect negative correlation) to +1.0 (perfect positive correlation). These are expressed using a two-decimal number, such as .84, .95, or .46. The closer to +1.0, the greater the validity or reliability. *Reliability* refers to the consistency of a test. The most common type of reliability is test–retest, which refers to the degree to which the test will yield the same or similar results if administered to the same population more than once. For example, to determine the test–retest reliability of a developmental test, it would be administered to a group of young children and then readministered in approximately 2 weeks. The two scores for each child would be correlated with the resulting coefficient providing an indication of how consistent the test results are. Although there is no absolute cutoff point, a correlation below .90 indicates that the test results should be interpreted with caution, particularly when using an individually administered test for evaluation purposes (Salvia & Ysseldyke, 1991). Another type of reliability is split-half, which refers to the test's internal consistency. This is determined by correlating the scores of the "odd" items on a test with the scores of the "even" items.

The *validity* of a test is the degree to which it measures what it purports to measure. For instance, does an intelligence test really measure "intelligence" or is it measuring something else? Types of validity include criterion-related, content, and construct validity. To establish the criterion-related validity of a developmental instrument, it would be administered along with another test (the criterion measure) to a group of children. Scores from the two tests would be correlated to yield the validity coefficient. A coefficient below .60 for an individually administered test indicates the results should be interpreted cautiously (Taylor, 1993). It is also important to remember that in determining criterion-related validity, the criterion measure itself must be valid. Another method of determining the validity of developmental tests is to demonstrate that there is a relationship between performance and chronological age. This is accomplished by showing that the performance (test scores) of the normative sample increase as the age of the subjects increase. This is a type of construct validity.

For norm-referenced tests, another important technical characteristic relates to the nature of the normative sample. In other words, what are the characteristics of the children in the sample to whom a given child's performance will be compared. An average score (i.e., 50th percentile) for a child would be interpreted quite differently if it were based on a test normed on children with severe disabilities compared to one normed on a large random or representative sample of all children.

SCREENING INSTRUMENTS

The screening instruments designed for children from birth to age 3 have limited use for a number of reasons. First, many screening instruments cover

TABLE 8.1. Additional Screening Instruments

Name	Type	Developmental area(s)	Subtest areas
Early Coping Inventory (Zeitlin, Williamson, & Szczepanski, 1988)	Criterion-referenced	Psychosocial, self-help Reactive behaviors	Sensory–motor organization Self-initiated behaviors
Milani-Comparetti Motor Development Screening Test (Milani-Comparetti & Gidoni, 1992)	Norm-referenced	Physical/motor Righting reactions Protective reactions Equilibrium reactions Postural control	Primitive reflexes Active movement
Receptive–Expressive Emergent Language Scale—2 (Bzoch & League, 1991)	Criterion-referenced (checklist)	Speech and language Expressive language	Receptive language
Rosetti Infant Toddler Language Scale (Rosetti, 1990)	Criterion-referenced	Speech and language	Interaction–attachment Pragmatic Gesture Play Language comprehension Language expression

a large age range (up to age 6 or 9 in some cases) resulting in fewer items designed for the young child (Taylor, 1993). Second, the technical characteristics are limited for the majority of these tests. For example, the size and representativeness of the standardization sample at the young ages are frequently inadequate. Screening for problems at this young age should include the gathering of information from a variety of sources, including input from parent and direct observation.

Each of the five instruments described in this section measures several developmental areas. Additional screening tests that measure more limited developmental areas are presented in Table 8.1.

Birth to Three Screening Test of Learning and Language Development

The Birth to Three Screening Test of Learning and Language Development (Bangs & Dodson, 1986) is a norm-referenced instrument that measures the developmental areas of cognition, physical/motor, speech and language, and psychosocial, although the number of items that measure cognition is limited. This instrument is part of an overall package called the Birth to Three Assessment and Intervention System that also includes a Checklist and an Intervention Manual. The areas involved in each of the three components are the same. The Screening Test includes 85 items that are also addressed in the Checklist and the Intervention Manual.

Age Range

Birth to 36 months.

Description of Areas

Language Comprehension: Measures prelinguistic awareness and comprehension of single and multiple word utterances.

Language Expression: Measures prelinguistic and word utterances.

Avenues to Learning: Measures problem-solving skills that are related to sensation, attention, perception, and memory.

Social/Personal Development: Measures self-concept and interpersonal skills.

Motor Development: Measures both gross motor and fine motor skills.

Technical Characteristics

Validity: No data are provided in manual.

Reliability: Interrater reliability coefficients ranged from .88 to .99. No other reliability data are reported.

Standardization Sample: Included were 357 children aged 4 months to 36 months from three states.

Types of Scores: T scores (standard score with mean of 50 and standard deviation of 10), percentile ranks, and stanines are available. A *T* score of 35 or less indicates the need for additional evaluation according to the authors.

In general, the information related to the technical characteristics of the Birth to Three Screening Test is very limited. Further, the available data (including the size of standardization sample) indicate the test is technically inadequate. Consequently, it appears to be more useful as an informal screening measure and should not be used as the only source of information to identify children in need of further evaluation. One criticism is that there are simply not enough items for each age group for each developmental area.

Denver-II

The Denver-II (Frankenberg et al., 1991) is a norm-referenced instrument that measures physical/motor, speech and language, and self-help skills. The Denver-II is a revised version of the popular Denver Developmental Screening Test (Frankenberg, Dodds, Fandal, Kazuk, & Cohrs, 1975). The four major areas have remained the same although some items were changed and added.

Age Range

Birth through 6 years.

Description of Areas

Personal/Social: Measures such skills as dressing and undressing, eating, relating to other people, and imitation.

Fine Motor—Adaptive: Measures drawing and other fine motor skills such as building with blocks and manipulating objects.

Language: Includes items measuring both receptive and expressive communication.

Gross Motor: Measures a variety of activities such as sitting up, standing, walking, and jumping.

Technical Characteristics

Validity: Limited validity data are available on the Denver-II.

Reliability: The test–retest reliability coefficient (.90) and interrater reliability coefficient (.99) were high, but were based on a sample of only 38 children.

Standardization Sample: Included were 2,096 children residing in Colorado. No disabled children were included in the standardization.

Types of Scores: Items are scored as advanced, normal, caution, delayed, or no opportunity. Profiles are subsequently determined and interpreted as being normal, questionable, abnormal, or untestable. Criteria are provided in the manual for the determination of the item scoring and the type of profile.

The scores of the Denver-II are used essentially to determine if further evaluation is necessary. According to the authors, the Denver-II should be used like a growth curve to compare a child to others. There are limited technical characteristics of this instrument, although the Denver-II is an improvement over the original Denver. The Denver-II includes more language items and has a special scoring system for identifying children who have mild disabilities. One of the problems with the original Denver was that it underidentified children needing further evaluation. It is too early to determine if the Denver II will have this same problem. Also, the length of the test is excessive given the limited amount of information it yields.

Developmental Profile II

The Developmental Profile II (DP-II) (Alpern, Boll, & Shearer, 1986) is a norm-referenced instrument that measures the developmental areas of cognition, physical/motor, speech and language, psychosocial, and self-help. There are 186 items in five scales included on the DP-II. The instrument uses an age scale in which there are approximately three items per age level in each developmental area. An age level usually covers 5–6 months for the 0–3 age range. Subsequently there are approximately six items per year per developmental area.

Age Range

Birth through 9 years.

Description of Scales

Physical Developmental Age Scale: Measures fine motor and gross motor areas such as walking, rolling, and riding a tricycle.
Self-Help Developmental Age Scale: Measures areas such as dressing and eating.
Social Developmental Age Scale: Measures the child's social skills and other areas such as exploration and following directions.
Academic Developmental Age Scale: Measures basic academic skills as well as some cognitive skills. For infants and toddlers, this involves copying, searching for objects, and pointing to body parts.

Communication Developmental Age Scale: Measures both receptive and expressive language skills.

Technical Characteristics

Validity: Although the authors provide an argument for the instrument's content validity, limited data are available.

Reliability: Limited reliability data are available.

Standardization Sample: Over 2,300 children were included, although the sample was not generally representative of the United States. There were significant restrictions related to geographic region and socioeconomic status of the children.

Types of Scores: Items are simply scored as passed, failed, or no opportunity. The age scores yielded are subsequently interpreted as either advanced or delayed based on the actual chronological age of the child.

The DP-II allows parent participation in the assessment process and is often used as an "icebreaker." The information can be obtained by interview or self-report. The DP-II, however, has very limited technical characteristics making its use as a norm-referenced instrument somewhat questionable. The DP-II contains a limited number of items for children from birth through age 3. It should not be used in isolation but might be helpful within a larger battery of tests. In other words, although the instrument does provide some meaningful information, the scores yielded by the instrument should be interpreted cautiously.

Minnesota Child Development Inventory

The Minnesota Child Development Inventory (MCDI) (Ireton & Thwing, 1974) is a norm-referenced instrument that measures the developmental areas of physical/motor, speech and language, psychosocial, and self-help.

Age Range

Birth through 6 years.

Description of Scales

The MCDI includes 320 items grouped into several developmental scales. There is also a Minnesota Infant Development Inventory (MIDI) that consists of 73 items designed for children aged 1 month to 15 months. Like the DP-II, the MCDI is administered through interview or questionnaire to the parent. There are scales available in the areas of General Development, Gross Motor, Fine Motor, Expressive Language, Comprehension Conceptual, Situation Comprehension, Self-Help, and Personal–Social.

Technical Characteristics

Validity: There are very little validity data available. The authors do discuss construct validity and data are presented that show the general developmental nature of the items.

Reliability: Split-half reliability coefficients are presented that range from the .50s to the .90s. No other type of reliability data are reported.

Standardization Sample: The sample included 796 children aged 6 months to 6½ years. The children were all white and the sample was not typical of the United States population.

Types of Scores: Results are placed on a profile that is scaled developmentally. The manual indicates that below-age expectation is defined as either below the 30% cutoff or within the 20–30% below-age range.

The technical characteristics of both the MCDI and the MIDI are very limited. Overall, this suggests that the norm-referenced aspects of the test should be downplayed because of these technical inadequacies. There is some evidence suggesting that the use of the MCDI results in overreferrals of children (Meisels, 1988). It should not be used as the sole criterion to determine if a child should be evaluated further. One interesting feature is an audiotape of the questions for use with parents who are nonreaders.

Rockford Infant Developmental Evaluation Scales

The Rockford Infant Development Evaluation Scales (RIDES) (Project RHISE, 1979), is a criterion-referenced instrument (developmental checklist) that measures the areas of physical/motor, speech and language, psychosocial, and self-help. The RIDES checklist consists of 308 developmental behaviors that are clustered into five specific skill areas.

Age Range

Birth to 4 years.

Description of Areas

Personal/Social/Self-Help: Measures skills such as self-awareness and self-responsibility.

Fine Motor/Adaptive: Measures such areas as manipulative tasks, imitative skills, and problem-solving skills.

Receptive Language: Measures the child's ability to attend to and understand the speech of others.

Expressive Language: Measures the child's ability to communicate effectively.

Gross Motor: Measures the development of the child's overall mobility skills.

The RIDES is a developmental checklist that can be used to identify strengths and weaknesses. It is probably best used by teachers who can complete the checklist over several sessions. The RIDES allows for the modification of items for children with different disabilities and also suggests the use of multiple methods of gathering the information. It might also be appropriate for the identification of general goals.

EVALUATION INSTRUMENTS

The majority of instruments for evaluation purposes measure single developmental areas. For example, some tests measure language skills, others motor skills, and others cognition. Depending on the eligibility criteria established by individual states, different combinations of these instruments might be used. Table 8.2 presents a brief description of several of these tests. There are, however, a few instruments that provide norm-referenced information in a number of developmental areas. Three of those are described next.

Battelle Developmental Inventory

The Battelle Developmental Inventory (BDI) (Newborg, Stock, Wnek, Guidubaldi, & Svinicki, 1984) is a norm-referenced instrument that measures the developmental areas of cognition, physical/motor, speech and language, psychosocial, and self-help. There are 341 items that are grouped within five domains that are further divided into several subdomains. Scores are available for each domain as well as for fine motor, gross motor, expressive communication, receptive communication, and the total test. A screening version of the BDI includes fewer items in each domain. The five domains and the corresponding subdomains are listed below.

TABLE 8.2.   Additional Evaluation Instruments

Name	Type	Developmental area(s)	Subtest areas
Peabody Developmental Motor Scales (Folio & Fewell, 1983)	Norm-referenced	Physical/motor	Gross motor Fine motor
Preschool Language Scale—3 (Zimmerman, Steiner, & Pond, 1992)	Norm-referenced	Speech and language	Auditory comprehension Verbal ability
Scales of Independent Behavior (Bruininks, Woodcock, Weatherman, & Hill, 1984)	Norm-referenced	Physical/motor Speech and language Psychosocial	Motor skills Social interaction and communication Self-help
Sequenced Inventory of Communication Development—Revised (Hedrick, Prather, & Tobin, 1984)	Norm-referenced	Physical/motor Speech and language	Receptive language Expressive language
Vineland Adaptive Behavior Scales (Sparrow, Balla, & Cicchetti, 1984)	Norm-referenced	Physical/motor Speech and language	Communication Daily living skills Socialization Motor skills

Age Range

Birth through 8 years.

Description of Domains

> *Personal/Social:* Measures the areas of adult interaction, expression of feeling/affect, self-concept, peer interaction, coping, and social role.
> *Adaptive:* Measures the areas of attention, eating, dressing, personal responsibility, and toileting.
> *Motor:* Measures the areas of muscle control, body coordination, locomotion, fine muscle, and perceptual–motor.
> *Communication:* Measures the areas of receptive and expressive communication.

Cognitive: Measures the areas of perceptual discrimination, memory, reasoning and academic skills, and conceptual development.

Technical Characteristics

Validity: Moderate concurrent validity coefficients with a variety of measures have been reported. The authors also provide arguments for the instrument's construct and content validity.

Reliability: Generally good reliability (test–retest and interrater) have been reported.

Standardization Sample: Included were 800 children from 24 states. Information related to age, race, and sex is presented in the manual.

Types of Scores: The BDI yields several types of scores including standard scores, percentile ranks, and age equivalents. A summary sheet is also available for a visual profile.

The BDI is one of the few norm-referenced developmental scales. It provides a profile of the child's ability in a number of areas. Overall, the technical characteristics appear to be adequate although there has been some question about the appropriateness of the items for younger children (Sheehan & Snyder, 1990). The advantage of the BDI over many other developmental instruments is that it does yield normative information. Suggestions for methods of extrapolating scores below the standard score of 65 also are provided in the manual.

Bayley Scales of Infant Development

The Bayley Scales (Bayley, 1969) is a popular norm-referenced instrument that measures the developmental areas of cognition and physical/motor. The three parts of the Bayley Scales are the Mental Scale (163 items); the Motor Scale (81 items); and the Infant Behavior Record. The Mental Scale includes items measuring sensory, perceptual, and discrimination skills as well as problem-solving abilities and abstract thinking. The Motor Scale measures both gross motor and fine motor skills. The Infant Behavior Record is completed by the examiner after the Mental and Motor Scales have been administered and is used to note the child's behavior during the testing.

Age Range

Two months to 30 months.

Technical Characteristics

Validity: The manual describes a criterion-related validity study between the Mental Scale and the Stanford Binet Intelligence Scale using 350 children (correlation = .57). Overall, there is general lack of validity data in the test manual itself to support the use of the Bayley Scales.
Reliability: Split-half reliability coefficients range from .81 to .93 for the Mental Scale and from .78 to .92 for the Motor Scale.
Standardization Sample: Approximately 1,250 children (nondisabled) stratified on the basis of the 1960 census.
Types of Scores Available: Raw scores are converted to a Mental Development Index (MDI) and a Psychomotor Development Index (PDI). These are standard scores with a mean of 100 and a standard deviation of 15. Although an age equivalent is also yielded, the examiner should not determine a ratio IQ by dividing the mental age by the chronological age.

The Bayley Scales of Infant Development has been perhaps the most widely used norm-referenced instrument for young children over the past 25 years. Although it is relatively easy to administer and score, there is some question about the independence of the Mental and Motor scales (Whatley, 1987). In addition, the norms are outdated although it should be noted that the Bayley Scales are undergoing a major revision (due in 1993). Among the changes proposed for the Bayley II are:

1. Increased age range (1 month to 42 months)
2. Content changes
   a. Adding new domains—Memory, Problem Solving, Cognitive Mapping, Habituation, and Attention
   b. Increased number of language and motor items
3. Materials and art work updates
   a. All manipulatives will be made from nonporous plastic
   b. All art work will be in four colors
4. Improved Infant Behavior Record—A more objective scoring system will be added

It is hoped that the new Bayley Scales will address the few shortcomings of the original instrument.

Infant Mullen Scales of Early Learning

The Infant Mullen Scales of Early Learning (IMSEL) (Mullen, 1989) is a norm-referenced instrument that measures the developmental areas of cognition, physical/motor, and speech and language. The theoretical basis for the IMSEL is in the area of neurodevelopment and intrasensory and intersensory learning. There are four mental ability scales and one motor scale.

Age Range

Birth to 36 months.

Description of Scales

Gross Motor Base: Measures large muscle movements.

Visual Receptive Organization: Measures visual discrimination, visual short-term memory, visual organization, visual sequencing, and visual spatial awareness.

Visual Expressive Organization: Measures bilateral and unilateral manipulation, copying, visual discrimination, and visual–motor control.

Language Receptive Organization: Measures auditory comprehension, auditory memory (one- and two-step commands), organization, auditory sequencing, and verbal–spatial concepts.

Language Expressive Organization: Measures verbal ability (both spontaneous and formal), language formulation, auditory comprehension, and auditory memory.

Technical Characteristics

Validity: The individual mental scales of the IMSEL correlated .50s to the .60s with the Bayley Mental Scale, whereas the Total Mental Scale correlated .97 with the Bayley Mental Scale. The Gross Motor Base Scale correlated .95 with the Bayley Scales' Motor Index. Other correlations with various preschool language measures and construct validity data are also presented.

Reliability: Test–retest reliability was quite high with correlations ranging from .98 to .99 for each of the individual scales. Interscorer reliability was .99 for each of the five scales.

Standardization Sample: The IMSEL was standardized on a stratified sample of 1,231 children. Stratification variables were geographic region, sex, race, and urban/rural residence.

Types of Scores: Raw scores from the Mullen Scales can be converted to *T* scores (mean = 50, standard deviation = 10) as well as "developmental stages" that range from 1 to 8.

The IMSEL is based on a neurodevelopmental approach and measures gross motor skills, visual reception and expression, and language reception and expression. The authors state that the child who scores two standard deviations or more below the mean should be considered for an early intervention program. Although the technical aspects appear to be adequate, the information should be supplemented before important decisions are made. It can be used to identify relative strengths and weaknesses in the motor areas, visual areas, and language areas. The IMSEL correlates relatively highly with cognitive measures and might be used by those individuals who follow more of a sensory integration approach to learning.

ASSESSMENT INSTRUMENTS

Assessment instruments that are used to establish specific educational objectives for infants and toddlers are primarily criterion-referenced developmental inventories. These instruments are usually quite comprehensive and follow a task-analytic model. In other words, a number of general areas are broken down into skill sequences with corresponding items. Because of their comprehensive nature, only portions of these instruments are administered. As a general rule, the teacher will pinpoint those areas that have been targeted for an early intervention program and will select the appropriate skill sequences to administer. By determining what the child can and cannot do within each skill sequence, the teacher has a good idea of not only where to start teaching, but also the sequential steps to teach. Several developmental inventories are described next. Table 8.3 provides information about other instruments used for assessment purposes.

Assessment Log and Developmental Progress Chart—Infants

The Assessment Log and Developmental Progress Chart—Infants (Johnson-Martin, Jens, & Attermeier, 1986) is a criterion-referenced test that measures the developmental areas of cognition, physical/motor, speech and language, and self-help.

Age Range

Birth to 24 months.

TABLE 8.3.   Additional Assessment Instruments

Name	Type	Developmental area(s)	Subtest areas
Callier-Azusa Scale (Stillman, 1978)	Criterion-referenced	Cognition Physical/motor Speech and language Psychosocial Self-help	Motor development Perceptual development Daily living skills Cognition communication and language Social development
Communication and Symbolic Behavior Scales (Wetherby & Prizant, 1990)	Informal (uses video tape of child's communicative behavior)	Speech and language Communicative means Reciprocity Social–affective signaling Verbal symbolic behavior Nonverbal symbolic behavior	Communicative function

Description of Areas

The Assessment Log and Developmental Progress Chart—Infants is one of the assessment components of the Carolina Curriculum. It was designed to identify appropriate instructional goals in 24 areas. Those areas are: Tactile Integration and Manipulative, Auditory Localization and Object Permanence, Visual Pursuit and Object Permanence, Object Permanence–Visual Motor, Spatial Concepts, Functional Use of Objects and Symbolic Play, Control Over Physical Environment, Readiness Concepts, Responses to Communication from Others, Gestural Imitation, Gestural Communication, Vocal Imitation, Vocal Communication, Social Skills, Self-Direction, Feeding, Grooming, Dressing, Reaching and Grasping, Object Manipulation, Bilateral Hand Activity, Gross Motor Activities—Prone, Gross Motor Activities—Supine, and Gross Motor Activities—Upright.

The Assessment Log is based on a well-researched model that includes numerous items in approximately 25 areas of development. Because of the number of items, the instrument is sensitive to small changes in behavior. The teaching suggestions that are related to the test items are helpful for teachers. One potential weakness is its heavy reliance on visually-based items that might be inappropriate for some children.

Brigance Inventory of Early Development—Revised

The Brigance Inventory of Early Development—Revised (Brigance, 1991) is a criterion-referenced instrument that measures the developmental areas of cognition, physical/motor, speech and language, psychosocial, and self-help. The Brigance—Revised includes over 1,000 items in 11 specific areas. These 11 areas include 84 skill sequences. For example, the area of speech and language skills includes 10 skill sequences such as prespeech, receptive language, and picture vocabulary. One feature of the Brigance—Revised is the inclusion of comprehensive skill sequences that can be used with children for whom a more detailed breakdown of the skills is warranted.

Age Range

Birth through 6 years.

Description of Areas

Preambulatory Motor Skills and Behaviors: Measures areas such as supine position and sitting.

Gross Motor Skills and Behaviors: Measures areas such as standing and walking.

Fine Motor Skills and Behaviors: Measures skills such as prehandwriting and cutting with scissors.

Self-Help Skills: Measures areas such as eating, dressing, and toileting.

Speech and Language Skills: Measures areas such as expressive language and sentence memory.

General Knowledge and Comprehension: Measures skills such as identifying body parts and classifying.

Social and Emotional Skills: Measures areas such as play skills.

Readiness—Reading, Manuscript, Writing, and Basic Math: These four areas are not appropriate for young children.

The Brigance—Revised is a criterion-referenced inventory designed to identify specific educational objectives. Like most inventories of this type, it is not designed to be administered in its entirety. Similarly, the developmental age equivalents yielded should be used for informal purposes only. The Brigance—Revised uses a task analytic model that includes 11 areas further broken down into 84 skill sequences and a number of other supplemental sequences. For very young children, the skill sequences do not have enough items to monitor small changes in behavior. Rather the comprehensive skill sequences should be used when available. For example the number of items increases from 37 to 67 when the comprehensive feeding/eating skill sequence is used instead of the regular skill sequence.

Early Learning Accomplishment Profile

The Early Learning Accomplishment Profile (LAP) (Glover, Preminger, & Sanford, 1988), is a criterion-referenced instrument that measures the developmental areas of cognition, physical/motor, speech and language, psychosocial, and self-help in children from birth to 36 months.. The Early LAP is a criterion-referenced developmental checklist that includes items in six areas. Those are: Social/Emotional, Gross Motor, Fine Motor, Cognitive, Language, and Self-Help.

The Early LAP is a comprehensive criterion-referenced inventory that was specifically designed for use with infants and toddlers who are disabled. The teacher should identify those areas in the instrument that have been targeted for early intervention for a particular child. There is also a LAP—Revised for children aged 36–72 months as well as a LAP—Diagnostic Edition.

Hawaii Early Learning Profile

The Hawaii Early Learning Profile (HELP) (Parks et al., 1988) is a criterion-referenced instrument that measures the developmental areas of cognition, physical/motor, speech and language, psychosocial, and self-help in children from birth to 36 months. There are 650 developmental items that are grouped together in six general areas. Those areas are: Cognitive, Expressive Language, Gross Motor, Fine Motor, Social/Emotional, and Self-Help.

Charts are included that can be used to provide a comprehensive profile of the child's developmental skills. There is also a checklist that lists the same 650 developmental skills. Finally, curriculum and intervention strategies are available in the form of an activity guide that provides numerous suggestions to teach each of the 650 skills.

The HELP is an overall package of assessment and instructional materials designed for children birth to age 3. The 650 items are grouped together to measure all the developmental areas noted in Part H. The instrument is usually administered through observation or parent interview. The teaching suggestions that accompany the HELP are valuable and can be used to involve parents in the educational process. Overall, the HELP appears to be a valuable instrument for making instructional decisions.

Vulpe Assessment Battery

The Vulpe Assessment Battery (Vulpe, 1979), is a very comprehensive criterion-referenced instrument that measures the developmental areas of cognition, physical/motor, speech and language, and self-help. There are eight major areas included in the Vulpe. Many of the items appear in more than one section and are cross-referenced on the test form. Some of the areas are further divided into subsections.

Age Range

Birth to 6 years.

Description of Sections

Basic Senses and Functions: Includes items measuring such areas as vision, hearing, and balance.

Gross Motor Behaviors: Measures skills such as lying down, standing, and kneeling.

Fine Motor Behaviors: Measures skills such as eye coordination, reaching, and manipulation.

Language Behaviors: Includes the subsections of Auditory Expressive Language and Auditory Receptive Language.

Cognitive Processes and Specific Concepts: Includes the subsections of Objects Concepts, Body Concepts, Color Concepts, Shape Concepts, Size Concepts, Space Concepts, Time Concepts, Amount and Number Concepts, Visual Memory, Auditory Discrimination, Auditory Attention, Comprehension, Memory, Cause/Effect or Means/End Behavior, Categorizing, and Combining Scheme.

Organization of Behavior: Includes the subsections of Attention and Goal Orientation, Internal Control to Environmental Limits, Problem-Solving and Learning Patterns, and Dependence/Independence.

Activities of Daily Living: Includes the subsections of Feeding, Dressing, Social Interaction, Playing, Sleeping, Toileting, and Grooming.

Assessment of Environment: Measures the interaction of the child with the environment.

The Vulpe is a very comprehensive instrument that measures a variety of developmental areas. As such, only very specific portions of the instrument should be administered. The Vulpe includes a scoring system that uses seven levels to indicate if the child can perform the skill as well as the conditions under which the skill can be performed. These levels are: no, attention, physical assistance, social–emotional assistance, verbal assistance, independent, and transfer. For instance, the verbal assistance score would indicate that the child could pass the item if verbal cues were used or if instructions were repeated. A transfer score would indicate that the child could pass the item and also could pass items of similar complexity in different environments.

SUMMARY

There are many instruments, both norm-referenced and criterion-referenced, available for use with infants and toddlers. It is important, however, that the instrument be chosen on the basis of its intended purpose or use. Described in this chapter were instruments used for screening, evaluation, and assessment, three distinct purposes noted in Public Law 99-457. In general, evaluation instruments, those used for eligibility purposes, are primarily norm-referenced. On the other hand, assessment instruments that are used to establish intervention objectives are primarily criterion-referenced. Screening tests are usually norm-referenced but many are also criterion-referenced. Table 8.4 provides a summary of the instruments described in this chapter.

Finally, it should be emphasized that the screening, evaluation, and assessment of young children must involve more than the administration and interpretation of tests. Test scores, particularly for this age group, are subject

TABLE 8.4. Developmental Areas Covered by Common Instruments

Name	Type		Purpose			Developmental areas covered				
	CRT	NRT	S	E	A	C	PM	SL	PS	SH
Birth to Three		×	×			×	×	×	×	
Denver-II		×	×				×	×		×
Developmental Profile II		×	×			×	×	×	×	×
Minnesota Child Development Inventory		×	×				×	×	×	×
Rockford Infant Developmental Evaluation Scales	×		×				×	×	×	×
Bayley Scales		×		×		×	×			
Battelle Developmental Inventory		×		×		×	×	×	×	×
Infant Mullen Scales		×		×		×	×	×		
Assessment Log	×				×	×	×	×		×
Brigance—Revised	×				×	×	×	×	×	×
Early Learning Accomplishment Profile	×				×	×	×	×	×	×
Hawaii Early Learning Profile	×				×	×	×	×	×	×
Vulpe Assessment Battery	×				×	×	×	×		×

Note. CRT, criterion-referenced test; NRT, norm-referenced test; S, screening; E, evaluation; A, assessment; C, cognition; PM, physical/motor; SL, speech and language; PS, psychosocial; SH, self-help.

to inaccuracy and misinterpretation. Although tests can be used to help guide an assessment, the process should be an active, dynamic one that includes information from a variety of sources. As Bagnato and Neisworth (1991) stated, "Early childhood assessment is a flexible, collaborative decision-making process in which teams of parents and professionals repeatedly revise their judgments and reach consensus about the changing developmental, educational, medical, and mental health service needs of young children and their families" (p. vi).

ACKNOWLEDGMENTS

Portions of this chapter were adapted, by permission, from other material written by the author. Those are:

Taylor, R. (1993). *Assessment of exceptional students: Educational and psychological procedures* (3rd ed.). Needham Heights, MA: Allyn & Bacon.
Florida Department of Education. (1992). *Prekindergarten assessment and training for the handicapped—Infants and toddlers: Screening, evaluation, and assessment*. Tallahassee, FL: Author.

REFERENCES

Alpern, G., Boll, T., & Shearer, M. (1986). *The Developmental Profile—II*. Los Angeles: Western Psychological Services.
Bagnato, S. (1992). Assessment for early intervention: Best practices with young children and families. *Child Assessment News, 2*, 1–10.
Bagnato, S., & Neisworth, J. (1990). *System to Plan Early Childhood Services*. Circle Pines, MN: American Guidance Service.
Bagnato, S. J., & Neisworth, J. T. (1991). *Assessment for early intervention: Best practices for professionals*. New York: Guilford Press.
Bangs, T., & Dodson, S. (1986). *Birth to Three Assessment and Intervention System*. Allen, TX: DLM Teaching Resources.
Bayley, N. (1969). *Bayley Scales of Infant Development*. San Antonio, TX: Psychological Corporation.
Brigance, A. (1991). *Inventory of Early Development—Revised*. North Billerica, MA: Curriculum Associates.
Bruininks, R., Woodcock, R., Weatherman, R., & Hill, B. (1984). *Scales of Independent Behavior*. Allen, TX: DLM Teaching Resources.
Bzoch, A., & League, R. (1991). *Receptive–Expressive Emergent Language Scale—2*. Austin, TX: PRO-ED.
Division for Early Childhood. (1993). *DEC Task Force on Recommended Practices: Indicators of quality in programs for infants and young children with special needs and their families*. Reston, VA: Council for Exceptional Children.
Folio, M., & Fewell, R. (1983). *Peabody Developmental Motor Scales*. Allen, TX: DLM Teaching Resources.

Frankenberg, W., Dodds, J., Archers, P., Bresnick, B., Maschka, P., Edelman, N., & Shapiro, H. (1991). *Denver-II*. Denver, CO: Denver Developmental Materials.

Frankenberg, W., Dodds, J., Fandal, A., Kazuk, E., & Cohrs, M. (1975). *Denver Developmental Screening Test, Reference manual* (rev. ed.). Denver: LADOCA Project and Publishing Foundation.

Glover, M., Preminger, J., & Sanford, A. (1988). *Early Learning Accomplishment Profile*. Chapel Hill, NC: Chapel Hill Training–Outreach Project.

Hedrick, D., Prather, E., & Tobin, A. (1984). *Sequenced Inventory of Communication Development—Revised*. Los Angeles, CA: Western Psychological Services.

Ireton, H., & Thwing, E. (1974). *Minnesota Child Development Inventory*. Circle Pines, MN: American Guidance Service.

Johnson-Martin, N., Jens, K., & Attermeier, S. (1986). *Assessment Log and Developmental Progress Chart*. Baltimore, MD: Paul H. Brookes.

Lerner, J., Mardell-Czudnowski, C., & Goldenberg, D. (1987). *Special education for the early childhood years*. Englewood Cliffs, NJ: Prentice-Hall.

Linder, T. (1989). *Transdisciplinary play assessment*. Denver, CO: Love.

Meisels, S. (1988). Developmental screening in early childhood: The interaction of research and social policy. *Annual Review of Public Health, 9*, 527–550.

Milani-Comparetti, A., & Gidoni, E. (1992). *Milani-Comparetti Motor Development Screening Test*. Omaha, NB: Meyer Rehabilitation Institute.

Mullen, E. (1989). *Infant Mullen Scales of Early Learning*. Cranston, RI: T.O.T.A.L. Child.

Newborg, J., Stock, J., Wnek, L., Guidubaldi, J., & Svinicki, J. (1984). *Battelle Developmental Inventory*. Allen, TX: DLM Teaching Resources.

Paget, K. (1983). *Psychoeducational assessment of preschool children*. New York: Grune & Stratton.

Parks, S., Furuno, S., O'Reilly, K., Hosaka, C., Inatsuka, T., & Zeisloft-Falbey, B. (1988). *Hawaii Early Learning Profile*. Palo Alto, CA: VORT.

Project RHISE. (1979). *Rockford Infant Developmental Evaluation Scales*. Bensenville, IL: Scholastic Testing Service.

Rosetti, L. (1990). *Rosetti Infant–Toddler Language Scale*. East Moline, IL: Lingui Systems.

Salvia, J., & Ysseldyke, J. (1991). *Assessment* (5th ed.). Boston, MA: Houghton-Mifflin.

Sheehan, R., & Snyder, S. (1990). Review of Battelle Developmental Inventory. *Diagnostique, 15*, 16–30.

Sparrow, S., Balla, D., & Cicchetti, D. (1984). *Vineland Adaptive Behavior Scales*. Circle Pines, MN: American Guidance Service.

Stillman, R. (1978). *Callier-Azusa Scale*. Dallas, TX: University of Texas.

Taylor, R. (1993). *Assessment of exceptional students: Educational and psychological procedures* (3rd ed.). Needham Heights, MA: Allyn & Bacon.

Vulpe, S. (1979). *Vulpe Assessment Battery*. Toronto, Canada: National Institute on Mental Retardation.

Wetherby, A., & Prizant, B. (1990). *Communication and Symbolic Behavior Scales*. Tucson, AZ: Communication Skill Builders.

Whatley, J. (1987). Bayley Scales of Infant Development. In D. Keyser & R. Sweetland (Eds.), *Test critiques* (Vol. VI, pp. 38–47). Kansas City, MO: Test Corporation of America.

Wolery, M., & Dyk, L. (1984). Arena assessment: Description and preliminary social validity data. *Journal of the Association for Persons with Severe Handicaps, 9*, 231–235.

Zeitlin, S., Williamson, G., & Szczepanski, M. (1988). *Early Coping Inventory*. Bensonville, IL: Scholastic Testing Service.

Zimmerman, I., Steiner, V., & Pond, R. (1992). *Preschool Language Scale—3*. San Antonio, TX: Psychological Corporation.

CHAPTER 9

Models of Service Delivery

DONNA M. BRYANT
MIMI A. GRAHAM

The ways in which early intervention services are provided to infants and toddlers with special needs vary widely in intensity, duration, setting, personnel, and cost. Conditions unique to each community influence the particular characteristics of the available early intervention programs. Conditions unique to each family influence the particular types of programs they chose. Differences in ways services have been provided have sometimes influenced the effectiveness of programs for young children.

Service delivery models are the combinations of philosophies, strategies, staff, and settings for providing intervention services at the program level. One traditional way of categorizing service delivery systems is by the type of setting in which the infant or toddler is served, for example, in his/her own home, in an integrated child care program, or in a medical foster home. For convenience we have adopted setting as a way of organizing the material in this chapter, although we acknowledge the great diversity within settings and models depending on the intensity and duration of services, the philosophy underlying the intervention, the expertise of the persons providing the services, and the characteristics of the children and families who are receiving them. The models are not necessarily exclusive and they may be used in combinations as desired by families.

Figure 9.1 arrays the major modalities of service delivery based on the typical intensity of supports or services that an infant or toddler would receive in a program of that type. For example, monitoring and tracking programs involve only occasional check-ups or visits. In a typical home visit program, an interventionist might see the child and family about once a week. In a hospital-based program, a child would receive specialized, 24-hour care. Within each of these models, specific additional services may be added (e.g.,

SERVICE INTENSITY

OUT-OF-HOME CARE		
Therapeutic or Medical Foster Care Out-of-home foster care for child whose special health needs cannot be met by family	**Residential Medical Care** Highly specialized developmental and health care for children not able to live at home	**Hospital** Full-time care in hospital (e.g.,"boarder babies") for children with special health needs

COMBINATIONS
Home and Center-based Programs Combination programs that include center-based child care and a home visiting component

CENTER-BASED PROGRAMS				
Parent-Child Centers Group activities to provide consultation and training for parents and intervention service for child	**Developmental Child Care** Child spends the day in a developmentally appropriate classroom in a community day care with many typically developing peers	**Reverse Mainstreaming** A specialized early intervention classroom that includes some children without special needs	**Traditional Specialized Intervention** Specialized classrooms and interventions serving only children with developmental needs	**Medical Child Care** Skilled nursing care in a group setting for children with complex health needs or children dependent on technology

HOME-BASED SERVICES AND SUPPORTS		
Family Supports Range of supports available, including materials, information, advice, instruction, and emotional support	**Home Visiting** In-home parent support and/or parent training; may include direct intervention with child	**Family Day Care Homes** Child care provider receives support and training to include child with special needs

SURVEILLANCE	
Tracking Regular monitoring of child's developmental status	**Health Monitoring** Accessible and frequent health check-ups

FIGURE 9.1. Continuum of early intervention service delivery options. Adapted, by permission, from Graham and Stone (1991).

occupational, physical, and speech therapy; health services; family support services), chosen by the family to meet their needs and priorities.

We begin this chapter with a brief discussion of general guiding principles, and then discuss different service delivery models, including a description of the kinds of services typically available within each model, the types of children and families usually served, and an examination of research on the effectiveness of different programs within or across models. We conclude with a discussion of the decision-making process that we believe should be used when policy makers develop new or expanded service programs.

GUIDING PRINCIPLES

While there are some quality indicators that are specific to certain service modalities, other indicators of best practice cut across all modalities. In the recent publication from the Division for Early Childhood (DEC) Task Force on Recommended Practices, McWilliam and Strain (1993) have identified five principles that should apply regardless of modality:

1. Whatever the service delivery model, it should be the least restrictive and most natural environment for the child and family.
2. Models should be family-centered and responsive to families' priorities.
3. Service delivery should be transdisciplinary for optimal child and family participation.
4. Empirical results and professional and family values should guide service delivery practices.
5. Each child's and family's services should be individualized and developmentally appropriate.

In addition to family-centered services, Hutchins and McPherson (1991) also emphasize the importance of community-based care as a guiding principle because, in the past, it has been difficult for children with disabilities or chronic health needs to receive day-to-day services in their own towns or communities. Community-based programs typically provide more normalizing experiences and are usually of lower cost than highly specialized or institution-based care. Several chapters in this volume address these issues specifically and in more detail (e.g., Hanline & Galant, Chapter 10, and Graham & Bryant, Chapter 11, on inclusive and developmentally appropriate environments, and Bailey & Henderson, Chapter 6, and Duwa, Wells, & Lalinde, Chapter 5, on family-centeredness). We mention these principles here as well because they should be at the core of any service delivery model for infants and toddlers with special needs.

SURVEILLANCE PROGRAMS

Developmental surveillance is early intervention at its simplest. Developmental screening will determine that some children may not need further assessment and Individualized Family Service Plan (IFSP) development, but may seem vulnerable in some way. Continued periodic monitoring of these children and provision of information to the parents may be all that is needed to prevent these children from potential developmental decline. Others, however, will clearly need assessment and referral (see Kochanek, Chapter 3, this volume).

Persons who regularly have contact with young children such as health care providers and child care personnel should be skilled in identifying signs of atypical development. Screening for developmental delays should be standard practice as part of each child's routine well-baby care, whether provided by private pediatricians or county public health nurses. If a visit is missed, the system should trigger someone to phone or attempt to reschedule (a "tickler-type" process). Such a system is crucial as it is not uncommon for children with severe vision and hearing impairments to be identified in child care at age 2 or 3. Good tracking systems can be the safety net for vulnerable young children as part of ongoing surveillance of risks. For example, in the first 6 months of Florida's Healthy Start universal prenatal and infant screening program, 40% of the 26,000 women screened were found to have risk factors that could adversely affect pregnancy outcome. Of the 55,000 infants screened, 12% were found to be at risk and in need of tracking and other supports.

Participation in Part H will be an incentive for states to systematically track vulnerable children. Although few systematic statewide tracking systems are in place, several states have systems targeted for specific populations such as drug-exposed children, or for high-risk areas such as subsidized housing. Hawaii's Healthy Start program, designed primarily for the prevention of child abuse, provides universal screening during pregnancy, at delivery, and when the child enters school. Children are systematically tracked and family support services provided as needed. West Virginia's innovative system gives families coupons that, when stamped after well-baby visits, can be redeemed for diapers, formula, and other supplies.

In North Carolina, the Child Service Coordination Program combines the tracking of high-risk children with targeted service coordination. Implemented through the 100 local health departments, hospital or health department staff complete an identification and referral form on every infant considered at risk at birth, based on biological characteristics of the infant and demographic and socioemotional characteristics of families. Identified infants are assigned a child service coordinator from the community agencies that have enrolled with the health department as program providers.

Several other states have tracking systems in place (Meisels & Provence, 1989). Identifying children who need early intervention services is a complex process; identifying those who most need services or would most likely benefit from services is more difficult. Matching children's and family's needs with the kinds of programs we can provide is an even greater challenge. But all start with a screening at the portal of entry and require monitoring to document and assure progress.

HOME-BASED SERVICES AND SUPPORTS

We include in this category of service delivery systems different home settings in which infants and toddlers with special needs and their families can be served—in their own home through a family support home visiting program or in the home of a family day care provider. Both settings are natural environments in which many children, both with and without special needs, spend their days. In what ways can effective programs be delivered within these settings?

Family Supports

Family supports are an important family-centered component along the continuum of service delivery options. Traditional means of providing early intervention have been limited to an array of predetermined, agency-provided services with decisions driven by service availability rather than family and child needs (Herrington, 1989). Families have been expected to fit into this professionally dominated system whether or not the services met their needs. This has often resulted in professionals' descriptions of families as uncooperative, not caring about their child, or unappreciative. A family-centered approach views the professional, the family, and other sources of support as equal contributors to the intervention.

In addition to the traditional early intervention services that are heavily emphasized in Part H, also included are "respite and other family support services" (Individuals with Disabilities Education Act, Section 303.12 [14 Note 2]). As described by Raab, Davis, and Trepanier (1993), a family support approach uses a broad-based definition of resources for children and families, including material, informational, and emotional support—whichever meet(s) the needs of the family. Table 9.1 identifies major resource categories.

In order to assist a family in identifying needed supports and resources, the family-directed assessment has been included as an optional part of the IFSP process. Thus, families can become part of the solution as they are strengthened in ways that help them be less, not more, dependent on professionals (Dunst, Trivette, & Deal, 1988). Research has shown that various forms of resources and support improve parent and family well-being and family functioning, enhance positive interaction with caregivers, improve parental perceptions of child functioning, and indirectly influence child behavior characteristics (Dunst & Leet, 1987; Dunst, Leet, & Trivette, 1988; Dunst & Trivette, 1986, 1987, 1988).

Both formal and informal support can be provided. Traditional formal sources of support have included hospitals, health care professionals, social

TABLE 9.1.   Major Resource Categories

Child education and development	Child care
Child development information	Routine child care (e.g., day care)
Learning opportunities	Nonroutine child care (e.g., drop-in)
Early intervention and therapy and	Emergency child care
instruction	Recreation
Adult education and enrichment	Information about recreation resources
Parenting education	Recreation facilities (e.g., pools, parks)
Instruction and learning	Cultural events
Information about parenting	Life necessities
Health care and education	Food and clothing
Medical and dental care	Housing and shelter
Health care supplies and equipment	Utilities
Health care information	Transportation
Economic	Personal transportation
Job	Public transportation
Money (for other resources)	

Source: Family Enablement Project, Family, Infant and Preschool Program, Western Carolina Center, Morganton, NC.

workers, educators, therapists, and early intervention programs. Informal supports include neighbors, clergy, clubs, relatives, and social groups (Dunst & Trivette, 1990). An innovative bartering system in Miami is a formal system that promotes informal support. For example, a retired person can provide child care for 2 hours and "bank" hours to receive later transportation to the grocery store. Wheelchairs can be exchanged for motors. Families provide respite for each other. The possibilities are endless and provide practical, low-cost supports for families.

Communities must strive to include both formal and informal supports in their array of early intervention services. Family supports are an important nonintrusive, cost-effective, family-centered means of providing services for children with disabilities and their families.

Home Visit Programs

Serving families in their homes is a practice of many professional groups, especially nurses, social workers, and educators (Wasik, Bryant, & Lyons, 1990). Literally thousands of home visit programs exist throughout the country (Wasik & Roberts, 1989). In a national survey of 1,904 home visit programs, 643 programs (34%) reported serving children from birth to age 3 with the primary reasons for service being developmental delay, physical handicap, specific learning impairments, low birth weight, or at risk (Roberts & Wasik, 1990). As reported on the survey, the two most frequently listed reasons for visiting were to provide support to parents or to teach parenting skills, with stress reduction a secondary reason. Many programs include modeling positive adult–child interactions, providing information, and teaching appropriate learning activities for the infant or young child.

Well-known programs that provide services in homes include public health departments, Association for Retarded Citizens, Easter Seals, and United Cerebral Palsy, which sponsor home visit programs for children with special needs. In these programs the early interventionist works in the home to promote the child's development, coordinate services needed by the child and/or family, involve the parent in the intervention, and be a source of support to the family. Head Start has long utilized home visiting (Wolfe & Herwig, 1986) and has recently established 34 Comprehensive Child Development Centers for infants and toddlers including a home component (Collins, 1993; Head Start Bureau, 1991).

Home visit programs have been conducted for low-birth-weight infants (Barrera, Rosenbaum, & Cunningham, 1986; Infant Health and Development Program, 1990), for children with Down syndrome (Bidder, Bryant, & Gray, 1975; Hanson & Schwarz, 1978), for moderate and severely delayed children (excluding Down syndrome) (Barrera et al., 1976; Brassell & Dunst, 1978), and for infants at risk for developmental delay due to impoverished environments (Gordon & Guinagh, 1978; Madden, O'Hara, & Levenstein, 1984; Scarr & McCartney, 1988; Wasik, Ramey, Bryant, & Sparling, 1990).

Home visiting is a very flexible, cost-effective strategy for observing, teaching, and supporting all families—first-time or teen parents and families with a child who has special needs or is at risk for delay. Especially in early infancy, when many working parents try to stay home for at least a few months with a newborn, the home is the primary environment for the infant and parent, and their needs at this time can best be met in the home. This is also the time when parents of a child with special needs are beginning to deal with their child's condition (Drotar, Baskiewicz, Irwin, Kennell, & Klaus, 1975), the special services they might need (Blackard & Barsh, 1982), the increased financial responsibilities that might occur (Beckman-Bell, 1981), and the social isolation that may ensue (Gabel & Kotsch, 1981). The need for support, especially from someone knowledgeable about the kinds of issues faced by families of infants with special needs as well as those faced by families of all infants regardless of need, can be met by a home visitor who stops by to help and listen at these critical times.

Although home visiting is a widely used strategy, home visit programs vary from one to another in scope, intensity, populations served, and staffing. As personnel, for example, home visit programs have utilized paraprofessionals, such as community resource workers, Head Start parents, and former migrant farmworkers, as well as professionals, such as nurses, social workers, and educators. The variety of personnel as well as the diversity among home visit components have made difficult any definitive evaluations of the effectiveness of services provided via home visits (Halpern, 1984). Some home visit interventions provided to high-risk infants and young children (primarily those from low-income families or those born at low birth weight) have shown gains in children's cognitive or social–emotional development (Powell & Grantham-McGregor, 1989; Resnick, Eyler, Nelson, Eitzman, & Buccizrelli, 1987) while others have not (Ramey, Bryant, Sparling, & Wasik, 1985; Scarr & McCartney, 1988). Similarly, some results from home visit programs to families of children with diagnosed developmental delays have shown child cognitive improvement (Brassell & Dunst, 1978) while others have not (Moxley-Haegert & Serbin, 1983). Factors such as frequency of visits (at least weekly) and training and supervision of visitors (intensive) seem to be important factors in the potential success of a home-based program (Powell & Grantham-McGregor, 1989).

Given the lack of an agreed-upon theoretical basis for home visiting (Powell, 1990) and the conflicting results regarding the effectiveness of home visiting (Halpern, 1984), we believe that home visiting should be just one component of a multifaceted approach to serving infants and young children with risks, developmental delays, or disabilities. Delivering services via home visits alone may not be a method potent enough to consistently alter children's developmental progress, but because it may help some children and it certainly has assisted parents in search of information and/or support, it should be included as a component of early intervention programs.

The home visit model has the capacity to serve a range of children with established conditions, delays, and risks, and to address a variety of family needs. However, some children need more frequent or specialized services than can be provided within home-based programs, such as therapies, health services, and adaptive equipment. Although other programs might deliver these services, home visiting can be an effective means of assisting parents to become the primary teachers of their children.

Family Day Care Homes

In the United States, the predominant form of nonrelative care for children under age 3 is a family day care home in which a female provider looks after other people's children in her own home. For employed mothers this type of arrangement serves 23% of infants and 27% of toddlers (12–36 months)

(Bureau of the Census, 1987). More than 5 million children are estimated to be in the care of 1.5 million providers (Kahn & Kamerman, 1987). Because many family day care providers operate in the underground economy and are unlicensed, these percentages and numbers are probably conservative. Parents tend to choose this form of care because generally the costs are lower, the hours more flexible, and the locations more convenient than most child care centers. In addition, parents who prefer family day care value the small group, the home-like atmosphere, and sense of shared values with the caregiver (Leibowitz, Waite, & Witsberger, 1988). However, family day care providers tend to be much less qualified than group care providers. On the average, family day care providers are older, have less post-high school education, and less experience in child care (Jones & Meisels, 1987).

Although family day care has also been the most frequently used form of child care for children with special needs (Fewell, 1986), it is an underutilized resource in providing effective intervention for children with special needs. This may have resulted from a concern about the quality of education, training, and skills of family day care providers for meeting the needs of children with disabilities or because family providers may be unable to address the needs of children who require special care. However, many family day care home providers *are* interested in learning to care for infants and toddlers with disabilities, but need training and support.

Several states have launched effective initiatives toward improving the capacity of family day care homes. North Carolina funds Partnerships in Mainstreaming, a program that employs four specialists around the state to recruit, train, and support family day care home providers to care for children with special needs (Wesley & Arnn, 1991). The Delaware FIRST Program gave 56 family day care providers specific training via preservice sessions and a home visitor twice monthly for the first 6 months, a toll-free advice number, newsletters, and a toy lending library. Research showed that this program improved the overall quality of these homes for infants and toddlers, increased the number of available placement slots for infants and toddlers with special needs in Delaware, and provided the families with support and respite (Deiner, Whitehead, & Peters, 1989).

If family day care providers receive the support, technical assistance, and encouragement needed to provide quality care, family day care homes can be good placements for children with a wide range of conditions, particularly children with mild to moderate levels of need. Family day care homes typically are not able to address other family needs, so additional components need to be added for this service model to be more family focused. Some children need more frequent or intense therapies or health services, supports that can be added to family day care. For a few children in the Delaware study, placement in a supported family day care home served as a bridge placement between a home-based early intervention program and a center-based intervention program. This progression might well meet the needs of many infants and toddlers with disabilities.

CENTER-BASED SERVICE SYSTEMS

Children with special needs and their families may be served in several different types of group care settings. These range from parent–child centers to regular child care to specialized child care such as developmental day centers and medical child care.

Parent–Child Centers

The history of the parent–child center as one way of serving infants, young children, and their families stems from the efforts of the Office of Economic Opportunity in the 1960s to teach and support parenting in low-income families through multipurpose family centers (Halpern, 1990). Over 30 centers were established to provide parent education, health, and social services to families of infants and toddlers up to 3 years of age. The premise of these services was two-fold: that families needed help in providing adequate care and stimulation for their infants and that extrafamilial obstacles such as poverty, unemployment, and low education also needed to be addressed.

Three Parent Child Development Centers (PCDCs) were studied quite extensively (Andrews et al., 1982). In these programs mothers spent from 6–20 hours weekly attending parent group meetings in the centers, child development classes, and workshops on community resources and interacting with infants in the infant nursery. Evaluation results showed that program mothers were more responsive and positive in their interactions with their children than were control mothers, but only one of three programs (Houston) found significant cognitive differences between program and control children. Follow-up results of the Houston children when they were in the second through fifth grades show that program children performed better than controls on achievement tests and were rated by their teachers as less hostile (Johnson & Walker, 1991).

Although the PCDC interventions clearly affected parenting skills and one had longer-lasting child effects, very high levels of parent and professional involvement were required. The PCDC attrition rates averaged 50%, with mothers who were returning to work or school especially likely to drop out. This illustrates the difficulty faced by intervention programs in balancing specific developmental needs of children, their parents' personal needs, and the family's survival needs (Weiss & Halpern, 1988).

Although the early parent–child programs faced obstacles, the results seemed positive enough to encourage others working with high-risk children and children with disabilities to follow and modify the model. Head Start now has Parent and Child Centers (PCCs) in every state, where parents in poverty can learn about parenting and child development. The PCCs serve pregnant women and children from birth to 3, providing an array of health, nutrition, and social services resources in addition to traditional parenting-skills training.

Parent–child programs also provide group intervention for infants and toddlers with disabilities and their caregivers. A skilled early interventionist leads the group in activities to promote the development of their babies and discussions to support the families. Groups generally meet once or twice a week for 1 to 2 hours. The primary intervention services offered are consultation and parent training for the caregivers and special intervention services for the child. Because parent–child centers are usually a part of an umbrella intervention program (e.g., an Easter Seals program), other intervention services such as therapies and evaluations are often available.

The parent–child center service delivery option has the capacity to serve children and families with a range of needs. Parent–child centers are the primary service delivery model for infants and toddlers with disabilities in some states (e.g., Massachusetts). Many children at risk for developmental delay are served in Head Start's demonstration PCCs. Delivering intervention via parent–child centers may be an effective means of enhancing parents' skills as the primary teachers of their children, but it does not address the child's needs intensively. Few effectiveness data exist on populations best served by this model.

Some children will need a higher intensity of services than can be provided within parent–child centers (e.g., therapies, health services). Working parents typically need full-day child care for their children and cannot leave their own jobs to attend daytime meetings. Parent–child programs do not generally have the capacity to provide the comprehensive array of other intervention services that a child/family may need (i.e., service coordination, transportation, health services). This model can provide parent training and support and some special intervention services to groups of caregivers and their children and may meet the needs of some families of children with special needs.

Developmental Child Care

In its idealized form, developmental child care is the nurturing care of children by competent, trained staff, in classes with low staff–child ratios, small group sizes, and developmentally appropriate environments. Developmental child care centers serve children from infancy through school age in most communities across the country. The types of programs and sponsoring agencies range dramatically. Settings include church-run nursery schools, private or nonprofit centers, Title XX subsidized settings, corporate-sponsored care, and intergenerational day programs. Recent survey data of generic child care programs such as these indicate that 19.2% of such programs throughout the country serve at least one child under age 2 with disabilities (Research Institute on Preschool Mainstreaming, 1990). The appropriateness of this model for infants and toddlers with special needs is dependent upon the basic quality of the child care and the ability to access the special intervention and support services needed to meet the individual needs of the child with disabilities.

First, however, is a problem of accessibility of high-quality developmental child care for children in general. This is really a set of three interrelated problems: the accessibility of any care at all, the cost of care, and the shortage of quality programs. With increasing numbers of mothers working, there is a shortage of center-based child care, particularly for infants and toddlers (Hofferth & Phillips, 1987). The cost of center-based care is more than care by relatives or family day care homes and represents a substantial expense for most families, averaging 10% of family income. For very low-income families, child care costs comprise 20–50% of incomes. The costs for some subgroups of children are even higher, especially infants (Grubb, 1988) and children with special needs (Brush, 1988; cited in Hayes, Palmer, & Zaslow, 1990). Finally, if the availability and affordability can be handled, it is not clear how many centers provide adequate, let alone high-quality, care. Salaries are low, staff turnover is high, and staff–child ratios do not often meet the standards that research and best practice guidelines indicate as best for infants and toddlers. Nevertheless, when they can find and afford center-based care, many parents prefer it because of a belief that more learning takes place (Atkinson, 1987).

Researchers have been advocating for expansion of child care services to encompass the needs of preschool children with disabilities for more than 15 years (Neisworth & Madle, 1975) for both social and economic reasons. The public need for early childhood services has increased as more than 55% of mothers of children younger than 3 are in the work force, about 70% full-time (Bureau of Labor Statistics, 1988). Klein and Sheehan (1987) estimated that about 40–50% of the mothers of infants with special needs were employed outside the home. This should not surprise us because there is no reason to believe that mothers of children with special needs have any less need to work than other women (Fewell, 1986). In fact, it seems reasonable to assume that families with exceptional children are more likely to have additional costs for diagnostic, therapeutic, or medical care and are therefore more dependent on two salaries (Bagnato, Kontos, & Neisworth, 1987), yet there is a negative relationship between maternal participation in the labor market and the severity of a child's disability (Breslau, Salkever, & Staruch, 1982).

In addition to providing care while parents work, other potential benefits exist in an inclusive center-based setting for children with special needs and children who are typically developing (see Hanline & Galant, Chapter 10, this volume). Full inclusion is appropriate for most children across a range of disabilities. It is also appropriate for cognitive and learning disorders, regardless of the severity of the disorder (Hanson & Hanline, 1989). Full inclusion has been successful in bilingual preschool programs serving Mexican-American children with and without special needs (Evans, 1976). A program run by the Arkansas Association for Retarded Citizens, Project KIDS (Kids in Integrated Daycare Services), provides inclusive services and supports to preschoolers with disabilities and their families at a per-child cost of one-third to one-half the cost of less effective services in a segregated program (Stone, 1989).

Even though many parents of children with special needs work outside the home, few early intervention programs provide full-day care. Most end at 2 or 3 P.M. Hence, there is a tremendous need for full-day and/or wrap-around care for children with disabilities. Parents need options. Some may only want several hours a week; others need full-time care. Currently, children usually have to pay and/or attend programs full-time to accommodate the reimbursement system. Settings in which children with special needs are served are most often determined by which program has opening or space. Choices regarding home-based or center-based, or segregated or integrated settings are usually made merely on availability, not on whether the placement is appropriate for the child.

Child care settings offer a tremendous capacity for becoming a model in which infants and toddlers with disabilities are served alongside their non-disabled counterparts. Families of children with special needs tend to choose the developmental child care model because of longer hours, convenient locations, lack of stigmatization, and the opportunities for their children to interact with nondisabled peers. Child care programs typically do not provide parenting education or support groups, so this model generally lacks the capacity for addressing family needs for special supports.

Children with mild to moderate developmental and/or health needs are best served in this model. There are mixed opinions about the appropriateness and the capacity for child care programs to meet the intensity of special needs required by children with profound disabilities or medical conditions. Special interventions and therapies can be provided by specialists working in the child care setting or through a consultative model in which professionals train the caregivers to provide needed services (Huefner, 1988; McWilliam,

1992). Especially needed are health services (nursing consultations and health monitoring) and family support services (parent training and counseling). Families must weigh the benefits of an integrated model against more specialized, intensive programs.

The major barrier to further expansion of this model is the shortage of high-quality child care programs. Nationwide, only 2,340 are accredited by the National Association for Education of Young Children. Many child care environments, including many currently receiving Child Care Block Grant subsidies, do not begin to approach the quality level described as developmentally appropriate. They typically fall short in the areas of recommended staff to child ratios, the facility and materials to meet children's needs, and staff competencies. This is largely because quality care, especially for infants and toddlers, is expensive.

The key to the utilization of child care settings for early intervention lies in facilitating the overlay of special intervention services onto quality child care. Child care settings can become viable settings for early intervention services given the appropriate technical assistance, training, access to consultative services, and incentives.

Reverse Mainstreaming

In the previous section, "regular" day care that included children with special needs was described as one model of providing early intervention services. The addition of nondisabled peers to programs previously serving only children with special needs, usually referred to as "reverse mainstreaming," is another model. Reverse mainstreamed programs usually serve somewhat more children with special needs, for example, 60% special needs and 40% typical needs (Peck, Apolloni, Cooke, & Raver, 1978). The teachers in these programs have often been trained in early childhood special education and have more experience with children with disabilities than traditional child care teachers, even those with degrees. This model has the double benefit of providing a high intensity of specialized intervention in addition to ongoing opportunities for interaction with nondisabled peers. Realizing these benefits, many previously segregated early intervention programs have recently converted to reverse mainstreaming models.

This model provides the level of intensity required for children with medium to high ranges of developmental needs. Additional health services may be required to meet more than minimal medical needs. The reverse mainstreaming model can provide high levels of support to families regarding their child (advocacy, parent training, service coordination, respite care), but such programs generally are limited in dealing with extenuating family needs (drug rehabilitation, vocational training, family therapy). Additional social work assistance might help the family obtain other needed services. Reverse mainstreaming models have many of the advantages of an integrated environment in addition to highly specialized staff and services.

Traditional Specialized Early Intervention Model

The traditional specialized early intervention model provides highly skilled staff experienced in providing interventions both with children with disabilities and with young children in segregated group settings. Both intensive educational interventions and therapies are usually available. Health resources are often needed and may be provided by nursing consultation, service, and training so that interventionists and caretakers can appropriately meet the health needs that often accompany a disability.

Children with a high level of developmental needs may be best served by the traditional specialized early intervention model. Many traditional specialized early intervention programs do not currently have the capacity to provide the medical expertise necessary for serving children who are technologically dependent or medically complex.

Like the reverse mainstreaming model, the trained professionals usually employed in specialized intervention programs can provide a high level of support to families regarding their children (advocacy, parent training, service coordination, respite care). Additional support to address other family needs may or may not be available (e.g., through a social worker also working with the intervention team).

Although specialized programs have the capacity to provide appropriate, intense, center-based intervention services, often the learning environment is not developmentally appropriate (Bailey, Clifford, & Harms, 1982). Many classes are too teacher-directed and highly structured, use didactic teaching methods, and provide limited opportunities for exploration, outdoor play, fantasy play, art, music, or other activities that can promote the child's normalization. Lack of opportunities for interactions with nondisabled peers limits socialization abilities and promotes stigmatization. The number of specialized programs is limited, creating long waiting lists for early intervention, sometimes as long as 3 years in Florida. In many rural areas, center-based interventions either are nonexistent or infants and toddlers must travel extensive distances.

Specialized programs can offer early intervention service of relatively high intensity, but they preclude the benefits of a more normalized environment. There may be circumstances when the family chooses this as the most appropriate model of service delivery.

Medical Child Care

To avoid unnecessary extended hospitalization or the isolation and cost of in-home nursing care, some children may be best served in a medical child care program, a group care center for children requiring skilled nursing care. For many families, this level of medical support may be the major enabling factor in discharging the child from the hospital or in a parent's returning to work. In Florida, there are several Pediatric Health Choice facilities that provide a therapeutic daytime environment for children requiring complex medical care. This model serves as a transitional setting that supports medically fragile children until they are healthy enough to enter nonmedical child care programs. However, some experts believe that if children can be in a center-based program, they can be in an integrated model with the opportunity for interactions with nondisabled peers.

Medical child care is a service that must be prescribed by a physician and is only for those children with extraordinary health needs requiring nursing interventions such as oxygen therapy, tracheotomy care, mechanical ventilation, and intravenous feedings. This model is also designed to provide the interventions and therapies to meet the developmental needs that so often accompany extensive health care needs.

Such programs can serve families with a wide range of needs. The model provides family supports, such as respite care and parent support groups, and educational opportunities to increase the family's ability to manage their child's medical needs. The availability of medical child care is limited in both urban and rural areas, but especially in smaller communities. Although medical child care is relatively expensive, it is cost efficient compared to the alternative of hospitalization or 24-hour nursing care. This model is one way of meeting a child's medical needs in a less clinical, more developmental setting.

COMBINATION PROGRAMS

Often families with infants or toddlers with special needs must choose between a daily center-based program or one offering a 1-hour home visit per week, or children may only be eligible for one type of program (based on their disability). However, some of the most effective interventions have resulted when center-based, child-focused interventions have been used in conjunction with home-based, family-focused services. The combination of home-based and center-based services is a powerful model of providing early intervention services.

Home visits and educational child care have been used in two very effective programs for at-risk children from low-income families. In the Milwaukee Project, families received many hours of home visits in the first 4 months after birth to help the mother with the newborn and to help make the transition into the center-based portion of the program (Garber, 1988). In Project CARE, families received home visits from their child's teacher from the time of program entry (around 6 weeks of age) until the child entered school (Bryant, Ramey, Sparling, & Wasik, 1985). Visits were weekly until the child was 3 years of age and then on a schedule selected by the mother (from weekly to every 6 weeks). Both these studies found significant cognitive differences (10–20 IQ points at various early ages) between the intervention children and those who had been assigned to a control group. Because both home visits and educational child care were received by the treatment groups, the gains cannot be attributed solely to either component of the programs, but one can conclude that both played a part.

The combination of health monitoring, home visiting, and full-day educational child care was a very effective intervention for preventing developmental delay in low birth weight infants (Infant Health and Development Program, 1990). The Infant Health and Development Program (IHDP) was an eight-site, randomized, controlled trial involving 985 low-birth-weight infants and their families. After 3 years, children in the intervention group demonstrated significantly higher intellectual performance and fewer problem behaviors as reported by their mothers. The level of children's participation in the program was positively related to their IQ scores at age 3, although participation was not related to any of the initial demographic or biological characteristics that were measured (i.e., maternal education and age, infant's sex, race, birth weight, and health status at birth) (Ramey et al., 1992). These findings are consistent with previous research linking intensity of intervention services with degree of positive cognitive outcomes for high-risk infants. The Centers for Disease Control is mounting a new effort to replicate the IHDP intervention in multiple, community-based settings around the country. The emphasis in the new research will be to reduce mental retardation in children of mothers with low educational levels through a combination of health services and developmental interventions.

The Pediatrics Branch of the National Cancer Institute offers a comprehensive intervention program for children with AIDS and their families (Wiener, Moss, Davidson, & Fair, 1992). Their services include a psychosocial support system and a case management approach particularly addressing health and mental health problems, including members of the extended family who often help care for children with AIDS. Another example of comprehensive intervention services—the Linda Ray Intervention Programs—has recently begun for substance-exposed children and their parents in Miami (K. Scott, personal communication, January 1993). The program calls itself a "full service preschool" with many services available: center-based preschool, home-based intervention, primary medical care, substance abuse treatment, literacy and vocational training, legal consultation, and on-site housing and WIC representatives. The progress and outcomes of this multiple service intervention will be of great interest to practitioners and policy makers.

The combination model offers the advantages of both center-based programs (intensity, child-focused, access to therapies, peer interactions) and home-based programs (family-focused, parent training, individualized interventions adapted to the home). Depending on the services within the center-based programs (i.e., health or developmental supports), this service delivery option has the capacity to serve children with a broad range of needs and has been found to be effective for infants and toddlers with established conditions, delays, or risks.

Funding priorities often do not allow the additional staff necessary to provide home visiting for children in center-based or clinic-based programs, especially with limited funding and waiting lists for both center- and home-based interventions. If center-based programs were half-day, the current staff could be utilized for home visiting in the remaining half-day. However, this option would not be viable for a large number of two-parent working families.

OUT-OF-HOME SERVICE SYSTEMS

Children with a high degree of both biological and environmental risks may be best served in out-of-home settings. When it is necessary to remove a child from the natural home, a safe, home-like placement is always preferable to residential, institutional settings.

Therapeutic or Medical Foster Care

Medical foster care is a model of short- or long-term care for a child outside the biological or adoptive family due primarily to special health care needs of the child and an inability of the family to meet these needs. Medical care providers are becoming increasingly aware of the negative effects of prolonged hospitalization on the child and family (Katz, 1993). With increasing incidences of "boarder babies" and orphans with health concerns, medical foster care offers an important alternative to extended hospitalizations or group residential care. It consists of a medical overlay of services and training on top of nurturing, quality foster care. Medical foster parents may be professionals (such as retired nurses) or paraprofessionals trained to care for children who have complex medical needs or are dependent on some sort of technology.

Foster parents should participate throughout the process of evaluations and IFSP development and implementation. They should be skilled in the daily caregiving for the child and responsible for seeing that the child's medical needs are addressed. Training manuals and procedures have been developed to help foster parents meet the needs of children with medical needs (Moffitt, Reiss, & Nackashi, 1991).

Obviously, children in foster care have experienced some family situation that seemed so serious as to require the child's placement out of the home. Children with moderate to high levels of health needs are best served by this model. Although medical foster care does not inherently address a child's developmental needs, a developmental component should certainly be provided.

A barrier to the expansion of medical foster care is its limited availability in both urban and rural areas. Many children with medical needs live in hospitals or residential group care situations although they would be more appropriately served in a home setting. A lack of trained foster care parents consigns them to "boarder baby" status. A major training initiative needs to be implemented to expand the number and skills of caregivers for children with medical complexities so that these children might be raised in a home setting.

SUMMARY OF THE SERVICE OPTIONS

Home visiting is a flexible, relatively low-cost (compared to center-based) approach to providing support or education for families of children with special needs. It is a method that meets the parent(s) at a place of their choice and on their level. Home visitors with different professional backgrounds can provide individualized help specific to each child's needs. However, a home visit program may not meet working families' needs for child care nor can it be a means of providing a very intensive intervention. Arranging for a child's placement in a quality family day care home through supporting the provider and the parent is a way to combine two options that are based in normalized settings—the home and a family day care home. An infant or toddler with disabilities may place special demands on a family provider, requiring additional training and perhaps better adult–child ratios than would otherwise have been offered in that family day care home. In North Carolina, family day care providers of children whose care is state and federally subsidized can receive up to 70% more than the typical fee, funds that should allow the provider to operate profitably with one fewer child (therefore, better ratios) or might allow an additional caregiver to be hired. Either way, the child with special needs benefits from better quality care.

Neither home visiting nor placement in specially trained, family day care homes can provide the breadth or intensity of services that children with moderate to severe disabilities sometimes need, such as special therapies, health services, or significant amounts of cognitive stimulation. Although these "extra" services could be added to ongoing programs, they are typically provided in other types of clinics or center-based programs, places where a parent might also more readily find additional support or counseling. Because home visiting and family day care homes so well achieve the principle of family-centeredness and because they are relatively inexpensive, continued enhancement and expansion of these models to meet the needs of infants and toddlers with established conditions or risks is recommended.

Parent–child centers typically provide a relatively low-intensity intervention via group activities with parents and infants for a few hours a week, but the group leader is usually a skilled interventionist, and ancillary therapies and counseling are often readily available through such programs. Thus, parent–child centers comprise a model that can adequately serve children with a range of disabilities and can enable their parents to be better teachers of the children. However, it is not a model that meets the child care needs of most working families and may be seen by some as yet another demand on their time rather than a support.

Developmental child care programs that include children with special needs provide a normalized experience for infants and toddlers and meet working parents' needs for child care. Whether serving just a few children with special needs in a general population child care center or a few children with typical needs in a reverse mainstreaming program, the real key is the developmental appropriateness of the program. Research shows that many typical child care programs and developmental day programs do not meet the best standards of care and education (Whitebook, Howes, & Phillips, 1989). When they do meet standards of developmental appropriateness, however, these programs can provide services to children with a broad range of disabilities. Some children with more severe or medically complex needs often require additional supports or attention if they are to succeed in child care programs.

Children whose fragile health makes them susceptible to infections are usually better served in smaller groups than those found in most center-based programs. Mechanisms to provide the needed ancillary services are often not available and funding such services becomes a problem. To meet family needs for support, information, and parenting-skills training, some center-based programs employ social workers, early interventionists, or others whose focus is on the families of children with disabilities. Many programs lack funding for coordinating or providing such services, so these family needs may go unmet.

Even if the availability of community-based and normalized options improves, some children may still need out-of-home services such as provided in hospital nurseries or medical foster care. Three conditions should be met when providing such services:

1. During the time of medical or specialized care, whether a short or extended period, opportunities for normal experiences should be provided when possible.
2. Parents should be involved as fully as possible in the decision making and supports should be provided to them as needed.
3. Movement of the child to less restricted surroundings should be a goal of the program, for example, through training the parents or foster parents to meet the child's medical needs in a home setting.

THE BEST OPTION: MAKING THE DECISION

Most children with special needs and their families could benefit from the general range of services as described so far in this chapter, although a few will need specialized, customized services. The services needed by some families will cost little, while other families will need services that are quite expensive. Some families will relocate in order to obtain the best services for their child, while others will be happy with a convenient, neighborhood program. Which options are best for particular children and families? And how can families be assured input in the decision-making process?

Decisions regarding our current early intervention service system have been built almost solely around the disability of the child and the funding available. This emphasis upon diagnosis of educational and behavioral deficits has produced programs designed primarily to eliminate the most obvious deficiencies. Assessment instruments focusing on children, with little, if any, consideration of the family context have led to interventions for the child provided in isolation from the family. University-based training programs related to early intervention have traditionally focused on fixing deficits in the child rather than enhancing competencies for their caregivers.

Family-driven decisions regarding early intervention are isolated cases rather than an established process. A recent Florida study of early intervention programs found that services offered were generally a result of the staff available rather than the needs of the child/family (Herrington, 1989). Available services tend to drive the service plan. For example, in many communities, options for infants and toddlers with sensory impairments are limited to home-based programs or twice-weekly intervention groups regardless of the family's need or preference for other options. Long waiting lists for services give families "choices" between the available service option or no services.

In many communities, funding sources do not allow for options of service delivery. For example, the funding of some educational programs has been jeopardized when integrated program options were planned, because children with disabilities are only allowed to be taught by special educators.

A New Decision-Making Process

How can the decision-making process be changed so that families can choose the service model? Ideally, interventions are chosen by the family to meet the needs of both the child and family, instead of services being chosen to fit the needs of service deliverers bound by the dictates of bureaucracy. Part H offers every state the opportunity to redesign the system to create more responsive, effective, and efficient services driven by both child and family need. New, or at least expanded, configurations or models of services must be developed as a result of the expanded population of children to be served, new etiologies of disabilities, an emphasis on prevention, and recognition of the impact of the family environment.

By definition of law, parent choice is a key element of the service system. The importance of this requirement is supported by recent research by Affleck and colleagues (Affleck, Tennen, & Rowe, 1991; Affleck, Tennen, Rowe, Roscher, & Walker, 1989). In a supportive, weekly home visit intervention for the parents of medically fragile infants as they made the transition to home, trained home visitors followed a consultation model of helping rather than a parent training or infant curriculum model. They listened to mothers talk about a wide range of concerns, provided support, and gave information about infant development and caregiving when needed. For mothers who had reported in the hospital that they desired a high level of support, the program improved their perceptions of control, sense of competence, and responsiveness to their infants. However, for mothers who said they needed little support, participation in the home visit program actually had negative effects on these outcomes. The authors surmise that for mothers reporting a low need for support, the information and support that they did not actively seek may have disrupted their positive view of their child's condition and caused them to question their parenting competence. Affleck concludes they would have been better served by being allowed full choice. And even if they never use a particular service system, perhaps parents derive some benefit just from knowing that help is available.

In an improved decision-making process, a child's developmental and health needs and the family's priorities would enter into decisions about the array of services, and these decisions would be made by the family and the intervention team. Children with severe impairments, autism, or spina bifida will need an intensive array of interventions whereas a relatively healthy low-birth-weight infant recently discharged from a neonatal intensive care unit (NICU) may need only routine stimulation and developmental monitoring. A child with complex medical needs may require a level of nursing care, but some medical routines, such as shunt monitoring, can be learned by parents and childcare providers. Some families can consistently and appropriately meet the needs of their child when provided information and minimal outside support. Other parents need significant help themselves, for example, counseling, job training, education, and drug or alcohol treatment. In planning individual child and family service delivery options, information should be integrated by the multidisciplinary team, with family input, into recommendations for a holistic plan of services, addressing issues of intensity, duration, and array of services needed. Other compelling factors might also be considered. The team and family would consider the options and the service coordinator would attempt to accommodate the family's preference of service delivery. One method for accomplishing this task is through the use of the *System to Plan Early Childhood Services* (SPECS) (Bagnato & Neisworth, 1990). This tool helps the evaluation team, including the family, convert assessment information into ratings in order to arrive at consensus regarding service priorities, intensity, and service delivery options (see Bagnato, Neisworth, & Munson, Chapter 7, this volume).

Array of Services

With input from the child's family and the multidisciplinary team, the IFSP must specify the "nature and extent of early intervention services that are needed" (Part H, Section 303.322[2][iii]). This may include the array of services (defined in Part H), the intensity, and duration of services needed. As listed in Figure 9.2, these services to be entitled are predominantly child-focused. However, from case studies and clinical experience, we know that the services required by Part H do not meet the holistic needs of the child/family. Meeting the environmental needs of the family and the biological conditions of the child must be addressed concurrently if intervention is to be most effective. Other services frequently identified as needed for families of children with disabilities are also listed on the chart. Provisions in Part H encourage that these other, related family supports also be identified on the IFSP.

Initiation and Duration of Services

Much debate has centered on the issue of when early intervention should begin. Research does show that the earlier the intervention—at birth or soon after—and the earlier the diagnosis of a disability or risk status, the greater the developmental gains and the less likelihood of later problems (Garland, Stone, Swanson, & Woodruff, 1981).

Experts generally agree that earlier is better and that prevention is always preferable to rehabilitation. Yet most of our programs require the condition to have manifested—whether it is abuse, HIV infection, or a specific disabil-

Part H Services (required by law)	Optional Part H Services	Other Services (not required)
• audiology	• developmental child care	• housing
• assistive technology	• medical child care	• educational opportunities and vocational training
• family training, counseling and home visits	• medical foster care	
• therapeutic foster care/shelter care	• family planning
• family assessment		• family therapy
• health services (only in order to benefit from other intervention)	• other health services	• culturally relevant special services
• family support (respite, homemaker, parent-to-parent)	• family unification services
• intake – screening		• environmental adaptations for special needs (i.e., wheelchair ramp)
• medical services (only for diagnostic or evaluation)	• play/psychosocial therapy for children with emotional problems	
• multidisciplinary evaluation		• legal services
• nursing services		• comprehensive drug treatment
• nutrition services		
• psychological services		• medications
• service coordination		• dental services
• service planning (IFSP, IEP)		• after-school care
• training and professional support for early childhood, early intervention, and social support staff
• special instruction		
• social work services		
• therapy services (occupational, physical and speech/language)		• outreach programs that make extended effort to locate children and families
• transportation services		
• vision services		

FIGURE 9.2. Definition of potential services for infants and toddlers and their families. Reprinted, by permission, from Graham and Stone (1991).

ity. An expanded view of the decision-making process includes not only treatment of established conditions but early identification of risk factors and preventative services.

The duration or length of intervention depends upon the condition of the child and the preferences of the family. Interventions provided for relatively short durations (1–6 months) might include short-term monitoring for health-related concerns such as NICU newborns, injuries, or other acute, temporary, or short-term conditions (e.g., to prevent delays following surgery, trauma, or injury). Other short-term interventions might include educating or intervening with families during periods of stress or crisis (e.g., pregnant teens) or monitoring substance-exposed babies and other children at risk for abuse or neglect. The primary purpose of such interventions is to improve outcomes and minimize developmental decline during a limited period.

Some children and families will require long-term interventions to minimize developmental decline and to maximize positive outcomes, for example, children with chronic conditions such as sensory impairments, brain damage, or AIDS, or children requiring complex medical or technological care. Some families will require long-term interventions as well, for example, parents with mental retardation or families with violence- or alcohol-related problems.

Duration or continuity of services is critical to the effectiveness of interventions as illustrated by Head Start and Follow-Through (the school-age follow-up of Head Start), which found that developmental gains are more likely to be sustained if some form of support continues. Often, however, interruptions of services occur in our current system at the end of the fiscal year when funds run low or during vacations in the traditional school calendar. Efforts should be made to prevent premature cessation of services.

Intensity of Services

The intensity of any given intervention must match each child's and family's needs. Intensity of early intervention services can be defined according to the purpose of the service, the level of expertise required, and the amount of service provided. The question of how much service is needed can be answered only by evaluating all variables, including the developmental needs, health-related concerns, and supports required. For example, a child with spina bifida may have a developmental need (physical therapy), health-related needs (orthopedic surgeries), and support needs (respite, family training). These needs are likely to be greatest in the first years of life, with intensity later tapering off. For another child with spina bifida, however, another combination of services may be required. Because of the wide diversity of impairments within a particular disability, the intensity of services needed must be determined individually.

Although services may be required in the long term, often the intensity will vary with the changing needs of the child and/or family. Similarly, families' levels of need for services will differ, according to their behavior, financial status, education, values, and social support system. Just as for children, families will have varying needs for support or education. The decision-making process must attempt to match these varying levels of need to the appropriate services, rather than assuming that all children and families with disabilities need the same level of service.

The purpose of a program affects intensity. The purpose may be to promote the child's development, coordinate the appropriate therapy, involve the parent in the treatment, and offer support to the family. Therefore, multiple services may be provided. For example, a home visitor may provide hands-on programming (early intervention services) with the child while demonstrating to the parent (parent education) and simultaneously coordinating services (case management). Of course, if the purposes of intervention are multiple, provision of a combination of services will increase intensity. For example, low-birth-weight babies born to teenage, drug-addicted mothers could benefit from many services, such as parent training, child care, respite care, drug rehabilitation, and vocational training, in addition to infant intervention.

The personnel necessary to provide early intervention services can vary widely in level of skill and expertise: from minimally trained but highly effective community resource mothers serving pregnant teens to skilled nurses providing daily care for a child dependent on a ventilator. Even within disciplines, a range of expertise (and correspondingly, cost) exists, such as levels of therapists, therapy assistance, and therapy aides.

Programs for high-risk infants that provide more contact time (actual hours with the child and/or family) generally tend to be more successful than programs with less contact time (Ramey, Bryant, & Suarez, 1987). For example, the Milwaukee Project, the Carolina Abecedarian Project, and Project CARE, intervention programs for high-risk children involving hundreds of hours of center-based intervention and contact time, all produced significant cognitive gains. However, a meta-analysis of 74 early intervention studies (Casto & Mastropieri, 1986; Casto & White, 1985) concluded that although contact time (either total hours or hours per week) is a critical variable for disabled populations, it is not for high-risk disadvantaged populations. Recent findings in a home visit program, however, show that outcomes are positively related to intensity with better results from weekly home visits than biweekly or monthly (Powell & Grantham-McGregor, 1989). Because the research does not provide definitive answers, it seems that the intensity and length of an early intervention program should be individualized according to the child's and family's needs and priorities.

Other compelling factors may also influence service decisions, including other child, family, or community conditions. These might include environmental factors such as living in a high-crime or violent neighborhood, being exposed to environmental toxins, or living in the same household with an abusive relative. A community-wide measles outbreak might become a compelling biological factor precluding, at least temporarily, the enrollment of a child with a suppressed immune system into a center-based intervention program.

Compelling factors could also be positive—a supportive extended family, an adoption, a move, or family reunification. The interaction of positive and negative family factors with child factors can codetermine a child's progress (see Kochanek, Chapter 3, this volume; Sameroff & Chandler, 1975). Cultural, ethnic, or religious factors may influence services as well. For example, Haitian healing beliefs may limit the usefulness of a conventional medical model of intervention.

Necessary Elements for a Coordinated Service System

The shift toward community-based care requires an organized network of coordinated services by private and voluntary agencies, federal, state, and local governments, and professional groups and associations. Because different agencies and organizations under different auspices operate hospitals, child care programs, family day care homes, and home visit programs, interagency collaboration and cooperation are critical to the success of an early intervention system (Garwood & Sheehan, 1989; Hutchins & McPherson, 1991). Formal interagency agreements need to identify specific expectations, roles, and responsibilities, as well as payment and administrative procedures (Elder, 1980).

Service coordination is a required component of the early intervention system and is the link between the child and family and the numerous programs that may be available to them. Even if the service system is fragmented, the case manager can overcome the complexity that would otherwise be daunting to the family (Miller, 1983). Service coordination involves assessing needs, developing service plans, coordinating and monitoring service delivery, and advocating on behalf of the needs and rights of the client (Minahan, 1987). Service coordinators work with families and local providers to help ensure comprehensive, responsive, and accessible services. Service coordination may also reduce gaps and duplicated services, and thus is a source of cost and quality control. Financing service coordination is a major challenge for families, communities, states, and the nation (see Clifford & Bernier, Chapter 14, this volume).

A comprehensive data collection system is required by Public Law 99-457. Although early intervention practitioners often grumble over the time required to complete paperwork, a high-quality data collection system can be efficient and extremely useful in documenting and identifying gaps in service programs, and, on the positive side, documenting progress towards meeting timetables of implementation and possibly identifying the successes of intervention. Past experiences should guide our current practices and the information system should be an ally of practitioners, not a burden. This requirement has been a difficult one for states to implement because of agency-specified forms and procedures, issues around confidentiality, and the sheer massiveness of a central reporting system.

SUMMARY

This chapter has described service delivery models, research on their effectiveness, and the level of needs best served by each. Service models are the result of the interactions of child health, development, family needs, services, and other compelling conditions. An inaccessible, separated service delivery system that forces families to go to multiple providers in order to meet their needs will not meet the letter or spirit of the law nor provide families with interventions that are likely to succeed.

In addition, the chapter described a new process for decision making so that early intervention services can integrate the full range of child *and* family needs and priorities. The hope is that by refining the decision-making process for intervention services, the lives of children will be improved, the choices for families increased, and the options for communities enhanced. Policy makers and providers will be better able to fulfill their desire to serve children effectively, and taxpayers will benefit through the improved cost-effectiveness resulting from matching need to service.

ACKNOWLEDGMENTS

This research was funded through Part H dollars in a grant from the Florida Department of Education, Bureau of Exceptional Students. This chapter is adapted from *Florida's Cost/Implementation Study: Vol. 7. Options for Delivery of Early Intervention Services: A New Approach to Decision-Making* by M. Graham as part of the Service Delivery Research Team headed by L. Stone. The research work was a collaborative project, interdependent upon the many individuals and groups that contributed their wisdom and guidance to this research effort.

REFERENCES

Affleck, G., Tennen, H., & Rowe, J. (1991). *Infants in crisis: How parents cope with newborn intensive care and its aftermath.* New York: Springer-Verlag.

Affleck, G., Tennen, H., Rowe, J., Roscher, B., & Walker, L. (1989). Effects of formal support on mothers' adaptation to the hospital-to-home transition of high-risk infants: The benefits and costs of helping. *Child Development, 60,* 488–501.

Andrews, S., Blumenthal, J., Johnson, D., Kahn, A., Ferguson, C., Lasater, T., Malone, P., & Wallace, D. (1982). The skills of mothering: A study of Parent Child Development Centers. *Monographs of the Society for Research in Child Development, 47*(6, Serial No. 198).

Atkinson, A. M. (1987). A comparison of mothers' and providers' preferences and evaluations of day care services. *Child and Youth Care Quarterly, 16*(1), 35–47.

Bagnato, S., Kontos, S., & Neisworth, J. (1987). Integrated day care as special education: Profiles of programs and children. *Topics in Early Childhood Special Education, 7*(1), 28–47.

Bagnato, S. J., & Neisworth, J. T. (1990). *System to Plan Early Childhood Services (SPECS).* Circle Pines, MN: American Guidance Service.

Bailey, D. B., Clifford, R. M., & Harms, T. (1982). Comparison of preschool environments for handicapped and non-handicapped children. *Topics in Early Child Special Education, 2,* 9–20.

Barrera, M. E., Rosenbaum, P. L., & Cunningham, C. E. (1986). Early home intervention with low-birth-weight infants and their parents. *Child Development, 57,* 20–33.

Barrera, M. E., Routh, D. K., Parr, C. A., Johnson, N. M., Arendshorst, D. S., Goolsby, E. L., & Schroeder, S. R. (1976). Early intervention with biologically handicapped infants and young children: A preliminary study with each child as his own control. In T. D. Tjossem (Ed.), *Intervention strategies for high-risk infants and young children* (pp. 609–627). Baltimore, MD: University Park Press.

Beckman-Bell, P. (1981). Child-related stress in families of handicapped children. *Topics in Early Childhood Special Education, 1,* 45–53.

Bidder, R. T., Bryant, G., & Gray, O. P. (1975). Benefits to Down's syndrome children through training their mothers. *Archives of Disease in Childhood, 50,* 383–386.

Blackard, M. K., & Barsh, E. T. (1982). Parents' and professionals' perceptions of the handicapped child's impact on the family. *TASH Journal, 7,* 62–70.

Brassel, W. R., & Dunst, C. J. (1978). Fostering the object construct: Large-scale intervention with handicapped infants. *American Journal of Mental Deficiency, 82,* 507–510.

Breslau, N., Salkever, D., & Staruch, K. (1982). Women's labor force activity and responsibilities for disabled dependents: A study of families with disabled children. *Journal of Health and Social Behavior, 23,* 169–183.

Bryant, D., Ramey, C., Sparling, J., & Wasik, B. (1986). The Carolina approach to responsive education: A model for day care. *Topics in Early Childhood Special Education, 7*(1), 48–60.

Bureau of Labor Statistics. (1988, September 7). *News.* Washington, DC: U.S. Department of Labor.

Bureau of the Census. (1987). *Who's minding the kids?* Current Population Reports, Series P-70, No. 9. Washington, DC: U.S. Department of Commerce.

Casto, G., & Mastropieri, M. A. (1986). The efficacy of early intervention programs: A meta-analysis. *Exceptional Children, 52,* 417–424.

Casto, G., & White, K. (1985). An integrative review of early intervention efficacy studies with at-risk children: Implications for the handicapped. *Analysis and Intervention in Developmental Disabilities, 5,* 7–31.

Collins, R. C. (1993). Head Start: Steps toward a two-generation program strategy. *Young Children, 48*(2), 25–33, 72–73.

Deiner, P. L., Whitehead, L. C., & Peters, D. L. (1989). *Delaware FIRST: Family/infant resources, supplemental training: Final report to the handicapped children's early education program* (Project No. 024MH70006, Grant No. GOO8630267). Washington, DC: U.S. Department of Education.

Drotar, D., Baskiewicz, A., Irwin, N., Kennell, J., & Klaus, M. (1975). The adaptation of parents to the birth of an infant with a congenital malformation: A hypothetical model. *Pediatrics, 56,* 710–717.

Dunst, C. J., & Leet, H. (1987). Measuring the adequacy of resources in households with young children. *Child: Care, Health and Development, 13,* 111–125.

Dunst, C. J., Leet, H., & Trivette, C. M. (1988). Family resources, personal well-being, and early intervention. *Journal of Special Education, 22,* 108–116.

Dunst, C. J., & Trivette, C. M. (1986). Looking beyond the parent–child dyad for the determinants of maternal styles of interaction. *Infant Mental Health Journal, 7,* 69–80.

Dunst, C. J., & Trivette, C. M. (1987). Enabling and empowering families: Conceptual and intervention issues. *School Psychology Review, 16,* 443–456.

Dunst, C. J., & Trivette, C. M. (1988). A family systems model of early intervention with handicapped and developmentally at-risk children. In D. Powell (Ed.), *Parent education as early childhood intervention: Emerging directions in theory, research, and practice* (pp. 131–180). New York: Ablex.

Dunst, C. J., & Trivette, C. M. (1990). Assessment of social support in early intervention programs. In S. J. Meisels & J. P. Shonkoff (Eds.), *Handbook of early childhood intervention* (pp. 326–349). New York: Cambridge University Press.

Dunst, C. J., Trivette, C. M., & Deal, A. G. (1988). *Enabling and empowering fmailies: Principles and guidelines for practice.* Cambridge, MA: Brookline Books.

Elder, J. O. (1980). Writing interagency agreements. In J. O. Elder & P. R. Magrab (Eds.), *Coordinating services to handicapped children: A handbook for interagency collaboration.* Baltimore, MD: Paul H. Brookes.

Evans, J. (1976). *Identification and supplementary instruction for handicapped children in a regular bilingual program.* Paper presented at the Annual Meeting of the American Educational Research Association, San Francisco. (ERIC Document Reproduction Service No. ED 123 891.)

Fewell, R. R. (1986). Child care and the handicapped child. In N. Gunzenhauser & B. M. Caldwell (Eds.), *Johnson & Johnson Pediatric Round Table Series: Vol. 12. Group care for young children: Considerations for child care and health professionals, public policy makers, and parents* (pp. 35–47). Skillman, NJ: Johnson & Johnson.

Gabel, H., & Kotsch, L. S. (1981). Extended families and young handicapped children. *Topics in Early Childhood Education, 1,* 29–36.

Garber, H. L. (1988). *The Milwaukee Project: Preventing mental retardation in children at risk.* Washington, DC: American Association on Mental Retardation.

Garland, C., Stone, N. W., Swanson, J., & Woodruff, G. (Eds.). (1981). *Early intervention for children with special needs and their families.* Monmouth, OR: WESTAR.

Garwood, S. G., & Sheehan, R. (1989). *Designing a comprehensive early intervention system: The challenge of Public Law 99-457.* Austin, TX: Pro-Ed.

Gordon, I. J., & Guinagh, B. J. (1978, March). *Middle school performance as a function of early stimulation: Final report to the Administration for Children, Youth and Families* (Project No. NIH-HEW-OCD-90-C-908). Gainesville, FL: University of Florida, Institute for Development of Human Resources; and Chapel Hill, NC: University of North Carolina, School of Education.

Graham, M. A., & Stone, L. (1991). Service delivery and design study: Options for delivery of early intervention services: New approach to decision making. In *Florida's cost/implementation study for Public Law 99-457, Part H, Infants and Toddlers: Phase II findings*. Tallahassee, FL: Florida State University Center for Prevention and Early Intervention Policy.

Grubb, W. N. (1988). *Choices for children: Policy options for state provision of early childhood programs*. Paper prepared for the Education Commission of the States. Palo Alto, CA: Stanford University School of Education.

Halpern, R. (1984). Lack of effects for home-based early intervention? Some possible explanations. *American Journal of Orthopsychiatry, 54*(1), 33–42.

Halpern, R. (1990). Community-based early intervention. In S. J. Meisels & J. P. Shonkoff (Eds.), *Handbook of early chidlhood intervention* (pp. 469–498). New York: Cambridge University Press.

Hanson, M. J., & Hanline, M. F. (1989). Integration options for the very young child. In R. Gaylord-Ross (Ed.), *Integration strategies for students with handicaps* (pp. 177–193). Baltimore, MD: Paul H. Brookes.

Hanson, M. J., & Schwarz, R. H. (1978). Results of a longitudinal intervention program for Down's syndrome infants and their families. *Education and Training of the Mentally Retarded, 13*, 403–407.

Hayes, C. D., Palmer, J. L., & Zaslow, M. J. (1990). *Who cares for America's children: Child care policy for the 1990s*. Washington, DC: National Academy Press.

Head Start Bureau, Administration on Children, Youth, and Families. (1991). *Comprehensive Child Development Program—A national family support demonstration* (First Annual Report) (DHHS Publ. No. [ACF] 92-31267). Washington, DC: CSR Inc.

Herrington, C. (1989). *A census of early intervention providers in Florida*. Tallahassee, FL: Center for Policy Studies in Education.

Hofferth, S. L., & D. A. Phillips. (1987). Child care in the United States: 1970–1995. *Journal of Marriage and the Family, 49*, 559–571.

Huefner, D. S. (1988). The consulting teacher model: Risks and opportunities. *Exceptional Children, 54*, 403–414.

Hutchins, V. L., & McPherson, M. (1991). National agenda for children with special health needs: Social policy for the 1990s through the 21st century. *American Psychologist, 46*, 141–143.

Infant Health and Development Program. (1990). Enhancing the outcomes of low birth weight, premature infants: A multisite randomized trial. *Journal of the American Medical Association, 263*, 3035–3042.

Johnson, D. L., & Walker, T. (1991). A follow-up evaluation of the Houston Parent–Child Development Center: School performance. *Journal of Early Intervention, 15*, 226–236.

Jones, S., & Meisels, S. (1987). Training family day care providers to work with special needs children. *Topics in Early Childhood Special Education, 3*, 1–12.

Kahn, A., & Kamerman, S. (1987). *Child care: Facing the hard choices*. Dover, MA: Auburn House.

Katz, K. S. (1993). Project Headed Home: Intervention in the pediatric intensive care unit for infants and their families. *Infants and Young Children, 5*, 67–75.

Klein, N., & Sheehan, R. (1987). Staff development: A key issue in meeting the needs of young handicapped children in day care settings. *Topics in Early Childhood Special Education, 7*(1), 13–27.

Leibowitz, A., Waite, L., & Witsberger, C. (1988). Child care for preschoolers: Differences by child's age. *Demography, 25*(2), 205–220.

Madden, J., O'Hara, J., & Levenstein, P. (1984). Home again: Effects of the Mother–Child Home Program on mother and child. *Child Development, 55*, 636–647.

McWilliam, R. A. (1992). Predictors of service delivery models in center-based early intervention. *Dissertation Abstracts International, 5309A*, 3171.

McWilliam, R. A., & Strain, P. S. (1993). Service delivery models. In *DEC recommended practices: Indicators of quality in programs for infants and young children with special needs and their families* (pp. 39–48). Reston, VA: Council for Exceptional Children.

Meisels, S. J., & Provence, S. (1989). *Identifying and assesing disabled and developmentally vulnerable young children and their families: Recommended guidelines.* Washington, DC: National Center for Clinical Infant Programs.

Miller, G. E. (1983). Case management: The essential service. In C. J. Sanborn (Ed.), *Case management in mental health services* (pp. 3–15). New York: Haworth.

Minahan, A. (Ed.). (1987). *Encyclopedia of social work* (18th ed.). Silver Spring, MD: National Association of Social Work.

Moffitt, K., Reiss, J., & Nackashi, J. (Eds.). (1991). *Special children, special care.* University of South Florida, Florida Diagnostic and Learning Resources System; University of Florida, Institute for Child Health Policy; and the Florida Developmental Disabilities Planning Council, Family Network on Disablities. (Available from University of South Florida Bookstore, 4202 E. Fowler Avenue, Tampa, FL 33620-6550.)

Moxley-Haegert, L., & Serbin, L. A. (1983). Developmental education for parents of delayed infants: Effects on parental motivation and children's development. *Child Development, 54*, 1324–1331.

Neisworth, J. T., & Madle, R. A. (1975). Normalized day care: A philosophy and approach to integrating exceptional and normal children. *Child Care Quarterly, 4*(3), 163–171.

Peck, C. A., Apolloni, T., Cooke, T. P., & Raver, S. (1978). Teaching retarded preschool children to imitate nonhandicapped peers: Training and generalized effects. *Journal of Special Education, 12*, 195–207.

Powell, C., & Grantham-McGregor, S. (1989). Home visiting of varying frequency and child development. *Pediatrics, 84*, 157–164.

Powell, D. R. (1990). Home visiting in the early years: Policy and program design decisions. *Young Children, 45*(6), 65–73.

Raab, M., Davis, M., & Trepanier, A. M. (1993). Resources versus services: Changing the focus of intervention for infants and young children. *Infants and Young Children, 5*(3), 1–11.

Ramey, C. T., Bryant, D. M., Sparling, J. J., & Wasik, B. H. (1985). Project CARE: A comparison of two early intervention strategies to prevent retarded development. *Topics in Early Childhood Special Education, 1*, 1–9.

Ramey, C. T., Bryant, D. M., & Suarez, T. M. (1987). Early intervention: Why, for whom, how, at what cost? In N. Gunzenhauser (Ed.), *Johnson & Johnson Pedi-*

atric Round Table Series: Vol. 13. Infant stimulation (pp. 170–180). Skillman, NJ: Johnson & Johnson.

Ramey, C. T., Bryant, D. M., Wasik, B. H., Sparling, J. J., Fendt, K. H., & LaVange, L. M. (1992). The Infant Health and Development Program for low birthweight, premature infants: Program elements, family participation, and child intelligence. *Pediatrics, 3,* 454–465.

Research Institute on Preschool Mainstreaming. (1990). *Policy and practice papers.* Pittsburgh, PA: Allegheny Research Institute.

Resnick, M. B., Eyler, F. E., Nelson, M. D., Eitzman, D. V., & Buccizrelli, R. L. (1987). Developmental intervention for low-birth weight infants: Improved early developmental outcome. *Pediatrics, 80,* 68–74.

Roberts, R. N., & Wasik, B. H. (1990). Home visiting programs for families with children birth to three: Results of a national survey. *Journal of Early Intervention, 14*(3), 274–284.

Sameroff, A., & Chandler, M. J. (1975). Reproductive risk and the continuum of caretaking casualty. In F. D. Horowitz, M. Hetherington, S. Scarr-Salapatek, & G. Seigel (Eds.), *Review of child development research* (Vol. 4, pp. 187–244). Chicago: University of Chicago Press.

Scarr, S., & McCartney, K. (1988). Far from home: An experimental evaluation of the Mother–Child Home Program in Bermuda. *Child Development, 59,* 531–543.

Stone, C. (1989, Fall). Kids are kids: Integrated day care works. *Family Support Bulletin,* 8–9.

Wasik, B. H., Bryant, D., & Lyons, C. (1990). *Home visiting: Procedures for helping families.* Newbury Park, CA: Sage.

Wasik, B. H., Ramey, C. T., Bryant, D. M., & Sparling, J. J. (1990). A longitudinal study of two early intervention strategies: Project CARE. *Child Development, 61,* 1682–1696.

Wasik, B. H., & Roberts, R. N. (1989). Home visiting with low income families. *Family Resource Coalition Report, 9,* 8–9.

Weiss, H., & Halpern, R. (1988). *Community-based family support and education programs: Something old or something new?* New York: Columbia University, National Resource Center for Children in Poverty.

Wesley, P., & Arnn, L. (1991). *Day care home training manual.* Chapel Hill, NC: Frank Porter Graham Child Development Center.

Whitebook, M., Howes, C., & Phillips, D. (1989). *Who cares? Child care teachers and the quality of care in America: Executive summary national child care staffing study.* Oakland, CA: Child Care Employee Project.

Wiener, L., Moss, H., Davidson, R., & Fair, C. (1992). Pediatrics: The emerging psychosocial challenges of the AIDS epidemic. *Child and Adolescent Social Work Journal, 9,* 381–407.

Wolfe, B., & Herwig, J. (Eds.). (1986). *The Head Start Home Visitor Handbook.* Portage, WI: Portage Project.

CHAPTER 10

Strategies for Creating Inclusive Early Childhood Settings

MARY FRANCES HANLINE
KIM GALANT

Young children with disabilities and developmental delays often receive early intervention services in center-based programs. When developed over 20 years ago, center-based programs usually were designed to serve only children who were developing atypically. However, in increasing numbers, children are receiving early intervention services in community child care/early education settings shared with nondisabled children. Opportunities for children with disabilities and developmental delays to learn alongside their nondisabled peers in such settings have been provided through a variety of mainstream and integration models. In general, "mainstreaming" refers to the placement of children in programs that primarily serve nondisabled children; "reverse mainstreaming" (or integrated special education) refers to including nondisabled children in programs designed for children with disabilities. The term "integration" is a more generic term that refers to any type of interaction between children with and without disabilities (McLean & Hanline, 1990; Odom & McEvoy, 1988).

In recent years, the concept of full inclusion has been replacing that of mainstreaming and integration for several reasons. According to Stainback and Stainback (1992),

> First, the concept of inclusion is being adopted because it more accurately and clearly communicates what is needed—children need to be included in the educational and social life of their neighborhood schools and classrooms, not merely placed in the mainstream. Second, the term integration is being abandoned since it implies that the goal is to integrate someone or some group back into the mainstream of school and community

life who has been excluded. The basic goal should be to not leave anyone out of the mainstream of school life in the first place, either education-ally, physically, or socially. (pp. 3–4)

Further, an inclusive setting does not focus solely on the child with dis-abilities, but builds a system in which "everyone belongs, is accepted, sup-ports, and is supported by his or her peers and other members of the school community in the course of having his or her educational needs met" (Stain-back & Stainback, 1990, p. 3).

For the very young child for whom the idea of neighborhood schools is inappropriate, inclusion may refer to children with disabilities and develop-mental delays being supported in community child care/early education pro-grams that are selected by families. That is, parents select a child care/early education program based on a number of factors including the reputation, location, cost, and philosophy of the program, and perhaps their past expe-riences with it. This process helps assure that child care/early education set-tings have a natural proportion of children with disabilities. Natural propor-tion means that the percentage of children with disabilities enrolled in each setting is similar to the proportion of persons with disabilities in the general population. The principle of natural proportion is a fundamental assump-tion of inclusive environments (Stainback & Stainback, 1992) and helps assure that a normalized environment is maintained when children with disabilities are integrated into typical settings along with nondisabled peers.

Educating young children with and without disabilities together has been supported by legal–legislative, social–ethical, and psychological–educational arguments (Bricker, 1978; Turnbull & Turnbull, 1990). Legal–legislative argu-ments center around judicial decisions and legislative acts that uphold the right of citizens with disabilities aged 3 to 21 to an appropriate public educa-tion in their least restrictive environment, the right of infants and toddlers to receive early intervention services in natural environments, and the right of persons with disabilities to participate fully in all aspects of society. The recent passage of the Americans with Disabilities Act (ADA) reaffirms these rights, prohibiting child care centers and family child care homes from discrimina-tion in enrollment based on a child's disability. Child care providers are now required to take "readily achievable" steps to accommodate the needs of chil-dren with disabilities (Surr, 1992).

Social–ethical arguments are based on the humane treatment of persons with disabilities, the detrimental effects of segregation, and the potential for changing negative societal attitudes toward persons with disabilities. Psycho-logical–educational arguments center around the benefits that children with disabilities and developmental delays could derive from observing and inter-acting with their nondisabled peers. Further, inclusive settings may encour-age the delivery of services that "promote the potential for 'normal' rather than 'disabled' routines," as suggested by the Division for Early Childhood (1993, p. 40).

Early intervention philosophy of the 1990s supports the provision of center-based services within full inclusion settings. According to Guralnick (1990), "early childhood mainstreaming is embedded well within a value system in which the terms inclusion, equity, full participation, and acceptance serve as a framework for program design" (p. 2). Providing specialized services within community child care/early education settings is supported by the principle of normalization, which maintains that any service provided to individuals with disabilities should be based on circumstances that are as culturally normative as possible (Wolfensberger, 1972). Further, services should be based on the doctrine of least restrictive alternative, which holds that government services must be provided in a way that results in the least infringement on individuals' rights (Taylor, 1988). In today's society, it is "normal" for parents to choose that their young children receive child care and to select the particular setting for their child. Thus, following the principles of normalization and least restrictive alternative, parent-chosen community child care/early education programs represent natural settings in which early intervention may occur. However, in order for community settings to be effective learning environments for children who are developing atypically, adaptations may need to be made.

The purpose of this chapter is to discuss programmatic variables and accommodations critical to creating inclusive child care/early education programs. Because there is no evidence that a child with a particular type or degree of disability is better suited for an integrated setting (Strain, 1990), inclusion refers to all children. Parental preference and sufficient child medical stability are the only prerequisites for inclusion (Chen, Hanline, & Friedman, 1989).

REVIEW OF RESEARCH

Over a decade of research has demonstrated that carefully planned, integrated early education programs resulted in increased learning opportunities for young children with disabilities and developmental delays and positive social, developmental, and attitudinal outcomes for young children without disabilities. In addition, when appropriate support and services are provided, parents and professionals report satisfaction with the integration process (Guralnick, 1990; McLean & Hanline, 1990; Odom & McEvoy, 1988).

Social Integration

Most preschool integration research has focused on social interactions between children with and without disabilities. The studies indicated that preschoolers with disabilities tended to be isolated from their nondisabled peers if inter-actions were left to chance. That is, nondisabled children communicated with nondisabled children more often than they communicated with peers with disabilities (e.g., Faught, Balleweg, Crow, & van den Pol, 1983) and chose nondisabled children as playmates and friends more often than they chose children with disabilities (e.g., Peterson, 1982; Strain, 1984). However, overt rejection of the children with disabilities is rare. In fact, nondisabled children adapt their verbal interactions in a way that ensures that children with devel-opmental delays will understand them (Guralnick & Paul-Brown, 1980) and are seen attempting to help and give affection to their peers with disabilities (Ipsa & Matz, 1978).

Despite potential positive outcomes of integration, physical integration of young children with disabilities does not necessarily result in their social integration. However, in most of the studies cited above, integration occurred only during certain times of the day and children with disabilities comprised more than half of the enrollment of each program. It may be that a full inclusion model that relies on the principle of natural proportion and/or that the shared experiences created by full inclusion provides the foundation for more social integration (Hanline, 1993a). Further, the current research knowl-edge base indicates that the greatest benefits to children in relation to social competence and friendship formation occur in programs serving primarily nondisabled children (Guralnick, 1990).

Developmental Outcomes for Children

Research has documented that both children with and without disabilities benefit from integration. That is, children with disabilities and developmen-tal delays make progress, and children without disabilities develop at the expected rate in integrated settings (Bricker, Bruder, & Bailey, 1982; Jenkins, Speltz, & Odom, 1985; Odom, Deklyen, & Jenkins, 1984). Further, studies have indicated that the learning that occurs in integrated settings may be more a function of the curriculum emphasis and quality of instruction than of integration alone (Cooke, Ruskus, Apolloni, & Peck, 1981; Jenkins, Odom, & Speltz, 1989).

Family Perspectives

Parents of children with disabilities and developmental delays, while able to identify potential positive outcomes of inclusion, often have concerns regard-ing the quality and provision of services, rejection of their child by both peers and adults, and the inability to share common interests with parents of nondis-abled children (Bailey & Winton, 1987; Hanline & Halvorsen, 1989; Winton,

Turnbull, & Blacher, 1985). Parents of nondisabled preschool children, while generally supportive of inclusion, express concern that regular educators may not be prepared adequately and that their children may imitate the child who is disabled. Parents of nondisabled young children also express the desire that their child's experiences be positive to facilitate the development of acceptance of individuals with disabilities (Green & Stoneman, 1989; Peck, Hayden, Wandschneider, Peterson, & Richarz, 1989).

Reactions of Service Providers

Service providers and parents tend to agree on issues related to inclusion. That is, they agree on the importance of integration to child development, of including parents in the process, and of careful planning for successful inclusion (Reichart, Lynch, Anderson, Svobodny, & Mercury, 1989). In addition, service providers tend to be supportive of the philosophical basis for inclusion (Blacher & Turnbull, 1982). Service providers who receive appropriate support and feel prepared and competent to meet the needs of children with disabilities and developmental delays generally report positive experiences with inclusion (Clark, 1974; Hanline, 1990).

CREATING INCLUSIVE CHILD CARE/
EARLY EDUCATION ENVIRONMENTS

The framework for creating inclusive environments includes (1) dedication to the philosophy that all children belong in the mainstream of community life, (2) an environment that reflects fair treatment of and mutual respect among children and adults, (3) instruction that accommodates the diverse characteristics and needs of all children, and (4) the provision of specialized services and supports within the mainstream. In addition, reliance on natural supports is fostered. That is, children are encouraged to learn through cooperative and collaborative ventures, assist and support each other, and share in decisions about their own learning. Further, service providers are encouraged to collaborate with each other, family members, and children to build a system that supports the development and competence of everyone (Stainback & Stainback, 1992).

The development and maintenance of inclusive learning environments presents challenges to everyone involved, and each setting presents a unique set of issues that must be addressed. Strategies that can be used to develop inclusive community child care/early education settings focus on gaining commitment to the service delivery model, establishing relationships with community agencies and professionals from a variety of disciplines, working in partnership with families, supporting child care providers/early educators, maintaining a learning environment that is developmentally appropriate, promoting respect for individual differences, developing adequate cost reimbursements, and accommodating the unique needs of each child. Many of these strategies are included as basic principles defining best practice in early intervention (Division for Early Childhood, 1993). That is, the use of family-centered approaches, transdisciplinary models, and interventions that are empirically and value driven, and developmentally and individually appropriate practices are indications of quality programs.

Appropriate Attitudes and Commitment

The commitment of parents and service providers to inclusion is critical (Striefel, Killoran, & Quintero, 1991). This commitment provides the foundation for the flexibility, creativity, and persistence often needed to explore and discover solutions to dilemmas. Strategies to help gain the commitment of involved persons include participation in workshops that include viewing videotapes of successful inclusion programs and discussions with individuals who have had positive experiences with inclusive settings. Opportunities to visit and to read about full inclusion child care/early education settings may be helpful. An open discussion about attitudinal and other potential barriers (ending with a plan of action to remove such barriers) may begin to establish commitment. In addition, personally meeting the children with disabilities and developmental delays who will be part of the inclusive setting may help persons unfamiliar with such children begin to accept and value the children.

Interagency Collaboration and Multidisciplinary Teaming

Creating inclusive environments for young children with disabilities and developmental delays requires the expertise and resources of service providers from a variety of disciplines and community agencies working in collaboration with families. Professionals who establish cooperative relationships with colleagues in their interagency network can serve as a resource to families by providing accurate information concerning the types of services and programs that are available in the community. They may also advocate for the rights of families within the service delivery system and set the stage for collaborative, responsive interactions with families. Cooperative interagency agreements help to alleviate frustrations that families often face when dealing with numerous agency personnel and may establish a continuum of service delivery options for families. Further, effective interagency collaboration allows for the redistribution of funds and services to meet the individual needs of the child and family (Hanline, 1993b; Sailor et al., 1989). In addition, by working together, agencies can join forces to educate and change community attitudes and values concerning the inclusion of people with disabilities in the mainstream of the community.

Quality services for all young children require programs staffed by well-trained personnel. Inclusive settings require staff to possess the knowledge and skills to work with both children with disabilities and children who are developing typically, as well as their families. The collaborative teaming of individuals from various disciplines brings expertise in different but complementary areas of service delivery that could provide a strong foundation for meeting the individual needs of children and families. As stated by Burton and colleagues, ". . . current service providers in each field could draw on the strengths of the other to gain competencies in providing early education services that are both age- and developmentally-appropriate and responsive to the unique needs of every individual child" (Burton, Hains, Hanline, McLean, & McCormick, 1992, p. 65).

However, effective interagency collaboration and multidisciplinary teaming requires commitment to the process and a willingness to work together to establish a climate of cooperation and trust. In addition, professionals must be willing to develop effective communication, problem-solving, and conflict-resolution skills, and demonstrate respect for the contributions of each discipline and agency (Flynn & Harbin, 1989; Spencer, 1989).

Supporting Child Care Providers/
Early Childhood Educators

Child care providers/early childhood educators are central in establishing quality inclusive early childhood settings (Allen, 1992; Hanline & Hanson, 1989). Inservice prior to the enrollment of a child with disabilities and developmental delays into a community child care/early education setting is often required. Regular early childhood educators have reported interest in learning about the developmental patterns of children with disabilities, the needs of the particular children who would be included in their setting, and how to manage the behavior of and teach children with disabilities (Hanline, 1990). Resources are available for inservice activities. Examples of resources include *Mainstreaming Works!* (Graham & Hanline, 1991), *Mainstreaming Young Children* (Wesley, 1992), *Special Children, Special Care* (Moffitt, Reiss, & Nackashi, 1991), and *Models of Interdisciplinary Training for Children with Handicaps* (Florida Department of Education, 1991). To be most effective, support should be ongoing, responsive to the needs of individual staff members, and directly address real-world concerns (Salend, 1984; Wang, Vaughan, & Dytman, 1985). Communication between family members, child care providers/early childhood educators, and other professionals can occur in a variety of ways, including (but not limited to) discussions at staff meetings, special scheduled meetings, staff development activities, brief daily conversations, and on-site demonstrations. Administrative support can help establish and facilitate time and resources for ongoing communication.

Collaboration with Families

An important ingredient in the successful inclusion of young children is partnerships between parents and service providers (Galant & Hanline, 1993). Partnership implies a long-term association between a professional and a family, whereby both contribute resources and expertise to enable them to make informed decisions to reach common goals (Paget, 1991). Creating partnerships with parents means encouraging them to be active participants in the process of assessment, intervention, and evaluation. To work collaboratively with parents, service providers must recognize parents' strengths, value their opinions and contributions, and support their role as decision-makers for the child and family. This approach to partnerships with families enables service providers to be sensitive to the needs, concerns, and priorities of all families, including those from diverse cultures. When parents and professionals work together, children benefit by having a comprehensive, appropriate, and consistent plan for services that is tailored to the individual strengths and needs of the child and family (see Duwa, Wells, & Lalinde, Chapter 5, this volume).

Shelton, Jeppson, and Johnson (1989) provided a comprehensive look at the components of collaboration with families and have developed checklists for implementation. Suggestions for effective partnerships include personal, agency, and policy commitments to the approach; conveniently scheduled meetings; reimbursement for parents' time, services, transportation, and child care expenses; meetings composed of equal numbers of parents and professionals; mechanisms for involving parents in inservice programs; training available for parents and professionals on collaboration and teaming; mechanisms for receiving information from parents and for disseminating information to them; and committees that represent parents of diverse cultural, economic, educational, and geographic backgrounds.

Developmentally Appropriate Environments

Learning environments that support the growth and development of all children begin with the premise that children learn through playful interactions with their physical and social environments. Play provides the context for discovery and practice of communication, social, cognitive, and motor skills. In play, children are free to master skills at their own rate, according to their interests and abilities, encouraging them to become self-motivated learners. In creating an environment to support children's play, professionals must plan activities with consideration for the developmental abilities of the children, while taking into account the unique experiences, learning styles, and preferences of each child. The role of the adult is to arrange the environment to support play, to encourage more sophisticated play, and respond to children's needs and attempts to communicate. Adults may provide guidance to assist children in making choices, provide assistance or prompts as needed to help children participate in an activity, or encourage social interactions (Bredekamp, 1991) (see Graham & Bryant, Chapter 11, this volume).

Service providers also must create an environment that celebrates diversity among children and that values and includes each child (Schaps & Solomon, 1990). Children with disabilities and developmental delays, children who are bilingual, children who are bicultural, and children who are different in other ways from the norm should find acceptance, respect, and understanding in their child care/early education setting. Adults must be conscious of their own views, aware of their own limited knowledge, and willing to explore with children the pluralistic nature of our society. In addition, nonsexist, antibias, and nonsterotyping materials and activities should be part of the daily activities and woven into all aspects of the curriculum. Children should have opportunities to learn about the diversity of human experience, as well as its common themes (Ramsey, 1983). Derman-Sparks and the A.B.C. Task Force (1989) provide excellent suggestions for implementing an antibias curriculum.

Facilitating Social Interactions

In inclusive child care/early education settings, nondisabled children and children with disabilities and developmental delays may need to be encouraged to play together. Social interactions between the two groups of children can be encouraged in many ways including teacher-mediated interventions, peer-mediated interventions, affection-training procedures, and correspondence training (McEvoy, Odom, & McConnell, 1992). In addition, various aspects of the social and physical environment may be organized to increase opportunities for social interactions (Hanline, 1985).

Teacher-mediated interventions require an adult to prompt and reinforce appropriate social behaviors. Some children may need assistance with basic social skills such as initiating interactions and/or responding to their friends' initiations. Other children may need to learn more advanced social skills such as sharing, helping, and playing cooperatively. When using teacher-mediated interventions, adults may praise social interactions that occur spontaneously with positive statements ("You two look like you are having fun playing together!"), touches, smiles, and other forms of reinforcement. In some situations, the teacher may need to set the stage for interactions to occur by asking specific children to play with each other, to take turns, or to share toys with each other. In other situations, a child may need adult assistance to gain entry into ongoing play activities. Adults can provide assistance at these times by modeling appropriate entry skills (e.g., asking to play with the others or offering a toy to the other children) or by asking the children who are already playing to invite the other child to join them. Although teacher-mediated interventions can be very effective, they must be used cautiously so that children do not develop reliance on adults. In addition, too much adult attention may interfere with the children's interactions, so adults must remember to remove themselves from the situation once the children have begun to play together.

Peer-mediated interventions utilize the skills of nondisabled children to provide instruction to the children with disabilities and developmental delays. Adults train the nondisabled children to assume this role, but do not actually intervene directly with the children who need assistance in learning social skills. When using this procedure, nondisabled children are taught (often through role playing with the adult) to initiate interactions with the children who have disabilities and to be persistent in obtaining a response. For example, they may be taught to offer a toy to a child with disabilities as a social initiation and taught to continue to offer the toy until the other child responds positively. Peer-mediated interventions have been effective in increasing social interactions of children with a variety of disabilities, but use of these procedures requires adults to spend time preparing the nondisabled children and to provide ongoing prompts and reinforcements to ensure that the nondisabled children are actually providing intervention.

Affection-training procedures are conducted during group activities that often occur in early childhood programs. Adults prompt children to display some type of affectionate behavior to other children. For example, children may play a game of Simon Says when children are told, "Simon says hug a friend." This type of training seems to result in increases in general social interactions in play situations and can be incorporated easily into the ongoing routine of a program. However, affection-training procedures seem to be most effective with children who already know how to interact socially, and they may be aversive to children who do not like physical contact with others.

"Say–do" correspondence training involves requiring children to state a behavior in which they plan to engage and then reinforcing them for engaging in the behavior. To encourage social interactions, nondisabled children may be requested to identify playing with a friend with disabilities as their behavior, then receive an appropriate reinforcement for engaging in that behavior.

In addition to the procedures described above, paying careful attention to various elements of the physical and social environment of a child care/

early education setting may encourage social interactions. For example, planning activities that require cooperation (e.g., painting a mural or making soup together), requiring children to share materials (e.g., a tub of crayons in the middle of the table rather than a separate box of crayons for each child), and serving snack and meals "family style" provides opportunity for interactions. Interactions also can be encouraged by being certain that children with disabilities and developmental delays are seated next to their nondisabled peers for group activities and that children who are unable to move independently are always positioned in ways that allow them to interact with nondisabled children. In addition, dolls and doll houses, blocks, balls, dishes, sectional trains, and other similar play materials promote more social interaction than do toys such as beads and string, puzzles, clay, and books.

Allowing the child who is disabled or developmentally delayed to lead activities, pass out materials, and be praised in front of peers helps the nondisabled children view the child with disabilities as a competent friend. Adults may need to teach and model appropriate ways of interacting with children with disabilities. For example, young children can learn to make eye contact with (or otherwise get the attention of) a child with a hearing impairment before speaking to her and to ask yes–no questions to a child who communicates through yes–no responses. In addition, adults promote an atmosphere of acceptance and respect through their own behavior. It is important that adults answer questions about disabilities honestly and openly, stress similarities (not differences) among the children, and convey the attitude that each child is equally appreciated.

MEETING INDIVIDUAL CHILD NEEDS

Individualized Planning Process

Federal legislation (Public Law 102-119) supports early intervention services for children birth through 5 years of age. The law requires a written plan detailing the goals or outcomes for a child and/or family. The Individualized Education Plan (IEP) for children 3 to 5 years of age and the Individualized Family Service Plan (IFSP) for children birth to 3 years of age are prepared through a process involving assessment of the child and family (if they choose) to identify concerns, priorities, and resources; development of goals and objectives; and identification of resources to accomplish the goals. Parents are an integral part of the team to assure that their concerns and priorities are addressed. In addition, service providers from multiple community agencies may be involved in the development and implementation of IEPs/IFSPs. For children receiving services in inclusive child care/early education settings, these documents will identify how the individual needs of children with disabilities and developmental delays can be met and families supported in the community settings. For example, the local school system may provide special education consultation to help determine instructional accommodations, a public health nurse may provide inservice regarding use and care of a catheter, Medicaid may pay for physical therapy, and the local chapter of The Arc (formerly called the Association for Retarded Citizens) may offer a parent support program.

Program Adaptations

Adapting to meet the individual needs of young children with disabilities and developmental delays in inclusive settings often requires few modifications to the curriculum for several reasons. First, materials for young children frequently can be used at varying developmental levels. Second, differences in the development of very young children who are developing atypically as compared to their nondisabled peers are often less obvious than when the children are older. In addition, children with disabilities and developmental delays usually follow the same sequence of development as nondisabled children and the majority experience mild to moderate disabilities and developmental delays thereby allowing them to benefit from and participate in the same activities as all other children. The challenge of making adaptations when needed, however, does not present a new challenge for early childhood teachers. Adjusting curriculum and teaching strategy to individual differences and developmental variations has long been the heart of early childhood education (Allen, 1992; Cook, Tessier, & Klein, 1992; Hanline & Hanson, 1989).

Accommodations most commonly needed to support the development of young children with disabilities and developmental delays center around adapting the physical environment, clarifying adult responsibilities, developing a flexible schedule, and adjusting adult–child interactions. In order to facilitate the inclusion of the children with disabilities, adaptations must be made with as little disruption to the regular curriculum as possible (Guralnick, 1981) and should be made in ways that do not isolate or stigmatize the child who is disabled (Hanline & Hanson, 1989).

Adapting the physical environment often involves using space differently and/or providing materials that children with disabilities can use as independently as possible. For example, additional space may be needed to accommodate adaptive equipment and children may need more space when using their equipment. If children are unsteady when walking, throw rugs and small items on the floor are dangerous. Ramps, bars in toilets, and special playground equipment may be needed to allow children access to and independence in the child care/early education setting. Children with visual disabilities may need additional or less lighting, depending on the type of visual impairment. Children with emotional disturbances may need a quiet place in which to be alone or in which to be held periodically throughout the day.

Larger crayons, puzzles pieces with knobs, extra water in the Play-Doh, and other adaptations may make participation by children with delays or differences in motor development easier. Boundaries between areas within a child care/early education setting may need to be highlighted to allow children with visual disabilities to see them and to allow children with behavior and learning difficulties to respond to them. In addition, space for teaming with family members and professionals from a variety of disciplines may need to be available.

Adults in inclusive settings may have to take on additional responsibilities, all of which must be clearly specified. For example, some children with disabilities and developmental delays are not toilet-trained as early as nondisabled children, may not eat independently, and may require medication throughout the day. Some children may not be able to hear a fire alarm, and some children will be unable to walk independently to a place of safety in an emergency. Well-developed emergency plans, as well as a daily schedule of responsibilities, are needed. For example, who is responsible for helping Cenon into a different position every hour? Who is responsible for Sally's 10 o'clock seizure medication? Which adult and peers will help Tamika during activity transitions? Who will feed Daniel? Who will turn the lights on and off to alert Lance that his snack is on the table if he is hungry?

Creative and flexible scheduling is also needed to accommodate the individual needs of all children. Some children with disabilities may need more rest time than other children and may need more time to eat, to walk from activity to activity, or to complete an activity. Often nondisabled peers or volunteers can assist when children with disabilities need assistance. Alternative activities may need to be available for some children as, for example, noisy activities may be painful or upsetting to children with neurological disabilities, bright environments may be painful to children with visual disabilities, and outdoor play in the summer may be too hot for children with certain health impairments. In addition, children with disabilities and developmental delays may not be able to tolerate group activities for the same length of time as nondisabled children. Creative and flexible scheduling also provides time for multidisciplinary teaming and for meeting with family members.

Interactions between adults and children may need to be adapted. Children with disabilities and developmental delays may need clearer and simpler directions (with verbal directions often combined with gestures) than nondisabled children of the same age, more repetitions of the same information in order to learn, and more time to process and respond to information. Adults may need to become familiar with alternative communication systems (e.g., sign language and computers) and may need to provide more language input to some children. For example, adults may need to identify the sound of footsteps in the hallway for children with severe visual disabilities and consistently label actions and objects for children with language and cognitive delays. In addition, adults must be alert and responsive to the nonsymbolic communicative attempts of children who do not yet communicate through verbalizations. Some children, particularly those with moderate to severe cognitive delays, may require systematic instruction to be embedded within the context of developmentally appropriate play-based activities (Hanline & Fox, 1993).

SUMMARY

Providing early intervention center-based services for young children with disabilities and developmental delays in inclusive child care/early education settings is supported by an extensive body of research, as well as by what has been defined as recommended practice by the Division for Early Childhood (1993). The effectiveness of such learning environments for promoting the growth and development of children with and without disabilities has been demonstrated repeatedly. The satisfaction of parents and service providers with such a service delivery model also has been documented through research. Values and principles surrounding the fair, humane, and respectful treatment of individuals with disabilities further support inclusion as a service delivery model. In inclusive settings, each child is viewed as an individual with needs for love, fulfillment, and respect. Building on natural supports available in a developmentally appropriate early childhood setting, all children are supported in their efforts to grow, learn, form relationships, and participate in the mainstream of community life.

REFERENCES

Allen, K. E. (1992). *The exceptional child: Mainstreaming in early childhood special education* (2nd ed.). Albany, NY: Delmar.

Bailey, D. B., & Winton, P. H. (1987). Stability and change in parents' expectations about mainstreaming. *Topics in Early Childhood Special Education, 7*(1), 61–72.

Blacher, J., & Turnbull, A. P. (1982). Teacher and parent perspectives on selected social aspects of preschool mainstreaming. *Exceptional Child, 29,* 191–199.

Bredekamp, S. (1991). *Developmentally appropriate practice in early childhood programs serving children from birth through age eight.* Washington, DC: National Association for the Education of Young Children.

Bricker, D. D. (1978). A rationale for the integration of handicapped and nonhandicapped preschool children. In M. Guralnick (Ed.), *Early intervention and the integration of handicapped and nonhandicapped children* (pp. 3–26). Baltimore, MD: University Park Press.

Bricker, D. D., Bruder, M. B., & Bailey, E. (1982). Developmental integration of preschool children. *Analysis and Intervention in Developmental Disabilities, 2,* 207–222.

Burton, C. G., Hains, A. H., Hanline, M. F., McLean, M., & McCormick, K. (1992). Early childhood intervention and education: The urgency of professional unification. *Topics in Early Childhood Special Education, 11*(4), 53–69.

Chen, D., Hanline, M. F., & Friedman, C. T. (1989). From playgroup to preschool: Facilitating early integration experiences. *Child: Care, Health and Development,* 15, 283–295.

Clark, E. A. (1974). Teacher attitudes toward integration of children with handicaps. *Education and Treatment of Children,* 11, 333–335.

Cook, R. E., Tessier, A., & Klein, M. D. (1992). *Adapting early childhood curricula for children with special needs* (3rd ed.). New York: Macmillan.

Cooke, T. P., Ruskus, J. A., Apolloni, T., & Peck, C. A. (1981). Handicapped preschool children in the mainstream: Background, outcomes, and clinical suggestions. *Topics in Early Childhood Special Education,* 1(1), 73–83.

Derman-Sparks, L., & the A.B.C. Task Force. (1989). *Anti-bias curriculum: Tools for empowering young children.* Washington, DC: National Association for the Education of Young Children.

Division for Early Childhood. (1993). *DEC Task Force on Recommended Practices: Indicators of quality in program for infants and young children with special needs and their families.* Reston, VA: Council for Exceptional Children.

Faught, K. K., Balleweg, B. J., Crow, R. E., & van den Pol, R. A. (1983). An analysis of social behaviors among handicapped and nonhandicapped preschool children. *Education and Training of the Mentally Retarded,* 18(3), 210–214.

Florida Department of Education, Bureau of Education for Exceptional Students. (1991). *Models of interdisciplinary training for children with handicaps: Modules 1–13.* Tallahassee, FL: Florida Department of Education, Exceptional Student Education.

Flynn, C. C., & Harbin, G. L. (1989). Evaluating interagency coordination efforts using a multidimensional, interactional, developmental paradigm. In B. E. Hanft (Ed.), *Family-centered care: An early intervention resource manual* (pp. 5.9–5.19). Rockville, MD: American Occupational Therapy Association.

Galant, K., & Hanline, M. F. (1993). Parental attitudes toward mainstreaming young children with disabilities. *Childhood Education,* 69(5), 293–297.

Graham, M. A., & Hanline, M. F. (1991). *Mainstreaming works!* Tallahassee, FL: Center for Early Intervention and Prevention Policy, Florida State University.

Green, A. L., & Stoneman, Z. (1989). Attitudes of mothers and fathers of nonhandicapped children toward preschool mainstreaming. *Journal of Early Intervention,* 13(4), 292–304.

Guralnick, M. J. (1981). Mainstreaming young handicapped children. In B. Spodek (Ed.), *Handbook of research on early childhood education* (pp. 456–500). New York: Free Press.

Guralnick, M. J. (1990). Major accomplishments and future directions in early childhood mainstreaming. *Topics in Early Childhood Special Education,* 10(2), 1–17.

Guralnick, M. J., & Paul-Brown, D. (1980). Functional and discourse analysis of nonhandicapped preschool children's speech to handicapped children. *American Journal of Mental Deficiency,* 84(5), 444–454.

Hanline, M. F. (1985). Integrating disabled children. *Young Children,* 40(2), 45–48.

Hanline, M. F. (1990). A consulting model for providing integration opportunities for preschool children with disabilities. *Journal of Early Intervention,* 14(4), 360–366.

Hanline, M. F. (1993a). The inclusion of preschoolers with profound disabilities: An analysis of children's interactions. *Journal of the Association for Persons with Severe Handicaps,* 18(1), 28–35.

Hanline, M. F. (1993b). Facilitating integrated preschool service delivery transitions for children, families, and professionals. In C. Peck, S. Odom, & D. Bricker (Eds.), *Integrating young children with disabilities into community implementation.* Baltimore, MD: Paul H. Brookes.

Hanline, M. F., & Fox, L. (1993). Learning within the context of play—Providing typical early childhood experiences for children with severe disabilities. *Journal of the Association for Persons with Severe Handicaps, 18*(2).

Hanline, M. F., & Halvorsen, A. (1989). Parent perceptions of the integration transition process: Overcoming artificial barriers. *Exceptional Children, 55*(6), 487–492.

Hanline, M. F., & Hanson, M. J. (1989). Integration considerations for infants and toddlers with multiple disabilities. *Severe Handicaps, 14*(3), 178–183.

Ipsa, J., & Matz, R. D. (1978). Integrating handicapped preschool children with a cognitively oriented program. In M. Guralnick (Ed.), *Early intervention and the integration of handicapped and nonhandicapped children* (pp. 167–190). Baltimore, MD: University Park Press.

Jenkins, J. R., Odom, S. L., & Speltz, M. L. (1989). Effects of social integration on preschool children with handicaps. *Exceptional Children, 55*, 420–428.

Jenkins, J. R., Speltz, M. L., & Odom, S. I. (1985). Integrating normal and handicapped preschoolers: Effects on child development and social interaction. *Exceptional Children, 52*, 7–18.

McEvoy, M. A., Odom, S. L., & McConnell, S. R. (1992). Peer social competence intervention for young children with disabilities. In S. L. Odom, S. R. McConnell, & M. A. McEvoy (Eds.), *Social competence of young children with disabilities* (pp. 113–134). Baltimore, MD: Paul H. Brookes.

McLean, M., & Hanline, M. F. (1990). Providing early intervention services in integrated environments: Challenges and opportunities for the future. *Topics in Early Childhood Special Education, 10*(2), 62–77.

Moffitt, K., Reiss, J., & Nackashi, J. (Eds.). (1991). *Special children, special care.* Tallahassee, FL: Florida Developmental Disabilities Council.

Odom, S., Deklyen, M., & Jenkins, J. R. (1984). Integrating handicapped and nonhandicapped preschoolers: Developmental impact on the nonhandicapped children. *Exceptional Children, 51*, 41–49.

Odom, S. L., & McEvoy, M. A. (1988). Integration of young children with handicaps and normally developing children. In S. L. Odom & M. B. Karnes (Eds.), *Early intervention for infants and children with handicaps* (pp. 241–268). Baltimore, MD: Paul H. Brookes.

Paget, K. D. (1991). Parent professional partnerships and family empowerment. In M. Fine (Ed.), *Collaboration with parents of exceptional children* (pp. 289–303). Brandon, VT: Clinical Psychology.

Peck, C. A., Hayden, L., Wandschneider, M., Peterson, K., & Richarz, S. (1989). Development of integrated preschools: A qualitative inquiry into sources of resistance among parents, administrators, and teachers. *Journal of Early Intervention, 13*(4), 353–364.

Peterson, N. L. (1982). Social integration of handicapped and nonhandicapped preschoolers: A study of playmate preferences. *Topics in Early Childhood Special Education, 2*(2), 56–59.

Ramsey, P. G. (1983). Multicultural education in early childhood. In J. F. Brown (Ed.), *Curriculum planning for young children* (pp. 131–142). Washington, DC: National Association for the Education of Young Children.

Reichart, D. C., Lynch, E. C., Anderson, B. C., Svobodny, L. A., & Mercury, M. G. (1989). Parental perspectives on integrated preschool opportunities for children with handicaps and without handicaps. *Journal of Early Intervention, 13*(1), 6–13.

Sailor, W., Anderson, J. L., Halvorsen, A. T., Doering, K., Filler, J., & Goetz, L. (1989). *The comprehensive local school: Regular education for all students with disabilities.* Baltimore, MD: Paul H. Brookes.

Salend, S. J. (1984). Factors contributing to the development of successful mainstreaming programs. *Exceptional Children, 5,* 409–416.

Schaps, E., & Solomon, D. (1990). Schools and classrooms as caring communities. *Educational Leadership, 48*(3), 38–42.

Shelton, T. L., Jeppson, E. S., & Johnson, R. H. (1989). *Family-centered care for children with special health care needs.* Washington, DC: Association for the Care of Children's Health.

Spencer, P. (1989). Team dynamics relative to exemplary early services. In B. E. Hanft (Ed.), *Family-centered care: An early intervention resource manual* (pp. 4.43–4.50). Rockville, MD: American Occupational Therapy Association.

Stainback, S., & Stainback, W. (1990). *Support networks for inclusive schooling: Interdependent integrated education.* Baltimore, MD: Paul H. Brookes.

Stainback, S., & Stainback, W. (1992). *Curriculum considerations in inclusive classrooms: Facilitating learning for all students.* Baltimore, MD: Paul H. Brookes.

Strain, P. S. (1984). Social behavior patterns of nonhandicapped–developmentally disabled friend pairs in mainstream preschools. *Analysis and Intervention in Developmental Disabilities, 4,* 15–28.

Strain, P. S. (1990). LRE for preschool children with handicaps: What we know, what we should be doing. *Journal of Early Intervention, 14*(4), 291–296.

Striefel, S., Killoran, J., & Quintero, M. (1991). *Functional integration for success— Preschool intervention.* Austin, TX: Pro-Ed.

Surr, J. (1992). Early childhood programs and the Americans with Disabilities Act (ADA). *Young Children, 47,* 18–21.

Taylor, S. (1988). Caught in the continuum: A critical analysis of the principle of the least restrictive environment. *Journal of the Association for Persons with Severe Handicaps, 13*(1), 41–53.

Turnbull, H. R., & Turnbull, A. P. (1990). The unfulfilled promise of integration: Does Part H ensure different rights and results than Part B of the Education of the Handicapped Act? *Topics in Early Childhood Special Education, 10*(2), 18–32.

Wang, M. C., Vaughan, E. D., & Dytman, J. A. (1985). Staff development: A key ingredient of effective mainstreaming. *Teaching Exceptional Children, 17*(2), 112–121.

Wesley, P. (1992). *Mainstreaming young children.* Chapel Hill, NC: Frank Porter Graham Child Development Center, University of North Carolina at Chapel Hill.

Winton, P. J., Turnbull, A. P., & Blacher, J. (1985). Expectations for and satisfaction with public school kindergarten: Perspectives of parents of handicapped and nonhandicapped children. *Journal of the Division for Early Childhood, 9,* 116–124.

Wolfensberger, W. (1972). *The principle of normalization in human services.* Toronto: National Institute on Mental Retardation.

CHAPTER 11

Characteristics of Quality, Effective Service Delivery Systems for Children with Special Needs

MIMI A. GRAHAM
DONNA M. BRYANT

One of the greatest challenges facing our society today is providing quality care and education for infants and young children. Extensive debate surrounds discussions of the best kind of child care environment for fostering growth and development for children with both typical and atypical needs. Educational practices used in early childhood education have traditionally varied from those utilized in early childhood special education. Although theoretically early childhood practices center around the developmental principles of Piaget, Erikson, and Montessori, early childhood special education is embedded in the behavioral constructs of Skinner, Pavlov, and Watson.

Although some themes are common to both orientations (e.g., independence, adaptation, contingent responsiveness, social competence, individualization) (Mallory, 1992), developmental and behavioral concepts have often been translated into polarized approaches toward teaching and learning for the child with atypical needs. For example, environments for children with disabilities are typically less stimulating and developmentally appropriate than those of their nondisabled peers (Bailey, Clifford, & Harms, 1982). Early childhood special education has been criticized for being too structured and too adult-directed (McWilliam & Strain, 1993). Behavioral learning strategies such as reinforcement, modeling, shaping, and prompting are more prevalent in programs for children with disabilities and have been shown to help them achieve developmental milestones (Mahoney, Robinson, & Powell, 1992). However, the applicability of skills generated by this method often does not extend beyond expected rates of maturation (Casto & Mastropieri, 1986; Dunst, 1986).

Guidelines for developmentally appropriate early childhood practices have been clearly defined and widely disseminated by the National Association for the Education of Young Children (NAEYC) (Bredekamp, 1987). Educational practices derived from this model emphasize play, discovery, and problem solving as the primary vehicles for mastery of developmental skills and fostering independence. The teacher's role is to facilitate and support child-initiated activities in an environment that enhances children's motivation to achieve through manipulation, discovery, exploration, and feedback.

The implicit assumption is that such programs are best for all children (Mallory, 1992), but consensus on this point is lacking. Some are concerned that the developmental approach does not improve self-sufficiency (Snell, 1987) and that children with certain behavioral conditions may not respond best to developmental approaches (Strain & Odom, 1986). However, Mahoney, Robinson, and Powell (1992) find support for developmental practices in studies relating child-oriented parent interaction with higher levels of progress in their children with disabilities (Bradley, 1989; Brooks-Gunn & Lewis, 1984; Mahoney, Finger, & Powell, 1985). The Division for Early Childhood's (DEC) Task Force on Recommended Practices suggests the inclusion of both developmentally and individually appropriate practices (McWilliam & Strain, 1993).

Concerns about the developmental appropriateness of "regular" child care environments for typically developing children (Whitebook, Howes, & Phillips, 1989) have heightened, with increasing emphasis on the inclusion of young children with special needs into child care settings. The NAEYC guidelines conceptually provide the basis of appropriate educational practices for all children, but alone are not sufficient for meeting the specific needs of children with disabilities and their families (Carta, Schwartz, Atwater, & McConnell, 1991; Wolery, Strain, & Bailey, 1992). Although basic needs such as physical safety, psychological well-being, and belonging are common to all children, those with disabilities usually have additional needs for development. Because of the child's disability, caregivers are needed who are skillful in adapting the environment and, particularly, in assessing and facilitating skills.

A multiplicity of labels has developed as a result of the various tracks of early education and care—early intervention, infant stimulation, family day care, nursery school, child care, early childhood, preschool, and early childhood special education. These labels continue to perpetuate a false dichotomy between the care and education of young children. Caldwell (1991) recommends the term "educare" to encompass both care and educational aspects of programs in early childhood. A broader, less exclusive term would help eliminate the artificial distinctions among programs and help move the nation toward more unified, inclusive environments for young children.

Toward this end, several groups have developed guidelines for quality practices (DEC, 1993; NAEYC, 1987). Following our work in developing and delivering a developmentally based educational intervention for low-birth-weight infants (Infant Health and Development Program, 1990; Ramey, Bryant, et al., 1992), we conducted more than 100 interviews and site visits with experts and their programs around the country. From these experiences and extensive review of the literature, we have attempted to make available the research about how infants and young children best learn and to offer strategies for adapting environments to meet the capabilities and needs of children with disabilities. Where appropriate, the excellent work of the recent DEC Task Force on Recommended Practices (1993) has been cited.

RATIOS AND GROUP SIZE

Among the most important structural variables affecting quality are child–teacher ratio and overall group size. One national study (Roupp, Travers, Glantz, & Goelen, 1979) showed that group size was associated with a measure of overall classroom quality and another study (Whitebook et al., 1989) found ratio, but not group size, to be significantly related to classroom quality. A more recent study showed that better ratios and smaller group sizes were related to better caregiving and more developmentally appropriate activities which, in turn, were related to more attachment security with caregivers and social competence with peers (Howes, Phillips, & Whitebook, 1992). Clearly, both ratio and group size are important.

The DEC Task Force on Recommended Practices suggests adult–child ratios that maximize safety, health, and promotion of identified goals (DEC, 1993). The NAEYC-recommended ratios (Bredekamp, 1987) (i.e., 1:3 or 1:4 for infants with group size no greater than 10) were derived with classes of normally developing children in mind. In an inclusive class where one or more of the children have special needs, the staff–child ratio should be even lower. Although research does not tell us the optimal ratio, it depends on the severity of the special needs condition(s).

Because personnel costs often comprise from 70 to 90% of a child care program's budget, ratios often get "pushed," especially early and late in the day. Maintaining workable ratios throughout the day should be an uncompromised condition. Many programs committed to high-quality care find creative ways to achieve better ratios through the use of foster grandparents, parent and student volunteers, and student interns.

Ratios interact with group size and age-grouping decisions. Some inclusive centers like Bank Street in New York City and the University of North Carolina's Frank Porter Graham Center (FPG) have chosen to have mixed-age groups of small numbers of children, an arrangement that promotes peer teaching and social interactions (Furman, Rahe, & Hartup, 1979). At FPG, this grouping began once children were old enough to leave the infant nursery (about 12–15 months). Bailey, Burchinal, and McWilliam (1993) found significant improvement in development across all domains for the youngest children when they spent time with older children, compared with those who were with same-age children. Grouping strategies may include a teacher responsible for one group of children or an adult assigned to an activity or learning area. This "zone" method was shown to increase children's participation in activities and reduce the amount of time spent in transitions (LeLaurin & Risley, 1972). Some centers combine different types of grouping, such as "family groups" for meal times and "developmental groups" for center time.

DEGREE OF STRUCTURE

The optimal amount of structure for children with special needs is a topic of much debate. In one meta-analysis, "structure" was defined as the degree to which the intervention activities were linked to a detailed set of outcome objectives and a specified curriculum. Using this definition of "structure," the authors concluded that highly structured programs were effective for high-risk disadvantaged children but not for children with disabilities (Casto & Mastropieri, 1986; Casto & White, 1985).

However, others believe that children with severe disabilities are better served in programs that are more structured and directive than programs designed for normally developing children (Alberto, Briggs, & Goldstein, 1983; Cicchetti & Sroufe, 1976; Warren & Rogers-Warren, 1982). This led to the development of traditional early intervention programs based on the belief that disabled children learn best through highly structured, didactic, teacher-directed instruction.

"Structure" has also been interpreted based on the philosophies of Piaget (1926) and Montessori (1964) in which both typical and atypical infants and young children learn best through exploration, manipulation, problem solving, sensory experiences, and social interactions. The caregiver carefully orchestrates the learning environment and facilitates, rather than directs, interactive learning. The learning environment is planned based on the application of a broad knowledge of child development in conjunction with understanding about the individual child's strengths, interests, and experiences. Learning is promoted by facilitating children's choices and their interactions with materials, and by asking questions that stimulate thinking (Elkind, 1986; Lay-Dopyera & Dopyera, 1986; Sparling, 1989). Because children with disabilities may be less spontaneous than nondisabled children in making choices, the environment should be stocked with inviting choices requiring thoughtful preparation by the caregiver. For example, Montessori programs, originally designed for children with mental retardation, create environments to support children's learning through allowing them to choose their own activities and using individualized, self-paced, and self-correcting materials. In addition, this method of learning fosters independence and self-reliance, thereby reducing the potential for behavioral problems because children are not forced into activities inappropriate for their developmental age (e.g., 20-minute circle-time for toddlers).

Children with special needs may interact with objects for less time than other children (Weiner & Weiner, 1974) and may be less tenacious at difficult tasks, less goal oriented, and more likely to give up (Jennings, Connors, Stegman, Sankaranarayan, & Mendelsohn, 1985). They may persist longer at activities of their own choosing, so many materials should be available on organized shelves at children's level; encouragement should be given when extended play is observed. Children with disabilities may also engage less in social play (Guralnick & Groom, 1987), so teachers should facilitate child–child interactions through prompting, modeling, and facilitating play. Structure is produced not through direct interaction with children but rather by the teacher's advance planning for activities.

Although both special education and early childhood practitioners concur that children learn best when their individual needs are met, individualization seems to be more of a concept than a practice as revealed in site visits we made to numerous programs throughout the nation. Children frequently spend the majority of the day in large group activities in which didactic instruction and materials are commonly used with little regard to individual child needs. Some programs have small groups of children with similar developmental levels to provide more individualized learning opportunities. With increasingly larger classroom sizes, varying exceptionalities within classrooms, and little time for planning, assimilation of individual learning modalities is difficult at best.

CURRICULUM

Curriculum has been defined as a "planned arrangement of experiences designed to bring about desired changes in the child's behavior" (Lerner, Mardell-Czudnowski, & Goldenberg, 1987). The curriculum is the anchor for any early childhood program as it integrates goals into a planned sequence of learning activities (Mori & Neisworth, 1983). All early childhood programs, with typical or atypical children, should follow a curricular plan for teaching, whether it is one developed by staff or adapted from commercial products. Curricula should be unbiased and nondiscriminatory concerning disability, sex, race, religion, and ethnic/cultural origin (McWilliam & Strain, 1993). No single curricular approach has been demonstrated to be more effective than another, although a strongly adult-directed, didactic program may have long-term negative effects (Bailey & Wolery, 1992; Schweinhart, 1989–1990; Spodek, Saracho, & Davis, 1991).

Most professionals agree that curriculum should contain at least three components: (1) content (sequence of skills for instruction), (2) methods for individualizing the content for each child, and (3) methods of teaching the individual content to each child (Wolery & Fleming, 1993; Wolery & Sainato, 1993).

Curricula need to be used with special attention devoted to the disability area but with equal emphasis placed on the whole child (Sparling, 1989). A child with speech delays may need additional focus on language development, but also requires age-appropriate activities promoting social and motor development as well as self-esteem. Children can participate in a wide array of activities without sacrificing the needed therapeutic interventions (and vice versa).

Because children with special needs often do not generalize well (Warren & Kaiser, 1986), curricula should focus less on traditional milestones and more on functionality. Because skills learned in isolation are of little use in alternative settings and future environments, curricula should provide a variety of activities for teaching the same skill. For example, stacking blocks is a common activity for enhancing hand–eye coordination. Applicability of this skill could be expanded by stacking cups and plates at meal time or sand buckets on the playground.

Although relatively few child development curricula have been empirically validated, several have been designed especially for infants and young children with disabilities. The majority of these are based on developmental tasks in cognition and language, motor, and social skills, with the assumption that infants and toddlers with disabilities follow developmental sequences similar to normally developing children. Curricula examples include *Early Partners* for preterm, low-birth-weight infants (Sparling, Lewis, & Neuwirth, 1993); *Learning through Play* for children with motor impairments (Fewell & Vadasy, 1983); the *SKI*HI Model* for children with hearing impairments (Clark & Watkins, 1985); and the cognitive–linguistic infant intervention strategy by Dunst (1981), the *Portage Guide to Early Education* (Bluma, Shearer, Frohman, & Hilliard, 1976), *The Carolina Curriculum* (Johnson-Martin, Jens, & Attermeier, 1986), and the *Hawaii Early Learning Profile* (HELP) (Furuno et al., 1985) for infants and toddlers with various disabilities.

In addition, many other curricula written for nondisabled children can be quite readily adapted for use by all children. Examples include *Learning Games for Birth through Three* and *Partners for Learning* by Sparling and Lewis (1979, 1985); *Active Learning for Infants* and *Active Learning for Ones* by Cryer, Harms, and Bourland (1987a, 1987b); *Infant/Toddler: Introducing Your Child to the Joy of Learning: A Parent/Caregiver Book* by Badger (1981); and *Learning Accomplishment Profile* and *Early LAP* by Sanford and Zelman (1981).

Curricular activities are generally used more purposefully with children with special needs than with typical children. Children's interactions, routines, and activities must be structured more intentionally, and effective instructional strategies should be embedded within them (Cooper, Heron, & Heward, 1987). This may necessitate the use of peers or more individual assistance (Wolery et al., 1991). Activities should also be integrated as naturally as possible into the care routines of the day (McWilliam & Strain, 1993). Diapering, feeding, and dressing are obvious opportunities for special one-to-one activities, in addition to the prescribed "therapy or activity time."

INTEGRATION OF SPECIAL THERAPIES

The way in which therapeutic services are delivered is a subject of much debate but with little empirical data (see Vergara, Adams, Masin, & Beckman, Chapter 12, this volume). Some treatments are delivered in an integrated fashion with the therapist interacting with the target child (and perhaps other children) in the classroom and providing consultation to the teacher so that there is greater continuity of therapeutic activities carried out throughout the course of the normal day. Some treatments are delivered in an individualized fashion where the therapist interacts with the child outside the classroom in a hands-on, one-on-one situation. However, no evidence exists to support the contention that one-to-one therapy is superior to integrated or group therapy except for children under 20 months, for whom therapies should be individually focused (Snyder-McLean & McLean, 1987).

When appropriate, therapies should be integrated within the regular routine. For example, fine motor skills can be developed through blocks and art. Speech and language can be improved through fantasy play and mealtime conversations. Gross motor skills can be addressed providing range of motion while changing an infant or on the playground or within dramatic play. A creative occupational therapist at Bank Street brought in her "treasure chest" full of exciting toys, which intrigued the target child as well as the other children gathered round to participate.

Although individualized, out-of-the-room treatment remains the predominant model in early intervention programs, integrated treatment is increasingly advocated by therapists and early childhood special educators. The DEC Task Force on Recommended Practices (1993) suggests that pull-out services should be used *only* when routine activity-based options have failed to meet identified needs (McWilliam & Strain, 1993). Some states, such as Connecticut, have required that therapies be delivered within the classroom.

The ultimate test of the effects of therapy should involve child change across all environments, not just the therapeutic setting. This implies that classrooms and other natural settings should be the primary locations of intervention.

INTEREST AREAS

A study by Bailey, Clifford, and Harms (1982) showed that settings for children with disabilities are less stimulating than those of their nondisabled peers, particularly in the areas of room arrangement for interest centers and for relaxation and comfort, and the opportunities for creative activities and social development. Art materials were limited or offered few choices. Few blocks or accessories were available. Very few programs organized storage areas to encourage independent use (e.g., pictures on shelves to show where blocks belong). Many programs for children with special needs had no provision for sand and water play, and those that did provided only limited access. Over half had no dramatic-play areas; the others generally focused on housekeeping roles with few provisions for pretend play involving work, transportation, or adventure. More than 75% of the classrooms for children with special needs had no "cozy area."

The design of the classroom spaces can facilitate children's interest in activities and their ability to explore, play, and learn through doing. Identifying and setting up interest areas requires attention to furniture size and placement, traffic patterns, the numbers of children who might be accommodated, the types of disabilities they might have, whether the area can be personalized by the children, and how the adult might "fit" in the area. Wesley (1992) has written detailed guidelines for organizing the environment to foster inclusion.

The activities in interest areas should be concrete, real, and relevant to the lives of young children (Evans, 1984; Piaget, 1972; Smith, 1985). For example, learning about apples should include drawings, photographs, and real apples (red, yellow, and green; big and small) that are smelled, tasted, and touched. Art projects should be open-ended, not worksheets to color or adult-made models to copy. Much of the "art" we observed in early intervention programs was adult-produced (e.g., precut or photocopied sheets that the children then color).

Children learn by doing rather than by being told and through active interaction with the physical environment (Piaget, 1952), yet many children with disabilities are constrained from exploring the environment because of the over-use of restrictive hook-on-table-top chairs and positioning chairs. Instead, it is simple to position the child in a specialized chair facing a shelf with choices within reach. If a child with disabilities cannot explore or learn through simple manipulation, more consistent structuring of the environment or reinforcement of experiences might be necessary (Bailey & Wolery, 1992).

The teacher's role is to prepare the environment for children to learn through active exploration and interaction with adults, peers, and materials (Fromberg, 1992; Lay-Dopyera & Dopyera, 1986). For example, the housekeeping corner should include a rich array of fantasy play clothes and should be changed at least monthly with additional props and themes such as doctors' offices, banks, space stations, zoos, post offices, grocery stores, and so forth. Furthermore, environments should be fun, thereby stimulating children's initiatives, promoting choices, and engaging the children with materials and peers (McWilliam & Strain, 1993).

ENVIRONMENTAL ASSESSMENT

Good measures are available to assess children's environments: the *Infant/ Toddler Environment Rating Scale* (ITERS) for classroom environments from birth to age 2 (Harms, Cryer, & Clifford, 1990); the *Early Childhood Environment Rating Scale* (ECERS) for children ages 2 through 5 (Harms & Clifford, 1980); and the *Family Day Care Rating Scale* (Harms & Clifford, 1989) are all reliable and valid instruments designed to give an overall picture of the environment for preschool settings, including the use of space, materials, and activities to enhance children's development, the daily program schedule, and the supervision of children. Although primarily created for normally developing children, these measures are all useful for early intervention programs because so many desirable characteristics of classrooms are similar for all children. Each of these measures includes some ratings concerning provisions for children with special needs, and an additional scale of items for the ECERS is available (Harms, Clifford, & Bailey, 1986).

FAMILY INFLUENCE ON DEVELOPMENT

Because the family is the central environment for the young child, interventions in the early years, particularly during infancy, must focus on the entire family unit—not solely on the child (Fewell & Vadasy, 1986; Turnbull & Turnbull, 1986). Family-centered interventions involve the family in all phases of diagnosis, planning, and treatment. A review of the effectiveness of more than 30 early intervention programs found that programs that adopted a joint focus on the child and the family were the most effective in achieving their goals (Shonkoff & Hauser-Cram, 1987). The underlying concept of family-focused intervention is that a child's functioning can be maximized by providing services in a manner designed to enhance the effectiveness of families. Family-centered services are an essential component of quality programs (McWilliam & Strain, 1993; Turbiville, Turnbull, Garland, & Lee, 1993; Vincent & Beckett, 1993). (For more specifics on family-centered services, see Duwa, Wells, & Lalinde, Chapter 5, this volume.)

MULTICULTURAL COMPETENCIES
AND PROGRAM ADAPTATIONS

Because of the critical impact of culture and families upon a child's development, culturally competent care must be a goal toward providing optimal intervention with different ethnic groups (Masin, 1991). Although no formal standards have been established related to cultural competence in early intervention, a recent survey of professionals identified competencies needed and the training experiences perceived as most effective for working with families from diverse cultural backgrounds in early intervention (Christensen, 1992).

Although minority children are often overrepresented in early intervention, materials, dolls, books, and pictures seldom reflect the cultural backgrounds of these children. In public school kindergartens, cultural awareness was the lowest-scored item in one recent study (Bryant, Clifford, & Peisner, 1991). Multicultural and non-gender-specific experiences, materials, and equipment should be provided for children of all ages in their educational environments (Ramsey, 1979; Saracho & Spodek, 1983). Assessments should also be adapted to a child's culture, such as testing in the child's language using nonverbal tests, parent report, observation, or otherwise adapting assessment instruments.

Several excellent resources are available specifically for early childhood programs: *Cultural Competence in Screening and Assessment* (National Early Childhood Technical Assistance System [NEC*TAS], 1991), *Roots & Wings: Affirming Culture in Early Childhood Programs* (York, 1991), *Serving Culturally Diverse Families of Infants and Toddlers with Disabilities* (Anderson & Fenichel, 1989), and *A Bibliography of Selected Resources on Cultural Diversity for Parents and Professionals Working with Young Children Who Have, or Are At-Risk for, Disabilities* (NEC*TAS, 1989).

PROMOTING SOCIAL INTERACTIONS

Social competence is important for all children and of special emphasis for children with special needs. Same-age, typically developing friends are what parents generally desire the most for their preschooler with disabilities (Strain, 1990).

Of all the factors that contribute to the social environment in which children are educated, the teacher is by far the most critical (Spodek, Saracho, & Lee, 1984) as social interactions between children with and without disabilities do not automatically occur. Children with special needs engage in less frequent and less sophisticated social play than their typical peers (Guralnick & Groom, 1987); thus, to create positive and reciprocal social interactions, the physical and social environment must be facilitated by the teacher (Hanson & Hanline, 1989) (see Hanline & Galant, Chapter 10, this volume).

Intervention strategies should encourage participation, initiative, autonomy, and age-appropriate abilities in many normalized situations (Wolery & Sainato, 1993). Effective strategies for promoting social interaction have included sociodramatic play, peer-mediated strategies (social interaction training, peer modeling, and peer reinforcement), and teacher prompts (Odom & McEvoy, 1988; Strain, 1990; Wolery & Sainato, 1993). Social interactions can be encouraged by carefully selecting activities and materials, grouping children, and providing appropriate teacher attention (Guralnick, 1982; Hanline, 1985; Strain & Odom, 1986). Toys such as wagons, doll houses, and blocks promote social interaction, while activities such as dramatic play and group art projects encourage cooperative play (see Hanson & Hanline, 1989, for other examples). Nearly all studies of social interaction or play behaviors for preschoolers with and without disabilities in integrated settings report positive effects (Cavallaro & Porter, 1980; Cormack, 1979; Edwards & Montemurro, 1979; Federlein, 1979; Furman, Rahe, & Hartup, 1979; Guralnick, 1980; Guralnick & Paul-Brown, 1980).

FACILITATING SOCIAL–EMOTIONAL DEVELOPMENT

Because some children with disabilities may be slower in developing social–emotional competencies, they may exhibit their frustrations and immaturity through an extended stage of undesirable behavior. Whether this is due to their primary disability or secondary to their often restricted environmental experiences and limited interpersonal relationships is unclear. Nevertheless, these behavioral needs must be addressed in the plan of therapy/education for young children with special needs (Guralnick, 1988).

It has long been known that children's behavior can be changed by the functional relationship between their behavior and environmental stimuli such as reinforcer or punishments (Bijou & Baer, 1961). Using contingent reinforcers for appropriate or positive behaviors, ignoring minor behavioral infractions, and restructuring the environment have all been shown to be effective ways of helping young children learn to control some of their impulses and negative behavior.

Caregivers of young children need more training on setting limits and positive strategies for incorporating many different aspects of learning theory with the conduct of their class. A negative tone is often seen in the rigid use of time-out, which is too often used inappropriately to control and punish young children in lieu of redirection or positive reinforcers.

HEALTH AND SAFETY

Nearly all infections causing common illness in young children have been associated with group child care settings (Goodman, Osterholm, Granoff, & Pickering, 1984). Increased exposure to a number of illnesses may limit the option of group care for children with significant medical or health risks (Kotch & Bryant, 1990; Hanson & Hanline, 1989). Medical risks should not, however, preclude other services and a range of service options must be available.

Often the care of children with disabilities may involve additional health procedures (e.g., managing seizures, tube feeding, suctioning, special diets) or the use of special equipment (e.g., hearing aids, walkers, wheelchairs). Parents are successfully taught these medical procedures, which staff can also learn so children can experience less clinical, more appropriate settings. Nurses can train teachers and be available for ongoing technical assistance. In addition, an affiliation with a pediatrician is recommended to contribute to policy making and staff development (American Academy of Pediatrics, 1987).

Checklists to monitor health and safety have been developed by Aronson and Nelson (1976) and NAEYC (1984). Guidelines for preventing infectious disease in child care settings have also been developed by the Centers for Disease Control (1984) and the American Public Health Association and the American Academy of Pediatrics (1992). All early childhood programs, those with or without children with special needs, should follow such standards, particularly universal precautions, because of the increasing incidence of hepatitis, pediatric AIDS, and other infections.

The importance of training staff cannot be overemphasized, both at orientation as well as continued training and occasional refreshers. In the Infant Health and Development Program, health and safety checklists were used on a weekly basis, rotating responsibilities among all staff to ensure continued awareness of issues. An excellent resource for practical application of health and safety practices in infant/toddler group care is available (Ferguson, Mulvihill, Spiker, & Bryant, in press).

OUTDOOR ENVIRONMENTS

Playgrounds are an important part of the young child's environment. However, a study by Aronson (1986) found that two-thirds of all child care injuries occurred there; slides and swings were often linked with accidents, while climbing equipment was most frequently associated with severe injuries. The U.S. Consumer Product Safety Commission (1992) reports that almost 70% of playground injuries result from falls. Playgrounds are often constructed with older children in mind, one factor that often results in accidents and lawsuits. The Commission recommends that all playgrounds be clearly separated based on preschool age (2–5) and school age (5–12).

Several general safety principles have been identified for playgrounds (Bowers, 1992): accessibility, avoiding steep slopes, limiting distance of falls to 18 inches, evaluating risky equipment, providing soft ground covering, matching size of equipment to ages, ensuring safe clearances, providing partially enclosed spaces, using interconnective play components, minimizing exposure to sun, using quality materials, inspecting equipment regularly, and increasing supervision. The U.S. Consumer Product Safety Commission's (1991) *Handbook for Public Playground Safety* provides guidelines for designing, purchasing, and maintaining playground equipment, and a playground safety checklist has been developed by the American Alliance for Health, Physical Education, Recreation and Dance, Committee on Play (Bowers, 1990).

In addition to safety, playgrounds should accommodate the needs for play of both typical and atypical children. The natural play of children involves active exploration, creativity, and mastery of physical challenges (Piaget, 1952), and children with disabilities generally select play activities similar to those of nondisabled children (Bowers, 1977). Basic movement abilities may develop more slowly in the child with a disability, but the sequence and pattern of motor development is basically the same for all children. The Americans with Disabilities Act requires that playgrounds be usable for individuals with disabilities, but offers no specific guidelines for what makes a playground "accessible." Dr. Louis Bowers of the University of South Florida has researched and designed safe and interesting playground modules for young children with disabilities. Other resources for playground accessibility include Steve King of Landscape Structures and Grounds for Play.

PERSONNEL PREPARATION AND STANDARDS

Merging of professional standards across early childhood special education and early childhood is consistent toward promoting the inclusion of children with disabilities in all aspects of society (Stayton & Miller, 1993). Many similarities exist between the required competencies for regular and special educators (Lowenthal, 1992); however, personnel preparation continues to be largely segregated despite the fact that it is "contradictory to legal, philosophical, empirical, economic, and moral reasoning for early childhood education" (Miller, 1992, p. 39). Segregated, unidiscipline teacher education programs are mostly the result of state certification requirements. Currently, only three states—Massachusetts, North Carolina, and Kentucky—have combined professional standards in the area of childhood (Miller, 1992). Personnel training practices continue to be cited as a major obstacle to mainstreaming efforts (Odom & McEvoy, 1988).

Efforts by several groups seem to be moving toward the merger of developmentally appropriate practices and professional standards—the NAEYC, the DEC Council for Exceptional Children, and the Association of Teacher Educators (Miller, 1992).

SUMMARY

Quality, research-based practices inspire excellence. We need to build on the most effective teaching and learning strategies from both early childhood and early intervention. The problem is that like so many "best practices," quality learning environments are not created solely by a new instructional technology, a better curricula, or an innovative approach to staff training. Successful learning environments depend on the director and teaching staff to create and orchestrate interesting and safe physical and social places in which children interact with materials, each other, and their caregivers. Researchers should continue to add information about the ways in which certain environmental provisions can affect children's learning or different dimensions of children's development (e.g., independence, social interactions, self-esteem). Each of us is part of the process of change that is shaping the future, integrating best practices from both early childhood and special education to develop a vision of the best possible future for infants and toddlers and their families.

ACKNOWLEDGMENTS

This work was supported in part by a grant from the Robert Wood Johnson Foundation and a contract from the State of Florida Department of Health and Rehabilitative Services. We wish to thank the directors and staff of the many programs we visited while reviewing this topic. An earlier version of this chapter was presented at the December 1991 conference of the National Center for Clinical Infant Programs.

REFERENCES

Alberto, P. A., Briggs, T., & Goldstein, D. (1983). Managing learning in handicapped infants. In S. G. Garwood & R. R. Fewell (Eds.), *Educating handicapped infants* (pp. 417–54). Rockville, MD: Aspen Systems.

American Academy of Pediatrics. (1987). *Health in day care: A manual for health professionals.* Elk Grove Village, IL: Author.

American Public Health Association and American Academy of Pediatrics. (1992). *Guidelines for day care for children with special needs.* Washington, DC: Author.

Anderson, P. P., & Fenichel, E. (1989). *Serving culturally diverse families of infants and toddlers with disabilities.* Washington, DC: National Center for Clinical Infant Programs.

Aronson, S. (1986). Maintaining health in child day care settings. In N. Gunzenhauzer & B. M. Caldwell (Eds.), *Johnson & Johnson Pediatric Round Table Series: Vol. 12. Group care for young children: Considerations for child care and health professionals, public policy makers, and parents* (pp. 137–146). Skillman, NJ: Johnson & Johnson.

Aronson, S., & Nelson, H. (1976). *Health power.* Philadelphia: Westinghouse Health Systems.

Badger, E. (1981). *Infant/toddler: Introducing your child to the joy of learning.* New York: McGraw-Hill.

Bailey, D. B., Burchinal, M. R., & McWilliam, R. A. (1993). Age of peers and early childhood development. *Child Development, 64,* 848–862.

Bailey, D. B., Clifford, R. M., & Harms, T. (1982). Comparison of preschool environments for handicapped and non-handicapped children. *Topics in Early Childhood Special Education, 2*(1), 9–20.

Bailey, D. B., & Wolery, M. (1992). *Teaching infants and preschoolers with disabilities* (2nd ed.). Columbus, OH: Merrill.

Bijou, S. W., & Baer, D. M. (1961). *Child development: A systematic and empirical theory* (Vol. 1). Englewood Cliffs, NJ: Prentice-Hall.

Bluma, S., Shearer, M., Frohman, A., & Hilliard, J. (1976). *Portage guide to early education.* Portage, WI: Cooperative Educational Service Agency.

Bowers, L. (1977, August). *Play learning centers for preschool handicapped children* (U.S. Office of Education, Research and Demonstration Project Report). Tampa, FL: College of Education, University of South Florida.

Bowers, L. (1990). National survey of preschool centers playground equipment. In S. C. Wortham & J. L. Frost (Eds.), *Playgrounds for young children: National survey and perspectives* (pp. 5–16). Reston, VA: American Alliance for Health, Physical Education, Recreation and Dance.

Bowers, L. (1992, March). Playground management and safety. In C. M. Hendricks (Ed.), *Young children on the grow: Health activity and education in the preschool setting* (Monograph No. 13, pp. 157–165). Washington, DC: ERIC Clearinghouse of Teacher Education.

Bradley, R. (1989). HOME measurement of maternal responsiveness. *New Directions for Child Development, 43,* 63–74.

Bredekamp, S. (1987). *Developmentally appropriate practice in early childhood programs serving children from birth through age eight.* Washington, DC: National Association for the Education of Young Children.

Brooks-Gunn, J., & Lewis, M. (1984). Maternal responsivity in interactions with handicapped infants. *Child Development, 55,* 782–793.

Bryant, D. M., Clifford, R. M., & Peisner, E. (1991). Best practices for beginners: An observational study of kindergarten. *American Education Research Journal, 28,* 783–803.

Caldwell, B. (1991). Educare: New product, new future. *Developmental and Behavioral Pediatrics, 12*(3), 199–204.

Carta, J. J., Schwartz, I. S., Atwater, J. B., & McConnell, S. R. (1991). Developmentally appropriate practice: Appraising its usefulness for young children with disabilities. *Topics in Early Childhood Special Education, 11*(1), 1–20.

Casto, G., & Mastropieri, M. (1986). The efficacy of early intervention programs: A meta-analysis. *Exceptional Children, 52,* 417–424.

Casto, G., & White, K. (1985). An integrative review of early intervention efficacy studies with at-risk children: Implications for the handicapped. *Analysis of Intervention for Developmental Disabilities, 5,* 7–31.

Cavallaro, S. A., & Porter, R. H. (1980). Peer preferences of at-risk and normally developing children in a preschool mainstream classroom. *American Journal of Mental Deficiencies, 84*(4), 357–366.

Centers for Disease Control. (1984). *What you can do to stop disease in the child day care center.* Washington, DC: U.S. Government Printing Office.

Christensen, C. M. (1992). Multicultural competencies in early intervention: Training professionals for a pluralistic society. *Infants and Young Children, 4*(3), 49–63.

Cicchetti, D., & Sroufe, L. A. (1976). The relationship between affective and cognitive development in Down's syndrome infants. *Child Development, 46,* 920–929.

Clark, T. C., & Watkins, S. (1985). *SKI*HI Curriculum* (4th ed.). Logan, UT: Utah State University, SKI*HI Institute.

Cooper, J. O., Heron, T. E., & Heward, W. L. (1987). *Applied behavior analysis.* Columbus, OH: Merrill.

Cormack, E. O. (1979, April). *Considerations for integration of physically handicapped and nonhandicapped preschool children.* Paper presented at the 57th Annual International Convention of the Council for Exceptional Children, Dallas, TX.

Cryer, D., Harms, T., & Bourland, B. (1987a). *Active learning for infants.* Menlo Park, CA: Addison-Wesley.

Cryer, D., Harms, T., & Bourland, B. (1987b). *Active learning for ones.* Menlo Park, CA: Addison-Wesley.

Division for Early Childhood. (1993). *DEC Task Force on Recommended Practices: Indicators of quality in programs for infants and young children with special needs and their families.* Reston, VA: Council for Exceptional Children.

Dunst, C. J. (1981). *Infant learning: A cognitive–linguistic intervention strategy.* Allen, TX: Teaching Resources/DLM.

Dunst, C. J. (1986). Overview of the efficacy of early intervention programs. In L. Bickman & D. I. Weatherfield (Eds.), *Evaluating early intervention programs for severely handicapped children and their families* (pp. 79–148). Austin, TX: Pro-Ed.

Edwards, E., & Montemurro, T. J. (1979, April). *The behavior of preschool handicapped children and their interaction with model children.* Paper presented at the 57th Annual International Convention of the Council for Exceptional Children, Dallas, TX.

Elkind, D. (1986, May). Formal education and early childhood education: An essential difference. *Phi Delta Kappan,* pp. 631–636.

Evans, E. D. (1984). Children's aesthetics. In L. G. Katz (Ed.), *Current topics in early childhood education* (pp. 73–104). Norwood, NJ: Ablex.

Federlein, A. C. (1979, April). *A study of play behaviors and interactions of preschool handicapped children in mainstreamed and segregated settings.* Paper presented at the 57th Annual International Convention of the Council for Exceptional Children, Dallas, TX.

Ferguson, J., Mulvihill, B., Spiker, D., & Bryant, D. (in press). Health and safety in infant and toddler daycare: Lessons from the Infant Health and Development Program. In R. T. Gross, D. Spiker, & C. Haynes (Eds.), *The Infant Health and Development Program.* Palo Alto, CA: Stanford University Press.

Fewell, R. R., & Vadasy, P. F. (1983). *Learning through play: A resource manual for teachers and parents.* Hingham, MA: Teaching Resources.

Fewell, R. R., & Vadasy, P. F. (Eds.). (1986). *Families of handicapped children.* Austin, TX: Pro-Ed.

Fromberg, D. (1992). A review of research on play. In C. Seefeldt (Ed.), *The early childhood curriculum: A review of current research* (pp. 42–84). New York: Teachers College Press.

Furman, W., Rahe, D. F., & Hartup, W. W. (1979). Rehabilitation of socially withdrawn preschool children through mixed-age and same-age socialization. *Child Development, 50,* 915–922.

Furuno, S., O'Reilly, A., Hosaka, C., Inatsuka, T., Allman, T., & Ziesloft, B. (1985). *Hawaii early learning profile (HELP)* (rev. ed.). Palo Alto, CA: VORT.

Goodman, R. A., Osterholm, M. T., Granoff, D. M., & Pickering, L. K. (1984). Infectious diseases and child day care. *Pediatrics, 74*(1), 134–139.

Guralnick, M. J. (1988). Efficacy research in early childhood intervention programs. In S. L. Odom & M. B. Kames (Eds.), *Early intervention for infants and children with handicaps* (pp. 75–88). Baltimore: Paul H. Brookes.

Guralnick, M. J., & Groom, J. M. (1987). Dyadic peer interactions of mildly delayed and nonhandicapped preschool children. *American Journal of Mental Deficiencies, 92,* 178–193.

Guralnick, M. J., & Paul-Brown, D. (1980). Functional and discourse analyses of nonhandicapped children. *American Journal of Mental Deficiencies, 84,* 444–454.

Guralnick, M. J. (1980). Social interaction among preschool handicapped children. *Exceptional Children, 46,* 248–253.

Guralnick, M. J. (1982). Programmatic factors affecting child–child social interactions in mainstreamed preschool programs. In P. S. Strain (Ed.), *Social development of exceptional children* (pp. 71–92). Rockville, MD: Aspen Systems.

Hanline, M. F. (1985). Integrating disabled children. *Young Children, 40*(2), 45–48.

Hanson, M. J., & Hanline, M. F. (1989). Integration options for the very young child. In R. Gaylord-Ross (Ed.), *Integration strategies for students with handicaps* (pp. 177–193). Baltimore, MD: Paul H. Brookes.

Harms, T., & Clifford, R. M. (1980). *Early childhood environment rating scale.* New York: Teachers College Press.

Harms, T., & Clifford, R. M. (1989). *The family day care rating scale.* New York: Teachers College Press.

Harms, T., Clifford, R. M., & Bailey, D. B. (1986). *Special needs items for the ECERS.* Chapel Hill, NC: FPG Child Development Center.

Harms, T., Cryer, D., & Clifford, R. M. (1990). *The infant/toddler environment rating scale.* New York: Teachers College Press.

Howes, C., Phillips, D. A., & Whitebook, M. (1992). Thresholds of quality: Implications for the social development of children in center-based child care. *Child Development, 63,* 449–460.

Infant Health and Development Program. (1990). Enhancing the outcomes of low birth weight, premature infants: A multisite randomized trial. *Journal of the American Medical Association, 263,* 3035–3042.

Jennings, K. D., Connors, R. E., Stegman, C. E., Sankaranarayan, P., & Mendelsohn, S. (1985). Mastery motivation in young preschoolers: Effect of a physical handicap and implications for educational programming. *Journal of the Division for Early Childhood, 9,* 162–169.

Johnson-Martin, N. M., Jens, K. G., & Attermeier, S. A. (Eds.). (1986). *The Carolina curriculum for handicapped infants and infants at risk.* Baltimore, MD: Paul H. Brookes.

Kotch, J. B., & Bryant, D. (1990). Effects of day care on the health and development of children. *Current Opinion in Pediatrics, 2,* 883–894.

Lay-Dopyera, M., & Dopyera, J. (1986). Strategies for teaching. In C. Seefeldt (Ed.), *Early childhood curricula: A review of current research*. New York: Teachers College Press.

LeLaurin, K. D., & Risley, T. R. (1972). The organization of day care environments: "Zone" versus "man-to-man" staff assignment. *Journal of Applied Behavioral Analysis, 5*, 225–232.

Lerner, J., Mardell-Czudnowski, C., & Goldenberg, D. (1987). *Special education for the early childhood years*. Englewood Cliffs, NJ: Prentice-Hall.

Mahoney, G., Finger, I., & Powell, A. (1985). Relationship of maternal behavioral style to the development of organically impaired mentally retarded infants. *American Journal of Mental Deficiency, 90*, 296–302.

Mahoney, G., Robinson, C., & Powell, A. (1992). Focusing on parent–child interaction: The bridge to developmentally appropriate practices. *Topics in Early Childhood Special Education, 12*(1), 105–120.

Mallory, B. L. (1992). Is it always appropriate to be developmental? Convergent models for early intervention practice. *Topics in Early Childhood Special Education, 11*(4), 1–12.

Masin, H. L. (1991). *Parental attitudes toward physical therapy services at the Debbie School Early Intervention Program*. Miami, FL: University of Miami.

McWilliam, R. A., & Strain, P. S. (1993). Service delivery models. In *DEC Task Force on Recommended Practices: Indicators of quality in programs for infants and young children with special needs and their families* (pp. 39–48). Reston, VA: Council for Exceptional Children.

Miller, P. S. (1992). Segregated programs of teacher education in early childhood: Immoral and inefficient practice. *Topics in Early Childhood Special Education, 11*(4), 39–52.

Montessori, M. (1964). *The Montessori method*. New York: Schocken.

Mori, A. A., & Neisworth, J. T. (1983). Curricula in early childhood education: Some generic and special considerations. *Topics in Early Childhood Special Education, 2*(4), 1–8.

National Association for the Education of Young Children. (1984). *Creditation criteria and procedures of the National Academy of Early Childhood Education: Position statement of the National Academy of Early Childhood Programs*. Washington, DC: Author.

National Early Childhood Technical Assistance System. (1989). *A bibliography of selected resources on cultural diversity for parents and professionals working with young children who have, or are at-risk for, disabilities*. Chapel Hill, NC: Author.

National Early Childhood Technical Assistance System. (1991). *Cultural competence in screening and assessment: Implications for services to young children with special needs ages birth through five* (prepared by M. Anderson & P. Goldberg in conjunction with NECTAS). Chapel Hill, NC: Author.

Odom, S. L., & McEvoy, M. A. (1988). Integration of young children with handicaps and normally developing children. In S. L. Odom & M. B. Karnes (Eds.), *Early intervention for infants and children with handicaps: An empirical case* (pp. 241–268). Baltimore, MD: Paul H. Brookes.

Piaget, J. (1926). *The language and thought of the child*. New York: Humanities.

Piaget, J. (1952). *The origins of intelligence in children* (M. Cook, Trans.). New York: W. W. Norton.

Piaget, J. (1972). *Science of education and the psychology of the child* (rev. ed.). New York: Viking.

Ramey, C. T., Bryant, D. M., Wasik, B. H., Sparling, J. J., Fendt, K. H., & LaVange, L. M. (1992). The infant health and development program for low birthweight, premature infants: Program elements, family participation, and child intelligence. *Pediatrics, 3*, 454–465.

Ramsey, P. G. (1979). Beyond "Ten Little Indians" and turkeys: Alternative approaches to Thanksgiving. *Young Child, 34*(6), 28–32, 49–52.

Roupp, R., Travers, J., Glantz, F., & Goelen, C. (1979). *Children at the center: Final report of the National Day Care Study.* Cambridge, MA: ABT Associates.

Sanford, A. R., & Zelman, J. G. (1981). The learning accomplishment profile, In D. B. Bailey, Jr. & M. Wolery (Eds.), *Assessing infants and preschoolers with handicaps* (p. 27). Columbus, OH: Merrill.

Saracho, O., & Spodek, B. (Eds.). (1983). *Understanding the multicultural experience in early childhood education.* Washington, DC: National Association for the Education of Young Children.

Schweinhart, L. S. (1989–1990). When the buck stops here: What it takes to run good early childhood programs. In J. S. McKee & K. M. Paciorek (Eds.), *Early childhood education 89/90* (10th ed., pp. 20–25). Guilford, CT: Duskin.

Shonkoff, J. P., & Hauser-Cram, P. (1987). Early intervention for disabled infants and their families—a quantitative analysis. *Pediatrics, 80*, 650–658.

Smith, F. (1985). *Reading without nonsense* (2nd ed.). New York: Teachers College Press.

Snell, M. E. (Ed.). (1987). *Systematic instruction of persons with severe handicaps* (3rd ed.). Columbus, OH: Merrill.

Snyder-McLean, L., & McLean, J. E. (1987). Effectiveness of early intervention for children with language and communication disorders. In M. J. Guralnick & F. C. Bennett (Eds.), *The effectiveness of early intervention for at-risk and handicapped children* (pp. 213–271). New York: Academic Press.

Sparling, J. J. (1989). Narrow- and broad-spectrum curricula: Two necessary parts of the special child's program. *Infants and Young Children, 1*(4), 1–8.

Sparling, J. J., & Lewis, I. S. (1979). *Learning games for the first three years: A guide to parent–child play.* New York: Walker.

Sparling, J. J., & Lewis, I. S. (1985). *Partners for learning.* Lewisville, NC: Kaplan Press.

Sparling, J. J., Lewis, I. S., & Neuwirth, S. (1993). *Early partners.* Chapel Hill, NC: Frank Porter Graham Child Development Center.

Spodek, B., Saracho, O. N., & Davis, M. D. (1991). *Foundation of early childhood education* (2nd ed.). Englewood Cliffs, NJ: Prentice-Hall.

Spodek, B., Saracho, O., & Lee, R. (1984). *Mainstreaming young children.* Belmont, CA: Wadsworth.

Stayton, V., & Miller, P. (1993). Personnel competence. In *DEC Task Force on Recommended Practices: Indicators of quality in programs for infants and young children with special needs and their families* (pp. 105–115). Reston, VA: Council for Exceptional Children.

Strain, P. S. (1990). LRE for preschool children with handicaps: What we know, what we should be doing. *Journal of Early Intervention, 4*, 291–296.

Strain, P. S., & Odom, S. L. (1986). Peer social initiations: Effective intervention for social skills development of exceptional children. *Exceptional Children, 52*(6), 543–551.

Turbiville, V., Turnbull, A., Garland, C., & Lee, I. (1993). IFSP's and IEP's. In *DEC Task Force on Recommended Practices: Indicators of quality in programs for infants and young children with special needs and their families* (pp. 29–38). Reston, VA: Council for Exceptional Children.

Turnbull, A. P., & Turnbull, H. R. (1986). *Families and special education.* Columbus, OH: Merrill.

U.S. Consumer Product Safety Commission. (1991). *Handbook for public playground safety.* Washington, DC: U.S. Government Printing Office.

U.S. Consumer Product Safety Commission/National Electronic Injury Surveillance System. (1992). *U.S. Consumer Product Safety Commission/Directorate for Epidemiology: National Injury Information Clearinghouse Report.* Washington, DC: Author.

Vincent, L., & Beckett, J. (1993). Related to family participation. In *DEC Task Force on Recommended Practices: Indicators of quality in programs for infants and young children with special needs and their families* (pp. 18–28). Reston, VA: Council for Exceptional Children.

Warren, S. F., & Kaiser, A. P. (1986). Generalization of treatment effects by young language-delayed children: A longitudinal analysis. *Journal of Speech and Hearing Disabilities, 51,* 239–251.

Warren, S. F., & Rogers-Warren, A. (1982). Language acquisition patterns in normal and handicapped children. *Topics in Early Childhood Special Education, 2*(2), 70–79.

Weiner, E. A., & Weiner, B. J. (1974). Differentiation of retarded and normal children through toy-play analysis. *Multivariate Behavioral Resources, 9,* 245–257.

Wesley, P. (1992). *Mainstreaming young children.* Available from author, FPG Center, CB#8180, UNC-CH, Chapel Hill, NC 27599.

Whitebook, M., Howes, C., & Phillips, D. A. (1989). *Who cares? Child care teachers and the quality of care in America. The national child care staffing study.* Oakland, CA: Child Care Employee Project.

Wolery, M., & Fleming, L. A. (1993). Implementing individualized curriculum in integrated settings. In C. A. Peck, S. L. Odom, & D. Bricker (Eds.), *Integrating young children with disabilities into community programs: From research to implementation* (pp. 109–132). Baltimore, MD: Paul H. Brookes.

Wolery, M., & Sainato, D. (1993). General curriculum and intervention strategies. In *DEC Task Force on Recommended Practices: Indicators of quality in programs for infants and young children with special needs and their families* (pp. 49–59). Reston, VA: Council for Exceptional Children.

Wolery, M., Strain, P. S., & Bailey, D. B. (1992). Applying the framework of developmentally appropriate practice to children with special needs. In S. Bredekamp & T. Rosegrant (Eds.), *Reaching potentials: Appropriate curriculum and assessment for young children* (Vol. 1, pp. 92–111). Washington, DC: National Association for the Education of Young Children.

York, S. (1991). *Roots & wings: Affirming culture in early childhood programs.* St. Paul, MN: Redleaf Press.

CHAPTER 12

Contemporary Therapies for Infants and Toddlers
Preferred Approaches

ELSIE R. VERGARA
SANDRA ADAMS
HELEN MASIN
DEBRA BECKMAN

The scope of early intervention therapy has changed dramatically in recent years. The expanding pluralistic society, the national emphasis on prevention, new etiologies of disabilities, new technological developments, partnerships with families, and incentives for teamwork have shifted the very nature of therapeutic assessment and interventions.

The emphasis on providing therapy services as early as possible in the life of a child has occurred in the last three decades. Prior to this contemporary trend, occupational, physical, speech and language, and other therapy services for infants and toddlers were provided only to children who exhibited established conditions such as cerebral palsy, congenital anomalies, or poliomyelitis. Mild conditions not overtly interfering with the child's development and daily functioning were often left untreated. Therapeutic procedures were generally limited to muscle strengthening and tone normalization, range of motion exercises, splinting, ambulation, and developmental stimulation. Therapists today provide a much wider scope of expertise as knowledge and technology have increased and as a primary focus on prevention has become stronger.

New etiologies of disabilities such as children with HIV or prenatal exposure to drugs and alcohol and changes in incidence of disabilities, such as increased numbers of surviving low-birth-weight infants, have resulted in a much more heterogeneous population of children in need of therapies. Assessment and intervention procedures have been developed or modified to address the needs of this newly emerging population of young children with disabilities.

The change toward early provision of therapy services has occurred concurrently with a recognition of the powerful influence of the environment, particularly of the family, on a child's developmental outcome (Dunst, Trivette, & Deal, 1988; Sameroff, 1982). The main goal of contemporary therapies is to optimize the child's environment as early as possible after a developmental delay is identified or suspected so as to further the child's developmental potential. The family is central in the determination of the child's therapy needs and is an active participant in the development of the child's intervention program.

Society's shift toward a more multicultural population has a major impact on the provision of therapies. The effectiveness of therapy can be enhanced if professionals are willing and able to modify their interventions to fit the beliefs and expectations of families with whom they work (Masin, 1992; Saunders, 1954). For example, professionals might establish better family communication with Hispanic-Americans if they were willing to include the extended family in the intervention program. Because of the critical impact of culture and families upon a child's development, culturally competent care must be a goal toward providing optimal intervention with different ethnic groups (Masin, 1992).

Another significant change in the provision of therapies has been the shift from a unilateral medical model of service delivery to a more holistic interdisciplinary or transdisciplinary team approach. The therapist is part of the team along with the family and other interventionists. The child's parents are encouraged to take an active role in the team's decisions. The emphasis on team services has resulted in new, different, and potentially more effective ways of serving children.

These rapid and expansive changes have left little time for consensus building in best practices for providing therapeutic interventions. High demand for direct care providers has further exacerbated the shortage of therapists in research positions resulting in limited empirical data proving the effectiveness of therapy practices. Recently, the Council for Exceptional Children, Division for Early Childhood (DEC) conducted an extensive survey to ascertain recommended practices in early intervention both from research literature and clinical practice (DEC, 1993). Although there is not widespread consensus on *best* practices in therapy, and although individualization continues to be endorsed, most concur on *preferred* practices from the neonatal period through infancy and toddlerhood. This chapter builds upon the DEC Recommended Practices to suggest interventions from the multidisciplinary perspective of therapists.

DEVELOPMENTALLY APPROPRIATE
NEONATAL INTERVENTIONS

Prior to the 1970s, only newborn infants with established developmental disabilities were offered therapeutic intervention. Technological and medical advances during the 1960s and 1970s significantly improved the survival rate of premature and sick infants. Neonatal intensive care units (NICUs) were established to provide special care to this increasing number of infants who, because of their fragility, were susceptible to developmental delays or dysfunctions. This section describes assessment and intervention strategies for newborns.

Neonatal Assessment

The infant's therapy needs should be thoroughly assessed prior to initiating intervention. NICUs with a full-time developmental staff (e.g., physical or occupational therapists) often screen all of the infants in the unit for potential developmental problems that may require intervention. Screening usually consists of systematic criterion-referenced observations that include aspects such as posture, muscle tone, reflex development, temperament (irritability), interactive abilities, self-organization, and feeding. In units with part-time developmental services, only the highest-risk infants, or those with conditions likely to affect development (e.g., intrauterine drug exposure, small for gestational age, HIV-positive, neurological insults), are screened. Commonly, nursing or medical personnel identify and refer the babies in need of developmental evaluation.

A neonatal assessment may include a number of domains; however, lengthy data collection that may increase the infant's stress level must be avoided when working with very small or sick infants (Als, 1986). To lessen stress, the assessment should rely as much as possible on observation rather than on hands-on procedures. Table 12.1 presents the domains frequently assessed in a comprehensive evaluation of newborn infants (Vergara, 1993a). The infant's medical stability and presenting problems usually determine which domains will be evaluated for a particular infant. Other factors that influence the domains to be evaluated are family concerns and priorities, time available for the assessment, expertise of the evaluator, role delineation of the institution, and financial reimbursement (Vergara, 1993a).

Of the few standardized neonatal assessment instruments available, no single tool evaluates all of the possible domains (see Taylor, Chapter 8, this volume). The Assessment of Preterm Infant Behavior (APIB) (Als, Lester, & Brazelton, 1982) is the most comprehensive test for assessing neurobehavioral functioning in premature infants. It gives a detailed picture of the infant's

TABLE 12.1.   Domains That May Be Included in a Comprehensive Neonatal Assessment

Domains	Components
Neurobehavioral organization and environmental modulation needs	Tolerance to stressful stimuli Self-regulation abilities State behavior Temperament Interactive abilities Sensory processing/deprivation Habituation
Reflex development	Hyper- or hyporeflexia Delays Asymmetries
Postural development	Predominant postures Need of external support Ability to adopt flexor postures Asymmetries Abnormal postures Postures that agitate the infant Best postures to reduce agitation
Motor activity	Quality, frequency, and range of spontaneous and facilitated motor activity Asymmetries Upper extremity versus lower extremity activity Flexor versus extensor activity Abnormal patterns
Oral motor functioning and feeding	Ability to lip seal Sucking quality and rhythm Sucking/swallowing/breathing synchrony Aspiration or reflux Hyper- or hypotonia of oral structures

response to stress, interactive abilities, physiological cost of stimulation, and other information. However, use of the APIB has been hindered by the complexity and length of its certification process. The Neurological Assessment of the Preterm and Full-Term Newborn Infant (Dubowitz & Dubowitz, 1981), the Neonatal Behavioral Assessment Scale (Brazelton, 1984), and the Neurological Evaluation in the Neonatal Period (Amiel-Tison & Grenier, 1986) give a less thorough overview of the infant's neurobehavioral functioning and require less or no formal training.

When using an assessment instrument other than the APIB, the evaluator often has to complement the evaluation findings with additional clinical observations regarding stress and interactive behavior. The Level 1 phase of the Neonatal Individualized Developmental Care and Assessment Program (NIDCAP) developed by Heidelise Als and Gretchen Lawhon (personal communication, October 1989) for training health care professionals in the use of the APIB is an excellent training program to gain observational skills and improve caregiving for high-risk newborns. Level 1 NIDCAP training is highly recommended for therapists who wish to learn to assess the infant's social and physical environment and to structure an environment that will be supportive to the individual infant's nervous system based on contemporary therapeutic approaches.

Types of Intervention

Among the most common referrals for neonatal intervention are environmental modulation and neurobehavioral organization, including caregiver–infant interaction, positioning, splinting, oral motor and feeding, and developmental and supplemental sensory stimulation (Vergara, 1993a). Intervention procedures such as environmental modulation and positioning are not intrusive and can be initiated even during the physiological instability stage. Assessment to begin these interventions can be done almost exclusively through observation.

Environmental Modulation and Neurobehavioral Organization

Originally, premature infants were believed to experience sensory deprivation as a result of their shortened intrauterine life and the isolation caused by the incubator environment. A number of sensory stimulation programs evolved in the 1970s to replicate the intrauterine environment so as to compensate for the sensory deprivation these infants were believed to be experiencing (Field, 1980; Linn, Horowitz, & Fox, 1985; Sweeney & Swanson, 1990). Although supplemental sensory stimulation programs were supported by research findings such as increased weight gain and improved development in some infants, it soon became obvious that only the larger, physiologically stable infants (the subjects selected for most research studies) were able to tolerate and benefit from the extra sensory stimulation. Younger and sicker premature infants were found to be frequently overwhelmed and distressed by increased sensory stimulation (Linn et al., 1985). Another theory emerged that described the neonatal intensive care atmosphere as a sensory-aversive, rather than sensory-deprived, environment (Gottfried, Wallace-Lande, Sherman-Brown, King, & Coen, 1981). Within this model, infants are believed to respond effectively to increased sensory stimulation only if their neurobehavioral system is sufficiently mature and stable to maintain its organization when exposed to the stimuli (Als, 1986).

Contemporary neonatal intervention models focus on modulating or adapting the infant's environment to decrease or eliminate unnecessary aversive stimuli likely to stress the infant and to encourage environmental stimuli that are safely tolerated and promote the infant's neurobehavioral organization. This type of intervention has resulted in improved modulation of the motor system, improved self-regulation, shorter hospitalization, shorter need of oxygen supplementation, and higher frequency of normal reflexes (Als & Duffy, 1989). Although environmental modulation allows for stable infants to be exposed to self-regulating stimuli as long as stress monitoring is provided, such stimuli may also need to be avoided when working with medically unstable infants.

Environmental modulation is also very important for fostering caregiver–infant interaction. Hussey (1988) is an excellent source for teaching parents to recognize and respond appropriately to their infant's signals. To enhance the quality of caregiver–infant interaction, parents need to learn to avoid exposing their infant to stressful stimuli, to offer time-out breaks when stress reactions occur, to employ strategies that improve their infant's neurobehavioral organization, and to time social interaction around the infant's best periods. Therapists should be supportive of positive parent–infant interactions and model more appropriate styles, when needed.

Positioning Intervention

Positioning intervention is indicated for infants who tend to adopt postures that may interfere with their development. Professionals and caregivers should frequently change the position of children unable to reposition themselves (DEC, 1993). The goals of neonatal positioning vary according to the type of problem presented. Premature infants often have low muscle tone and tend to adopt postures that may disrupt the development of rolling over and crawling (Semmler, 1989; Vergara, 1993b). To alleviate this problem, a boundary is formed around the infant with foam, rolled towels, sandbags, or other positioning devices to help the child maintain a flexor posture until muscle tone increases. This technique is typically used in the prone position because prone is most favorable for the development of flexor tone, longer and deeper sleep, and respiration rates. However, in the supine position, the technique can be used by creating a cradle or nest (supine nesting) around the baby to flex the extremities. To prevent breathing difficulties, the neck is flexed only slightly

(Semmler, 1989; Vergara, 1993b). Supine positioning has become emphasized because of the recently reported association of prone positioning with increased incidence of Sudden Infant Death Syndrome (American Academy of Pediatrics Task Force on Infant Positioning in SIDS, 1992). Prone continues to be used for positioning premature infants whose vital signs are continually monitored.

Sidelying positioning poses a different problem in that it promotes development of hyperextended postures, especially in infants with breathing difficulties who tend to extend the neck to breathe. Posterior head and trunk support are helpful to prevent neck hyperextension when prolonged sidelying positioning is necessary (Vergara, 1993b).

Other positioning intervention involves preventing head flattening and gastroesophageal reflux or aspiration. The use of water mattresses and eggcrate foam seem to reduce head flattening, but no studies have formally assessed their effectiveness. Intervention to prevent reflux consists of positioning in prone over a 30° incline (head elevated). Harnesses and reflux wedges help prevent sliding from the slant.

Splinting

Infants who have limitations of range of motion or joint deformities require a specialized form of positioning that is best accomplished through splinting. Splinting involves positioning of a specific body part. The type of splint required is determined on an individualized basis according to the infant's needs. In general, splinting materials for neonates should be soft (foam is frequently preferred) and should mold at low temperatures. Special care must be taken to protect skin integrity. Detailed recommendations regarding infant splinting are found in Anderson and Anderson (1988).

Oral Motor Intervention and Feeding

Oral motor and feeding training are also common reasons for neonatal intervention. Oral motor interventions are specific procedures provided outside mealtime to enhance the functional response to pressure and movement on the face and within the mouth, including range, strength, variety, and control of movements for the lips, cheeks, jaw, and tongue. Sucking, chewing, swallowing, and speech depend on the development of specific controlled movements. Sucking with adequate strength and duration for breast or bottle feeding is obviously important for a newborn.

Nervous system immaturity is the most prevalent cause of feeding disorders in newborn infants (Braun & Palmer, 1985). Studies suggest that infants are not ready for nipple feedings until after 35–36 weeks postconception (Gryboski, 1969). Common feeding problems in premature infants include weak or arrhythmic sucking; poor lip seal; inadequate intraoral suction; poor coordination of sucking, swallowing, and breathing; low endurance; oral hypersensitivity; abnormal muscle tone; abnormal postural patterns; and decreased oxygen saturation during feedings (Braun & Palmer, 1985; Vergara, 1993b). Other neonatal feeding problems include Failure to Thrive, cleft lip or palate, Pierre Robin, Prader–Willi syndrome, and severe irritability (Vergara, 1993b).

Great concern results when an infant has difficulty with oral intake because of either failure at breast feeding or other feeding problems. Infants referred for nipple-feeding (bottle or breast) training should be physiologically stable. Those who fail to gain weight or who exhibit aspiration when orally fed may require enteral (intravenous), gavage (oral or nasal), or gastric tube feeding. In the initial stages of feeding training, feeding types may be combined (e.g., nipple and supplemental gavage) especially if the infant takes more than 20–30 minutes to eat.

The specific factors interfering with a child's ability to feed should be determined prior to and throughout any feeding intervention. Although most therapists prefer to use criterion-referenced feeding assessments, two standardized instruments are available specifically for neonates: the Neonatal Oral Motor Assessment Scale (NOMAS) (Braun & Palmer, 1985) and the Nursing Child Assessment Feeding Scale (NCAF) (Barnard, 1980). The NOMAS evaluates many of the oral motor components required for feeding whereas the NCAF assesses parent–infant interaction during feeding.

Feeding training should begin with proper structuring of the environment to optimize the infant's feeding abilities. Minimal stimulation environments considerably improve feeding efficiency (Lawhon & Melzar, 1988). Proper nipple selection is also a very important element of feeding training (Morris & Klein, 1987). Nutritive sucking has been found to improve when preparatory nonnutritive sucking and intraoral stimulation are given. Stress signals need to be monitored to avoid stress reactions as the infants are fed.

During breast feeding, infants are traditionally positioned in a sidelying position. This position may enhance sucking for an infant with a weak suck receiving fluids from a bottle. A reclined position in which the child is more supine requires more strength and control to bring cheeks, lips, and jaw toward midline. Increased spillage, reduced intake, increased fatigue, and incoordination of swallowing and breathing may result. Maintaining the head in alignment with the trunk, with the head in slight flexion (the chin is aimed slightly toward the chest, rather than toward the ceiling), may enhance oral control during sucking. Additional handling techniques may be needed to stabilize and support the head, cheeks, jaw, and lips.

The following are suggestions to correct some of the most common feeding problems of neonates (Vergara, 1993b):

- Jaw and cheek support improves lip seal, sucking rhythm, and decreases liquid loss.
- Oral hypersensitivity is decreased by progressively applying perioral and intraoral stimulation, moving toward the inside of the mouth as sensitivity decreases; hand-to-mouth exploration and nonnutritive sucking also tend to decrease hypersensitivity.
- Swaddling, proper postural support, and inhibitory techniques help prevent abnormal extensor postures that cause jaw thrusting likely to interfere with feeding.
- Limiting the amount of liquid to be swallowed at one time improves coordination of sucking, swallowing, and breathing; this is achieved by using slow-flowing or Haberman nipples (Campbell & Trenouth, 1987), keeping the bottle as horizontal as possible, and feeding from a syringe (liquid may be thickened to decrease its flow for older infants).
- Oral intake for infants with cleft palates can be improved with the use of squirt bottles.
- Infants with gastroesophageal reflux must be fed as upright as possible to prevent aspiration.

Developmental and Supplemental Sensory Stimulation

Neurobehavioral stability is a prerequisite to begin developmental or supplemental sensory stimulation intervention. Infants must have achieved a high tolerance to stimulation and be free of major stress reactions, particularly those that affect their physiological (autonomic) system. Developmental stimulation involves the use of a series of therapeutic handling techniques to normalize muscle tone and reflexes and to promote more advanced functioning (Anderson & Auster-Liebhaber, 1984). It is usually reserved for older infants (beyond 3 months of age). Development is encouraged according to the normal developmental sequence. Supplemental sensory stimulation programs are geared to somewhat replicate the intrauterine sensory experiences that were shortened because of premature birth (Cole, 1985; Gorga, 1989; Heriza & Sweeney, 1990). Tactile, vestibular, and proprioceptive input are offered according to a preestablished protocol. Readiness for supplemental stimulation intervention is determined by absence or low incidence of stress reactions. Other sensory stimulation programs involve visual and auditory stimulation to promote development of sensory processing. Although these programs may be beneficial for some infants, stress reactions always need to be closely monitored while offering extra sensory stimulation.

Developmental Follow-Up after Neonatal Intensive Care

Most NICUs have multi- or interdisciplinary follow-up programs to monitor children and meet the needs of high-risk infants after discharge through at least the second year (often through age 5 years). The main purpose of these programs is to identify potential developmental problems that may require immediate preventive or early remedial intervention (Taeusch & Ware, 1980). Other purposes of infant follow-up include providing specialized management of complex medical conditions and enhancing the family's caregiving skills through education and support. Atypical development is determined through periodic neurological and/or developmental evaluations commonly assessing the domains of gross motor, fine motor, oral motor, self-help, social–emotional, cognitive, and sensory processing and perceptual–motor skills. Infants with established conditions known to affect their developmental potential are often referred for preventive therapy before developmental delays emerge. Home programs to teach the family to optimize their child's development may be designed and implemented as part of the follow-up programs. Follow-up schedules vary from center to center. Many institutions evaluate these children at certain transitional ages: 3–4 months, 9 months, 1 year, 18 months, and 2 years. Other programs follow infants more closely, every 2 to 3 months during the first year, every 6 months for the second year, and annually thereafter. Because there is no research evidence to indicate that following infants more frequently is more beneficial, the American Academy of Pediatrics recommends that follow-up visits should be determined by the needs of the individual infant and family (American Academy of Pediatrics, 1992). This organization further states that "it may be necessary to examine some of these infants weekly or bimonthly at first" (p. 113), and that to ensure early identification of problems and referrals for remediation in high-risk infants, "neurologic, developmental, behavioral, and sensory status should be assessed more than once during the first year" (p. 113).

Follow-up often includes screening such as the Denver-II (Frankenburg et al., 1990) or other measures described by Taylor in Chapter 8 of this volume. However, comparing a child's performance to established norms does not assess quality of function. Assessing quality of function is important because quality and age appropriateness vary independently—a child's performance may be age appropriate, although abnormal in quality. Quality of function is best assessed through skilled observation and criterion-referenced methods. Neurological assessments such as the Amiel-Tison and Grenier Neurological Evaluation in the Neonatal Period (1986), the Milani-Comparetti Motor Development Screening Test (Stuberg, 1992), and the Movement Assessment of Infants (Chandler, Andrews, & Swanson, 1980) are useful to detect abnormal muscle tone, reflexes, and motor development.

The Early Intervention Developmental Profile (EIDP) (Rogers, D'Eugenio,

Brown, Donovan, & Lynch, 1981) and the Hawaii Early Learning Profile (HELP) (Furuno et al., 1979) have been designed to facilitate program planning in a very practical and simple format. These two tests can be used with parents and other caregivers to help them understand the child's needs and identify appropriate activities to promote the child's development.

More specific assessments (e.g., oral motor, range of motion, muscle strength, or speech/language), when needed, are usually administered by therapists upon consultation with the follow-up team. Results from these tests are analyzed within the context of the child's developmental level to establish the basis for intervention through infancy and toddlerhood.

INTERVENTION BEYOND THE NEONATAL PERIOD: INFANTS AND TODDLERS

The concept of early intervention beyond the neonatal period and its importance in enhancing the developmental potential of children began to gain popularity approximately three decades ago. A number of studies conducted in the late 1960s suggested that children who exhibited a number of conditions known to cause developmental delays could benefit from initiation of therapy during their infancy. Early intervention physical and occupational therapy programs emerged around the nation in response to these findings. However, most of these programs were geared to provide intervention for children who had been diagnosed with a condition likely to cause atypical development. It was not until the 1970s that the provision of services to infants at risk for disabilities without obvious established conditions was given serious attention. The latter occurred simultaneously with the national efforts to enhance the developmental outcome of children from deprived environments through programs such as Head Start.

Passage of the Individuals with Disabilities Education Act in 1986 promoted the development of early intervention programs. Despite increased awareness and legal efforts, early intervention services have not grown as anticipated. It is estimated that the number of early intervention programs available throughout the nation is insufficient to address the needs of the current at-risk population of children. Most early intervention programs are still focused on secondary prevention, to optimize the developmental potential of children with established conditions likely to cause developmental disabilities. Within the next few years, it is anticipated that many states will expand early intervention initiatives to also address the needs of the children at risk for developmental problems.

Gross motor, fine motor, and oral motor interventions constitute the areas of major focus in early intervention programs. Other areas of focus include provision of therapy services for infants of special populations such as those exposed to cocaine *in utero* and those with AIDS. This section presents a summary of the early intervention practices currently in use within the major areas of intervention.

Gross Motor

Gross motor delays are among the most common disorders of high-risk infants and toddlers. Infants with developmental delays progress along the developmental sequence at a slower pace (Ellison, 1984; Sweeney & Swanson, 1990). Preventing or ameliorating gross motor delays early in the life of an infant is extremely important because functional skill acquisition in other developmental domains is believed by many to be dependent on a gross motor foundation.

Developmental Sequence

Gross motor development progresses in a sequential and predictable order, but its pace can vary between children. Extensor control emerges first in the neck, moving gradually along the spine to the pelvic and hip region. Antigravity flexor control begins to emerge as the infant gains control over the back (extensor) muscles. This control also progresses from the center of the body toward the extremities (proximal–distal and medial–lateral). Adequate postural stability is achieved when the infant develops balanced extensor and flexor control. The ability to bear and shift weight improves as extensor–flexor control is gained and, in turn, greater control is gained as the infant bears and shifts weight. The infant's ability to extend the neck promotes a weight shift toward the elbows that allows progression to the next stage: prone on elbows. As control moves distally, the infant becomes able to bear weight on extended arms. Simultaneously, control progresses caudally enabling the infant to adopt the quadruped and sitting positions. Further caudal and distal progression of control enables the infant to stand and eventually to walk while development of trunk rotation enables the infant to move smoothly between different positions (Bly, 1983).

Intervention to Improve Gross Motor Delays

Intervention for children with gross motor delays involves providing activities and situations that foster the necessary motor control to achieve skills according to this developmental sequence. Several instruments are available for determining the child's performance level in the developmental sequence (Chandler, Andrews, & Swanson, 1980; Folio & Fewell, 1983; Furuno et al., 1979; Rogers et al., 1981).

Therapists foster the acquisition of foundation skills, including the development of trunk, spine, shoulder, and hip/pelvic stability and control; development of antigravity flexion; ability to coordinate extensor and flexor muscles; integration of primitive reflexes; development of righting and equilibrium reactions; development of trunk rotation; and ability to bear and shift weight in different positions. Acquisition of foundation skills promotes the development of more advanced adaptive gross motor skills.

Children whose development is progressing somewhat slowly but who have no neurological involvement often do not need direct intervention from a therapist. These children usually respond to gross motor intervention programs provided through indirect (consultation) services. In this case, the occupational or physical therapist evaluates the child in collaboration with the family and other interventionists to determine the child's gross motor needs and the family's priorities for the child. A program to enhance the child's acquisition of gross motor skills is then developed by the team, implemented by the family, educators, or paraprofessionals, and monitored by the therapist. Programs such as the Developmental Programming for Infants and Young Children (Schafer & Moersch, 1981) are particularly practical and effective for helping families and paraprofessionals foster gross motor skill development. These children may also receive intervention in groups with the parents serving as treatment coproviders under the ongoing direction of the therapist.

Intervention for Neurologically Based Gross Motor Problems

Infants who have neurological abnormalities along with developmental delays require more complex intervention. Assessment for these infants involves determining the quality of the children's movements in addition to determining their developmental performance level. Soon to be available, Miller's Toddlers and Infants Motor Evaluation (TIME) test (developed by the author of the Miller Assessment for Preschoolers) promises to become a key instrument for the assessment of quality of function in this age group. Miller's TIME test assesses quality of gross as well as fine motor performance (Ricardo Carrasco, personal communication, October 28, 1992).

Intervention to ameliorate or improve neurologically based gross motor problems and to improve quality of movement typically involves a series of neurodevelopmental procedures administered by specialized personnel (Bobath, 1980; McCormack, 1990). Such procedures focus more on the acquisition of the foundation skills previously described than on practice and repetition of specific delayed skills. Frequency and intensity of the treatment program are determined through neurological assessment done in collaboration with the family. The physical therapist is frequently the primary service provider for these children, particularly when development of ambulation is an issue. Occupational therapists also become involved in the treatment of gross motor dysfunctions as necessary to optimize the child's functional skill development and advanced upper extremity gross motor skills such as ball throwing. Parents, teachers, and paraprofessionals participate with the therapists in the implementation and carry over of the intervention goals outside the therapy sessions.

A developmental intervention perspective for children with neurologically based developmental delays also involves the application of specific therapeutic handling procedures to normalize abnormal reflexes and muscle tone and to promote more normal movement patterns. Examples of specialized procedures to inhibit abnormal patterns and facilitate normal functioning include placing, tapping, and pressure techniques, and facilitation of key points of control, movement, rotation, and weight bearing. Righting and equilibrium reactions are often elicited to facilitate flexion, extension, elongation of certain muscle groups, and shortening of muscles opposite to the ones being elongated (Andersen, 1991). Proper positioning and handling at home and in the classroom (when indicated) are essential to extend the benefits of therapy beyond the intervention period.

Intervention may also involve selection and use of adaptive seating and standing arrangements as well as wheelchair mobility training and use of technological devices. The therapist works in collaboration with the parents and teachers to determine proper positioning to optimize the child's functional skills. Although parents are responsible for overseeing that positioning recommendations are followed at home, teachers provide therapeutic continuity in the classroom.

Fine Motor

A gross motor foundation is believed by many to be essential for skilled fine motor performance. Postural neck and spinal stability allow the child to develop the necessary trunk control to move the extremities freely away from the body and shoulder control to support the arms in order to use the hands efficiently. Adequate upper extremity range of motion, muscle tone, muscle strength, and coordination are also essential components for fine motor skill development. The ability to use the hands to manipulate tools (e.g., spoons, pencils, crayons) is the ultimate purpose in the development of fine motor skills in children. Understanding the developmental sequence and the underlying components of function of fine motor skills is essential for parents and personnel engaged in helping infants and toddlers to achieve their optimal potential in the use of their hands.

Development of Reaching

Development of purposeful reaching is the first step in the acquisition of fine motor skills (Sugden, 1990; Vinter, 1990). Purposeful reaching emerges in normal infants around 3 to 4 months of age (Erhardt, 1982). Random arm activity precedes this stage. At about 4 months, infants begin to reach while momentarily grasping light objects with the ulnar aspect of the palm (Erhardt, 1982). At this stage, reaching is bilateral, where the child approaches the target object with both hands simultaneously. Unilateral reaching begins to emerge around 5 to 6 months of age and continues to refine throughout the first year.

Disorders in any of the gross and fine motor foundation components can cause reaching difficulties, with inadequate postural stability being one of the most common causal factors. Intervention is often geared to enhance gross motor control rather than specifically to foster fine motor skills. Children with neurologically based reaching problems such as increased tone or uncoordinated movements often require the use of procedures to normalize tone and inhibit abnormal movements.

Orthopedic limitations and muscle weakness may also interfere with a child's ability to reach. Problems such as these are usually treated through conventional methods of muscle strengthening and range of motion exercises. Splinting may be indicated for positioning or stabilizing a body segment, or to stretch tight muscles or contractures. Graded age-appropriate activities are used to reinforce the gains achieved through traditional exercise. Collaboration with parents and teachers through follow-up at home and in the classroom is essential to accelerate therapy benefits.

Development of Grasping

Grasping patterns become more radial (toward the thumb side), gradually incorporating the use of the thumb to completely enclose objects in the palm. This occurs throughout the second half of the first year as the grasp reflex becomes fully integrated and as muscle control and stability progress distally toward the wrist, fingers, and palm (Erhardt, 1982). As stability in the palmar arches improves, the child begins to use the fingers to grasp objects more distally, no longer requiring objects to be held against the palm for stability (Boehme, 1988; Erhardt, 1982).

In using the thumb and fingers, infants first attempt to grasp a small object such as a pellet by using the thumb against the curled index finger. This type of grasp is usually unsuccessful. Then, as thumb opposition and interphalangeal stability improves, they begin to grasp pellets between the finger pads. Achievement of this skill reflects the distal progression of motor control. Near age 1 year, infants develop the ability to grasp a pellet between the thumb and the fingertips. By this age, the child's grasping ability is as mature as it will ever be. The ability to release objects voluntarily emerges only after the entire repertoire of grasping patterns is present and forearm supination is fully developed (Erhardt, 1982).

Development of Object Manipulation

Although the ability to grasp objects does not change much after age 1 year, the ability to manipulate or purposefully use objects continues to improve throughout at least early and middle childhood. Crude object manipulation and exploration (within the hand) begins at about 6 months of age, but is not refined until after the first year when stability of the palmar arches is well established and the sequence of prehension has been completed (Boehme, 1988). By 7 months, infants demonstrate primitive object manipulation in activities such as banging and transferring objects between the hands (Erhardt, 1982). Between 1 and 3 years, the child begins to use objects such as a crayon or a spoon, still with an immature grasping pattern. The ability to use tools requires acquisition of cognitive and perceptual–motor skills along with fine motor control. Interaction with the environment, particularly through play, enables infants and toddlers to develop the cognitive and perceptual foundations for later academic and play skills. Tool use becomes refined after the toddler period as fine motor, cognitive, and perceptual–motor functions become further refined.

Intervention to Accelerate Skill Acquisition

Appropriate intervention in motor development addresses all aspects of movement. This includes but is not limited to strength, physical and motor fitness, postural control, eye–hand coordination, object manipulation, positioning, mobility, adaptation, generalization, sensory motor integration, and spatial awareness. Specific techniques for the instruction of these motor attributes can be found in motor curricula such as BodySkills (Werder & Bruininks, 1991) and the Peabody Developmental Motor Activity Cards (Folio & Fewell, 1983).

Given that movement is a constant body activity, it is appropriate that facilitation of quality movements be incorporated into all daily routines. For example, it is just as important to focus on walking while going to a table for a meal as on walking a straight line. Without the generalization of effective movement patterns to all situations, the taught skill is of little value. Likewise, it is important that all family members concerned about a young child's development recognize the need to facilitate efficient motor skills and contribute to the development of these skills.

Children with nonneurological fine motor problems or delays usually respond well when exposed to developmentally graded activities and practice of emergent patterns (Schafer & Moersch, 1981). After age 1 year, therapy should be directed to foster more advanced prehensile patterns, finger isolation, and in-hand manipulation and exploration in preparation for preschool activities (Corbetta & Mounoud, 1990; Erhardt, 1982; Klein, 1982). Play activities and self-help tasks are always useful for enhancing fine motor skill development. Families and other caregivers can contribute greatly to the selection of activities that are appealing and relevant to the child and are thus likely to improve function more effectively. Incorporating the family in the development of the intervention program helps ensure that the program responds to their priorities, concerns, and needs; enhances their compliance; and ultimately results in greater developmental benefit for the child.

Neurologically Based Intervention

Neurological dysfunctions are the most common cause of fine motor problems in high-risk infants (Boehme, 1988). Intervention is focused on neurodevelopmental procedures geared to normalize muscle tone and to promote normal movement patterns. Activities to improve the stability of the palmar arches and to improve forearm rotation and coordination are useful to improve finger dexterity and hand function (Boehme, 1988). A number of procedures focused on the development of the gross motor foundation for fine motor skills are routinely used to improve neurologically based fine motor problems. Further discussion of specific neurodevelopmental principles to address fine motor dysfunctions are beyond the scope of this chapter.

Oral Motor

Oral motor problems are very common in children with developmental delays, particularly in infants who have neurological involvement. Low muscle tone is one of the most common oral motor problems in these children.

Oral Motor Characteristics of the Low-Tone Face

Eruption of the deciduous teeth may be delayed in infants with low tone. Drooling may occur more frequently than in a typical child age birth to 3 years. Facial expressions may be reduced because the lips and cheeks have limited strength and range of movement. Progression from bottle to cup drinking and from pureed foods to table foods may be delayed and frustrating to both the child and the parent. Speech development from vowels to consonants to syllables, words, and phrases may be delayed and/or disordered, adversely affecting development of communication as a result. As the child grows, alignment of the orofacial muscles may not develop, with a resulting "different" appearance from other members of the family and peers.

Knowing that these problems exist is not the challenge. The challenge is to impact these areas at a precognitive level for the child, so that maximum function can develop from the beginning. Because the children cannot follow commands, the therapist works with the family or caregiver to plan, implement, and monitor specific interventions during mealtime and outside mealtime to improve oral motor skills.

Assessment

To best determine the individual child's oral motor needs, parents or caregivers, in partnership with the therapist, evaluate the child's skills during eating to note normal, primitive, and abnormal patterns of movement. The patterns noted are compared to age-specific criteria such as the Pre-Speech Assessment Scale (Morris, 1982). In addition, the areas of strength and of concern for the individual child are determined. The function and symmetry of the facial structures are assessed while the child is at rest and during functional movements (facial expressions, vocal play, eating). Further assessment of oral motor skills involves the child's response to pressure and movement (Howard, Fetters, & MacDonald, 1978; Jaffe, 1980; Morris, 1989; Strominger, Winkler, & Cohen, 1984; Zlatin, 1967).

Range (distance) of movement for passive and active muscle elongation of the lips, cheeks, jaw, and tongue also affects the development of more mature patterns, and must be assessed through observation and directed movements. Reduced variety and strength of movement may result if range of movement is impaired. Control of orofacial movements for eating and management of oral secretions is impacted by the response to pressure and movement, range of movement, variety of movement, and strength of movement of the lips, cheeks, jaw, and tongue. By assessing each of these components, the family and therapist have a detailed baseline from which to plan intervention.

Intervention Plan

Intervention strategies during feeding may include positioning, utensils, food type and consistency, and handling techniques, in addition to changes in the environment in general (Beckman, Roberts, & Tencza, 1992; Morris & Klein, 1987). Specific intervention strategies to improve bottle and breast feeding are discussed earlier in this chapter. Children receiving nonoral intake also need a specific management plan regarding intake that includes the above mentioned areas. If the child is learning to eat pureed foods, the management plan must include all of the following components: positioning, utensils needed, handling techniques, control of placement and flow of food, and food consistency.

In addition to mealtime strategies, the parents and therapist must also address interventions outside mealtime to enhance functional response to pressure and movement as well as range, strength, variety, and control of movement of the lips, cheeks, jaw, and tongue. For children receiving nonoral intake, these interventions are extremely important for oral development. The orofacial structures may easily become overstimulated or fatigued; thus, controlling input to a specific muscle without overflowing to other areas is a challenge. More consistent opportunities for orofacial movement can occur throughout the day and week if the caregiver is a partner in this treatment.

Mealtime and nonmealtime intervention plans may look wonderful on paper, but if the strategies are not consistent with real-life demands of the family's daily schedule, the plan is frequently not implemented. The caregiver(s) and therapist must work together to find the best plan to address the needs of the child. Issues not specific to the child such as availability of resources (time, people, utensils, equipment), continuity of caregivers and therapists, and the skills of the caregiver and therapists should also be considered when implementing an intervention plan.

Over time, as the child's needs change, the intervention strategies must be modified. Ongoing communication between the family and treatment providers is essential, as is ongoing and informal assessment in addition to more formal data gathering.

Progression through a feeding intervention program is constantly monitored to determine modifications needed in response to the child's functional improvement. Provision of external support should be decreased as the child gains stability and control of the postural muscles and oromotor structures. Food texture, density or consistency, and type (e.g., liquids or solids) are modified or introduced as oral hypersensitivity decreases and as the child gains more maturity and coordination of the oromotor structures. More mature eating patterns are also introduced as reflex development progresses and more mature skills emerge. Emergence of the following skills may require a modification in the intervention program:

- Improved lip closure.
- Improved postural stability (neck and trunk).
- Improved jaw stability.
- Decreased intraoral hypersensitivity (tolerance of coarser textures).
- Stronger or more mature sucking.
- Rhythmic sucking.
- Use of the upper lip for cleaning the spoon.
- Moving the food laterally inside the mouth for chewing.
- More mature chewing patterns.

A therapist's sensitivity and response to a child's minor improvements is likely to result in faster and more efficient gains in the child's feeding skills.

INTERVENTIONS FOR SPECIAL POPULATIONS

The alarming rise in the use of cocaine and the incidence of HIV virus and AIDS in pregnant women has led to increased concern about the potential deleterious effects of *in utero* exposure on the infant. The following section discusses common problems presented by newborn infants exposed intrauterinely to either cocaine or the HIV virus and the most common intervention approaches to address the complex needs of these infants and their families.

Cocaine-Exposed Infants and Toddlers

Effects of Gestational Cocaine Exposure

Chasnoff (1989) estimates that 11% of the infants born nationwide are exposed to cocaine. A variety of effects on fetal development have been reported, including relative or absolute microcephaly and a high incidence of intra-uterine growth retardation (Cherukuri, Minkoff, Feldman, Parekh, & Glass, 1988, Hadeed & Siegel, 1989). Neurological problems include perinatal cerebral infarction, cranial ultrasound abnormalities (such as intraventricular hemorrhage, brain necrosis, and cavitary lesions), and transient electroencephalographic changes (Chasnoff, Bussey, Savich, & Stack, 1986; Dixon & Bejar, 1989; Doberczak, Shanzer, Senie, & Kendall, 1988). In addition, some researchers have found significant increases in congenital malformations (Bingol, Fuchs, Diaz, Stone, & Gromisch, 1987; MacGregor et al., 1987). Controversy exists as to whether a cocaine withdrawal syndrome exists in newborns or whether newborn symptoms of drug exposure, such as irritability, tremulousness, jitteriness, and startles, are indicators of more lasting central nervous system changes (Chasnoff et al., 1985; Schneider, Griffith, & Chasnoff, 1989).

Neurobehavioral effects in cocaine-exposed newborns as measured by the Brazelton Neonatal Behavioral Assessment Scale (Brazelton, 1984) have also been reported. Some studies have found significantly poorer interactive, state regulation, and motor control capabilities in full-term cocaine-exposed infants than in nonexposed infants (Griffith, 1989; Chasnoff, Burns, Schnoll, & Burns, 1985; Chasnoff, Burns, & Burns, 1987). In a study matching substance-exposed preterm infants with nonexposed preterm infants, they differed on measures of autonomic regulation and motor control from the Dubowitz and Dubowitz Neurological Assessment of the Preterm and Full-Term Newborn Infant (Adams, 1992; Dubowitz & Dubowitz, 1981). Signs of autonomic instability include high heart and respiration rates, color changes, tremulousness, jitteriness, and startles in response to low threshold stimulation (Newald, 1986; Oro & Dixon, 1987). These infants often vacillate between extreme states, moving from deep sleep states to frantic crying states with minimal stimulation, or they may enter deep sleep states and remain completely unresponsive to stimulation (Griffith, 1988; Schneider et al., 1989).

Although the majority of cocaine-exposed infants will fall within normal limits on standardized developmental testing, such as the Bayley Scales of Infant Development (Bayley, 1969), qualitative differences in behavioral organization and motor control, including social interaction and perceptual–motor development, are often noted in these children (Poulsen, 1990). Schneider (1988) has reported increased muscle tone and retention of primitive reflexes beyond the neonatal period. Problems in attachment and representational play have also been reported in cocaine-exposed toddlers (Beckwith & Howard, 1989). In one of the few longitudinal studies done on this population, Griffith (1991) has also reported speech and language delays and/or attention deficits. Self-regulation problems present at birth may also be demonstrated in the first few years of life in the form of impulsiveness and less goal-directed behavior, resulting in increased risk for learning and behavior problems (Kopp, 1982).

Feeding disorders are also very common in cocaine-exposed newborns and may reflect poor oral motor control as well as hypersensitivity to oral stimulation. Abnormal extensor tone and disorganized motor patterns can contribute significantly to poor oral motor control (Schneider, 1990). Increased crying due to irritability and poor state control may also interfere with their ability to suck and swallow. In addition, they may be unable to relax enough to reach an adequate state of alertness to suck efficiently or may demonstrate a hyperactive suck that lacks coordination with respiration (Vergara, 1993b).

The most pervasive adverse effect of gestational cocaine exposure may be the strain it places on the developing mother–infant relationship. The fragile, irritable, tremulous infant who cries frantically or does not respond at all to stimulation requires adaptive, sensitive handling. Difficult to feed and difficult to console, these behaviors generate feelings of frustration and inadequacy in the mother and are often perceived as rejection (Burns & Burns, 1988). Consequently, many mothers respond with inappropriate patterns of detachment, hostility, or overstimulation that can place these infants at higher risk for abuse and neglect (Griffith, 1988).

In contrast to their findings, other researchers have found only minimal effects of cocaine on behavioral outcomes of infants (Coles, Platzman, Smith, James, & Falek, 1992).

Specialized Interventions

Therapeutic intervention beyond the infancy period will depend on the problem areas that are identified by the family, formal assessment, and clinical observation. Generally, many cocaine-exposed infants and toddlers will require more sensitive handling than that normally required of a growing infant in order to stimulate development in all domains (i.e., cognitive, social–emotional, gross and fine motor, language development) without exceeding the infant's threshold of overstimulation. The child's reaction to stimulation (gaze aversion, erratic eye movements, yawns, hiccups, and sneezes) should be a cue of overload (Griffith, 1991).

The following intervention goals target the most common problems in cocaine-exposed newborns:

- Facilitate mother–infant interaction.
- Improve infant's self-regulatory abilities, particularly self-quieting.
- Increase tolerance of external stimuli and decrease irritability.
- Increase quality and quantity of quiet alert periods.
- Normalize tone and promote relaxed, calm state for interaction.
- Improve feeding patterns.

Primary goals of intervention with cocaine-exposed infants and toddlers are continued facilitation of self-regulation and organization, especially the ability to quiet self. Occupational therapy may focus on promoting sensory integration as a basis for self-organization, motor control (including oral motor control), and emotional stability (Ayres, 1980).

External structuring and soothing techniques can be taught to the mother, which will allow her to take an active role in improving the overall organization and, consequently, responsiveness of her infant. Swaddling in flexion enhances the infant's self-organization and breaks up abnormal extensor tone. Slow rocking, including vertical rocking, is also helpful to calm the infant and to allow more efficient mother–infant interaction. Use of a pacifier can soothe and also reduce frantic sucking behavior. Initially, sensory stimulation should be limited to one sensory modality at a time to avoid sensory overload. Handling should be done gently but firmly to decrease hyper-excitability and to improve state control and motor patterns. The family should be taught a variety of positioning and handling techniques to decrease their infant's stress and promote caregiver–infant interaction (Schneider et al., 1989; Vergara, 1993b).

Physical therapy intervention during this period will also enhance nor-mal movement patterns in order to improve the infant's ability to move in his/her surroundings (Schneider, 1990). Speech therapy may focus on oral motor control and improving suck/swallow coordination in addition to development of prelanguage and early speech and language skills (Beckman, 1991).

Although many cocaine-exposed toddlers may not require intensive ther-apy, monthly sessions may be helpful to demonstrate to the caregivers new handling skills and developmentally appropriate activities needed to promote further development (Schneider et al., 1989). For those youngsters demon-strating delay in one or more domains of development, therapeutic interven-tions would incorporate sensory integration, neurodevelopmental, and play therapy principles appropriate for use with children in the early sensori-motor period of development. A family-centered approach, as well as trans-disciplinary teamwork, will be necessary to help each child achieve maximum potential.

Infants and Toddlers with AIDS

Pediatric AIDS is rapidly becoming one of the major conditions requiring early intervention services. Conservative estimates suggest its incidence is already exceeding that of Down syndrome and meningomyelocele. Most ther-apists who work in early intervention programs or in the school system are currently treating HIV-infected children and children with AIDS, many times unknowingly (Anderson, Hinojosa, Bedell, & Kaplan, 1990). Thus, therapists and caregivers should follow universal precautions with all infants as recom-mended by the Centers for Disease Control (1988).

Clinical Course of HIV

Emergence of clinical signs of AIDS may take weeks to years after the initial signs of HIV infection. Central nervous system involvement, particularly encephalopathy, is frequently the first indication associated with HIV infec-tion in the newborn infant.

Signs of central nervous system dysfunction appear in early infancy even prior to or concomitantly with the development of immunological abnor-malities (Belman, 1990). Clinical signs in the newborn infant (present only in infants whose clinical course begins *in utero*) may include neurological, physical, cognitive, and psychosocial deficits (Anderson et al., 1990). Impaired brain growth, atrophy, and microcephaly are also prevalent (Belman, 1990; Diamond, 1989).

Additionally, the effects of HIV in the newborn infant may be confounded with the effects of other neonatal factors such as drug exposure, prematurity, low birth weight, and poor environment (Coulter & Chase, 1990). Developmental delays, however, are rarely present at birth.

The majority of children with symptomatic HIV infection present with a variety of neurological manifestations that require early intervention (Anderson et al., 1990; Belman, 1990; Coulter & Chase, 1990; Diamond, 1989). Neurological deterioration, unfortunately, prevails in approximately 62% of the cases (Diamond, 1989). Common neurological problems include acquired microcephaly (slow brain growth), cognitive impairment, developmental delays, motor abnormalities, corticospinal tract signs, and neuropsychological deficits (Belman, 1990). Functional skill development in the areas of self-care, learning, and play is also likely to be affected to the extent that the child's encephalopathy may be progressing. Neurological deterioration may include a decline in mental development, deterioration of play, and loss of previously acquired language and social adaptive skills.

Motor involvement in some children is markedly progressive, severe, and incapacitating, involving all of the extremities. In other children, cognitive and social skills may be more impaired, albeit with more stable motor involvement. The infant may initially become hypotonic but, as the disease progresses, spasticity appears (Belman, 1990).

Assessment and Intervention

Individual intervention for newborn infants with AIDS will depend on the specific problems manifested. Areas that may require intervention include muscle tone normalization, positioning, feeding, environmental modulation, caregiver–infant interaction, reflex development, and development of sensory processing abilities.

The Neonatal Behavioral Assessment Scale (Brazelton, 1984) and the Dubowitz and Dubowitz Neurological Assessment of the Preterm and Full-Term Newborn Infant (Dubowitz & Dubowitz, 1981) are sensitive instruments to identify early signs of neurological involvement in newborn infants as well as potential ways to enhance infants' neurobehavior. The Neurological Evaluation in the Neonatal Period (Amiel-Tison & Grenier, 1986) may be more sensitive to detect muscle tone abnormalities and early signs of spasticity. Standardized assessment should be complemented with criterion-referenced assessments because, as previously stated, no neonatal assessment can identify all of the potential problems in infants with complex disorders such as AIDS. Both assessment and intervention measure the integration of services across disciplines needed to meet the complex needs of HIV-infected infants (Anderson et al., 1990).

Intervention for HIV-exposed infants must also be family-oriented. Team members responsible for providing psychological support to the family will play an important role from the beginning. Learning about the child's diagnosis is a crisis even for the most stable of families (Tasker, 1992; Wiener & Septimus, 1991) and is even more stressful if the biological mother learns about her own infection at the same time. Comprehensive family support and follow-up are essential because learning to cope with the medical and neurological consequences of HIV in their infant is an exhausting task for parents. Feelings of helplessness, guilt, sadness, and anticipatory mourning are common (Wiener & Septimus, 1991). Dealing with feelings such as these while attempting to interact with an infant who may be irritable and difficult to console is likely to affect development of caregiver–infant interaction (Anderson et al., 1990).

Parental collaboration in the development and implementation of the assessment and intervention plan is highly recommended, although not always possible, particularly if the infant is pending assignment of legal custody or if parents are unavailable because they are sick, which is rather common. Highlighting the child's strengths to the parents is often a good method to enhance caregiver–infant interaction. Engaging the parents in their child's intervention program through play and self-care activities helps them recognize the child's skills and limits and also to discover and practice ways to realistically optimize the child's development within his or her potential and limitations.

As the disease progresses, specific intervention for children with AIDS should address the following areas: psychosocial intervention, sensorimotor intervention (gross, fine, and oral motor), cognitive intervention, perceptual–motor intervention, self-care intervention, and work with caregivers. Intervention is most effective when an integrated approach is used (Anderson et al., 1990). Psychosocial intervention should be geared to maximizing environmental interactions that are pleasurable to the child to increase the child's engagement in play and socialization activities and to help the child cope with the illness (Anderson et al., 1990; Dayley, 1992; Wiener & Septimus, 1991).

Sensorimotor intervention should be based on theoretical principles such as neurodevelopmental treatment and sensory integration. Enjoyment of movement, however, may at times be more important for these children than experiencing normal patterns of movement. Play activities are ideal for development of perceptual–motor and cognitive skills. Self-care intervention should foster age-appropriate independence, within the child's stress tolerance limits. Feeding should be an area of primary emphasis to maintain optimum health and nutrition (Anderson et al., 1990).

Intervention during the neonatal period typically does not differ from that of infants with similar problems not exposed to HIV (Anderson et al., 1990); however, long-term intervention goals should take into consideration a potential deterioration of the condition. Knowing how the disease can progress helps therapists in developing realistic intervention programs for individual children. Intervention goals for children in a progressive stage of infection should be short term and based on frequent assessments of their developmental and neurological status (Anderson et al., 1990; Diamond, 1989). Intervention should focus primarily on providing psychological support to the child and the family as the disease progresses and in preparation for death (Anderson et al., 1990; Dayley, 1992; Tasker, 1992; Wiener & Septimus, 1991). Children should be allowed and encouraged to achieve the maximum level of mobility and functional independence possible within their gradually deteriorating potential (Anderson et al., 1990). Play and social activities should allow the child to express fears, anger, anxiety, depression, and other negative feelings (Anderson et al., 1990; Dayley, 1992; Wiener & Septimus, 1992). Providing activities to improve the child's self concept may also help strengthen the child's coping power and attitude toward the disease process. This is even more important when caretaking is inconsistent or when the home environment is stressful (Anderson et al., 1990). Treatment priorities need to be flexible and respond to how the child is feeling, physically as well as psychologically. Due to the medical fragility of most of these children, especially those who are approaching the terminal stages of the disease, intervention should remain well within their physical, medical, and emotional tolerance limits.

Intervention goals for children with static encephalopathy and those whose AIDS disease is progressing slowly or is arrested can be more invasive and demanding. The limits in the latter will depend on the severity of the neurological involvement and the child's medical status.

In summary, the complexity of AIDS in infants and toddlers makes it necessary to plan the intervention program from a holistic, integrated perspective in which the child as well as the family are included. Discretely treating the child's developmental delays or neurological signs will likely fail to address the myriad of problems that these children manifest.

THERAPY SERVICE DELIVERY MODELS

A variety of service delivery models are commonly used in providing therapy services. Among these are individual therapy, group therapy, consultative therapy, and integrated therapy. Each type of therapy can be conducted in a variety of settings (e.g., hospitals, child care centers, early intervention programs).

Individual Therapy

Individual therapy is one-on-one intervention in which the therapist provides service to a single child at a time. This option is based on the traditional medical model used in hospitals and requires the hands-on expertise of the therapist. The advantage of this type of service is the individual attention of the therapist. Individual therapy is usually recommended when the treatment is complex and cannot be taught to other members of the staff (Diaz, 1990a); when the child is under 12 months of age; and when funding sources require individual therapy. The disadvantage of individual therapy is that it is time intensive for the therapist and therefore costly. If individual therapy occurs out of the classroom, there is loss of other instructional opportunities, interruption of classroom scheduling, and possible stigmatization because of removing the child from class (Cole, Harris, Eland, & Mills, 1989).

Group Therapy

Group therapy is provided when two or more children are treated together. Other intervention staff usually participate with the therapist in the group treatment. This therapy is recommended when the children are able to function as part of a group (generally over 24 months old) and are making steady progress, but progress is not occurring rapidly. The advantages of group therapy include a cost-effective use of the therapist's time; an opportunity for modeling and training with other staff (e.g., teachers and assistants), family, and community resources (Diaz, 1990a); and the opportunity for inclusion of nondisabled children and a more naturalistic learning environment. The disadvantages of group therapy are that each child does not receive individual hands-on treatment from the therapist during each treatment session and it is not billable under certain funding sources, for example, Medicaid.

Therapists may adapt or use different types of groups to meet the needs of a wide range of children and their families. One may focus on children functioning at the same developmental level. A second type of group may target children at varying levels so that higher functioning children can serve as models for lower functioning children. A third type of group integrates the services of physical, occupational, and speech and language therapists simultaneously. Group size may vary depending on the activity being introduced. For example, small groups may focus on specific strengthening activities while large groups may participate in activities related to food preparation. In addition, parent groups may function to provide hands-on training for parents under the supervision of a therapist.

Consultation

The consultative or indirect service model is used when the therapist advises and assists families, other caregivers, teachers, and other interventionists in settings including homes, child care centers, family day care homes, or in the classroom setting. The caregivers, rather than the therapist, are the actual providers of the intervention, under the guidance of the consulting therapist. Therapists help caregivers to observe and correct abnormal motor patterns and to use appropriate techniques, activities, or adapted equipment. This model is becoming more popular in response to the increasing shortage of therapists.

Integrated Therapy

Integrated therapy is also known as transdisciplinary therapy or collaborative therapy. It refers to two or more individuals of different disciplines who share information and expertise across traditional discipline boundaries to assist children to attain intervention goals. Therapists combine their methods with those of other disciplines, with the intent that the combined efforts will result in more consistent, comprehensive programming and more functional outcomes. With input from the family, various disciplines incorporate their objectives into the daily routine of the child as suggested by McWilliam and Strain (1993). One advantage of the integrated therapy approach is that there is consistency of input and control of environmental stimulation. A second advantage is that the interventions are integrated into the child's daily activities, rather than needing separate time for therapies. Third, there is encouragement for transition and generalization from the safety of home and center into the demands of the environment and the community.

Disadvantages of the transdisciplinary model include the difficulty of getting professional staff to relinquish traditional service roles (Diaz, 1990b). A second difficulty involves the need to develop a mature team that can work effectively and efficiently together. A third difficulty is changing people's attitudes regarding the process of change necessary to implement this model.

Effectiveness and Efficiency of the Models

The criteria for the use of these different models vary depending on the intervention setting. In most cases, therapists and teachers tend to use a combination of two or three of these intervention approaches. Research regarding the different models has resulted in variable findings. Cole et al. (1989) compared in-class therapy service delivery with out-of-class therapy. No significant differences in performance between the two groups were found although a trend favoring the in-class model was noted. The authors suggested that additional research needed to be done with a larger sample size before the trends toward greater motor gains in the in-class model could be substantiated.

The developmental outcomes of children with severe mental retardation and cerebral palsy who received either individual therapy or no therapy were compared in a study by Sommerfield, Fraser, Hensinger, and Beresford, (1981). No significant differences in development of mature developmental reflexes, improved gross motor skills, or improved range of passive joint motion among similar students in the two groups were found. In another study, Palisano (1989) compared progress in students with learning disabilities who were treated either in therapist-directed large-group and small-group therapy or in a consultation group receiving large-group therapy and teacher-led follow-up sessions. Both methods of service delivery were found to be effective based on student progress, the therapy needs of each group, teacher satisfaction, and utilization of available resources. Both types of services enabled more children to be seen in less time as compared to individual therapy.

Given the diversity of research results, it appears that there is considerable need for additional research in the area of effective and efficient therapy service delivery. With health care costs increasing nationwide, it behooves therapists to conduct research that provides guidelines for optimal service delivery at reasonable cost.

SUMMARY

Recommended practices for therapy have changed dramatically in recent years in response to technological improvements, the family partnership movement, a national shift toward prevention, expanded etiologies of disabilities, funding restrictions and a nationwide shortage of therapists. This chapter has reviewed the major aspects of current research findings regarding therapeutic interventions as a basis for recommending strategies for most effectively intervening with special populations of infants and toddlers. Thus, preferred practices have been summarized from a multidisciplinary perspective of therapists.

REFERENCES

Adams, S. (1992). *An analysis of neuromotor and neurobehavioral organization in preterm, cocaine-exposed neonates.* Unpublished doctoral dissertation, University of South Florida, Tampa, FL.

Als, H. (1986). Synactive model of neonatal behavioral organization: Framework for the assessment and support of the neurobehavioral development of the premature infant and his parents in the environment of the neonatal intensive care unit. In J. K. Sweeney (Eds.), *The high-risk neonate: Developmental perspectives* (pp. 3–53). New York: Haworth Press.

Als, H., & Duffy, F. H. (1989). Neurobehavioral assessment in the newborn period: Opportunity for early detection of later learning disabilities and for early intervention. *Birth Defects, 25*(6), 127–152.

Als, H., Lester, B. M., & Brazelton, T. B. (1982). Toward a research instrument for the assessment of preterm infant's behavior. In H. E. Fitzgerald, B. M. Lester, & M. W. Yogman (Eds.), *Theory and research in behavioral pediatrics* (Vol. 1, pp. 35–132). New York: Plenum Press.

American Academy of Pediatrics. (1992). *Guidelines for perinatal care* (3rd ed.). Elk Grove Village, IL: Author.

American Academy of Pediatrics Task Force on Infant Positioning in SIDS. (1992). *Pediatrics, 89*(6, Part 1), 1120.

Amiel-Tison, C., & Grenier, A. (1986). *Neurological assessment during the first year of life—The neurological evaluation in the neonatal period.* New York: Oxford University Press.

Andersen, R. (1991). Gross motor early intervention. In E. R. Vergara (Ed.), *Training for occupational and physical therapy services in early intervention: Unit 3— Physical therapy early intervention beyond the neonatal period* (pp. 69–143). Tallahassee, FL: Florida Department of Education.

Anderson, J., & Auster-Liebhaber, J. (1984). Developmental therapy in the neonatal intensive care unit. *Physical and Occupational Therapy in Pediatrics, 4*(1), 89–107.

Anderson, J., Hinojosa, J., Bedell, G., & Kaplan, M. (1990). Occupational therapy for children with perinatal HIV infection. *American Journal of Occupational Therapy, 44,* 249–255.

Anderson, L. J., & Anderson, J. M. (1988). Hand splinting for infants in the intensive care and special care nurseries. *American Journal of Occupational Therapy, 42,* 222–226.

Ayres, A. J. (1980). *Sensory integration and the child.* Los Angeles, CA: Western Psychological Services.

Barnard, K. (1980). *Nursing Child Assessment Feeding Scale.* Seattle, WA: NCAST.

Bayley, N. (1969). *Bayley Scales of Infant Development.* New York: Psychological Corporation.

Beckman, D. (1991, November). *Oral motor assessment and intervention seminar.* Seminar presented by Arkansas Children's Hospital Neonatology Group, Little Rock, AK.

Beckman, D., Roberts, L., & Tencza, C. (1992). *Mealtime challenges: Eating assistance for individuals with severe oral motor challenges.* Produced for the Oklahoma Department of Human Services by Therapeutic Concept, Inc., Winter Park, FL.

Beckwith, L., & Howard, J. (1989). The development of young children of substance-abusing parents: Insights from seven years of intervention and research. *Zero to Three, 9*(5), 8–12.

Belman, A. L. (1990). Neurologic syndromes associated with symptomatic human immunodeficiency virus infection in infants and children. In P. B. Kozlowski, D. A. Snider, P. M. Vietze, & H. M. Wisniewski (Eds.), *Brain in pediatric AIDS* (pp. 45–63). Basel, Switzerland: Karger.

Bingol, N., Fuchs, M., Diaz, V., Stone, R. K., & Gromisch, D. S. (1987). Teratogenicity of cocaine in humans. *Journal of Pediatrics, 110,* 93–96.

Bly, L. (1983). *The components of normal development during the first year of life.* Chicago: Neurodevelopmental Treatment.

Bobath, K. (1980). *A neurophysiological basis for the treatment of cerebral palsy.* Philadelphia: J. B. Lippincott.

Boehme, R. (1988). *Improving upper body control: An approach to assessment and treatment of tonal dysfunction.* Tucson, AZ: Therapy Skill Builders.

Braun, M., & Palmer, M. M. (1985). A pilot study of oral–motor dysfunction in "at-risk" infants. *Physical and Occupational Therapy in Pediatrics, 5*(4), 13–25.

Brazelton, T. B. (1984). *Neonatal Behavioral Assessment Scale.* Philadelphia: J. B. Lippincott.

Burns, W. J., & Burns, K. A. (1988). Parenting dysfunction in chemically dependent women. In I. J. Chasnoff (Ed.), *Drugs, alcohol, pregnancy and parenting* (pp. 159–171). Hingham, MA: Kluwer Academic.

Campbell, A. N., & Trenouth, M. J. (1987). A new feeder for infants with cleft palates. *Archives of Disease in Childhood, 62,* 1292–1293.

Centers for Disease Control. (1988). Update: Universal precautions for prevention of transmission of Human Immunocare settings. *Morbidity and Mortality Weekly Report, 37*(24), 462–464.

Chandler, L. S., Andrews, M. S., & Swanson, M. W. (1980). *Movement assessment of infants: A manual.* Rolling Bay, WA: Authors. (Available from Infant Movement Resarch, P.O. Box 4631, Rolling Bay, WA 98110.)

Chasnoff, I. J. (1989). Drug use in women: Establishing a standard of care. *Annals of the New York Academy of Science, 52,* 208–210.

Chasnoff, I. J., Burns, K. A., & Burns, W. J. (1987). Cocaine use in pregnancy: Perinatal morbidity and mortality. *Neurotoxicology and Teratology, 9,* 291–293.

Chasnoff, I. J., Burns, W. J., Schnoll, S., & Burns, K. A. (1985). Cocaine use in pregnancy. *New England Journal of Medicine, 313,* 666–669.

Chasnoff, I. J., Bussey, M. E., Savich, R., & Stack, C. M. (1986). Perinatal cerebral infarction and maternal cocaine use. *Journal of Pediatrics, 108,* 456–459.

Cherukuri, R., Minkoff, H., Feldman, J., Parekh, A., & Glass, L. (1988). A cohort study of alkaloidal cocaine ("crack") in pregnancy. *Obstetrics and Gynecology, 72*(2), 147–151.

Cole, J. G. (1985). Infant stimulation reexamined: An environmental and behavioral-based approach. *Neonatal Network, 3*(5), 24–31.

Cole, K. N., Harris, S. R., Eland, S. F., & Mills, P. E. (1989). Comparison of two service delivery models: In-class and out-of-class therapy approaches. *Pediatric Physical Therapy, 1,* 49–54.

Coles, C. D., Platzman, K. A., Smith, I. E., James, I., & Falek, A. (1992). Effects of cocaine, alcohol and other drug use in pregnancy on neonatal growth and neurobehavioral status. *Neurotoxicology and Teratology, 14*(1), 23–33.

Corbetta, D., & Mounoud, P. (1990). Early development of grasping and manipulation. In C. Bard, M. Fleury, & L. Hay (Eds.), *Development of eye–hand coordination across the life span* (pp. 188–216). Columbia, SC: University of South Carolina Press.

Coulter, D. L., & Chase, C. (1990). Neurological assessment of infants and young children with HIV infection. In P. B. Kozlowski, D. A. Snider, P. M. Vietze, & H. M. Wisniewski (Eds.), *Brain in pediatric AIDS* (pp. 80–90). Basel, Switzerland: Karger.

Dayley, A. A. (1992). Terminal care for the child with AIDS. In P. A. Pizzo & C. M. Wilfert (Eds.), *Pediatric AIDS: The challenge of HIV infection in infants, children, and adolescents* (pp. 619–629). Baltimore, MD: Williams & Wilkins.

Diamond, G. W. (1989). Developmental problems in children with HIV infection. *Mental Retardation, 27*(4), 215–217.

Diaz, I. (1990a). *Physical therapy service delivery model in an educational setting.* Unpublished manuscript.

Diaz, I. (1990b). *Physical therapy in an early intervention program.* Unpublished manuscript.

Division for Early Childhood. (1993). *DEC Task Force on Recommended Practices: Indicators of quality in programs for infants and young children with special needs and their families.* Reston, VA: Council for Exceptional Children.

Dixon, S. D., & Bejar, R. (1989). Echoencephalographic findings in neonates associated with maternal cocaine and methamphetamine use: Incidence and clinical correlates. *Journal of Pediatrics, 115,* 770–778.

Doberczak, T., Shanzer, S., Senie, R., & Kendall, S. (1988). Neonatal neurologic and electroencephalographic effects of intrauterine cocaine exposure. *Journal of Pediatrics, 113,* 354–358.

Dubowitz, L., & Dubowitz, V. (1981). *The neurological assessment of the preterm and full-term newborn infant.* Philadelphia: J. B. Lippincott.

Dunst, C. J., Trivette, C. M., & Deal, A. G. (1988). *Enabling and empowering families— Principles and guidelines for practice.* Cambridge, MA: Brookline Books.

Ellison, P. H. (1984). Neurologic development of the high-risk infant. *Clinics in Perinatology, 11*(1), 41–58.

Erhardt, R. P. (1982). *Developmental hand dysfunction: Theory, assessment, treatment.* Tucson, AZ: Therapy Skill Builders.

Field, T. (1980). Supplemental stimulation of preterm neonates. *Early Human Development, 4*(3), 301–314.

Folio, M. R., & Fewell, R. R. (1983). *Peabody Developmental Motor Scales and Activity Cards.* Hingham, MA: Teaching Resource.

Frankenburg, W. K., Dodds, J., Archer, P., Bresnick, B., Maschka, P., Edelman, N., & Shapiro, H. (1990). *Denver II Screening Manual.* Denver, CO: Denver Developmental Materials.

Furuno, S., O'Reilly, K. A., Hosaka, C. M., Inatsuka, T. T., Allman, T. L., & Zeisloft, B. (1979). *Hawaii Early Learning Profile.* Palo Alto, CA: VORT.

Gorga, D. (1989). Occupational therapy treatment practices with infants in early intervention. *American Journal of Occupational Therapy, 43,* 731–736.

Gottfried, A., Wallace-Lande, P., Sherman-Brown, S., King, J., & Coen, C. (1981,

November 6). Physical and social environment of newborn infants in special care units. *Science*, p. 214.

Griffith, D. R. (1988). The effects of perinatal cocaine exposure on infant neurobehavior and early maternal infant interaction. In I. J. Chasnoff (Ed.), *Drugs, alcohol, pregnancy and parenting* (pp. 105–114). Lancaster, UK: Kluwer Academic.

Griffith, D. R. (1989). Neurobehavioral effects of intrauterine cocaine exposure. *Ab Initio: An International Newsletter for Professionals Working with Infants and Their Families, 1*(1).

Griffith, D. R. (1991, December). *Developmentally appropriate interventions for substance-exposed infants and their families.* Paper presented at the National Center of Clinical Infant Programs Training Institute, Washington, DC.

Gryboski, J. D. (1969). Suck and swallow in premature infants. *Pediatrics, 43,* 96–102.

Hadeed, A., & Siegel, S. (1989). Maternal cocaine use during pregnancy: Effect on the newborn infant. *Pediatrics, 84,* 205–210.

Heriza, C. B., & Sweeney, J. K. (1990). Effects of NICU intervention on preterm infants: Part 1—Implications for neonatal practice. *Infants and Young Children, 2*(3), 31–47.

Howard, R. B., Fetters, L., & MacDonald, D. M. (1978). The nervous system and handicapping conditions. In R. B. Howard & N. H. Herbold (Eds.), *Nutrition in clinical care* (pp. 462–492). New York: McGraw-Hill.

Hussey, B. (1988). *Understanding my signals.* Palo Alto, CA: VORT.

Jaffe, M. B. (1980). Neurological impairment of speech production: Assessment and treatment. In K. M. Yorkston & D. R. Beukelman (Eds.), *Recent advances in clinical dysarthrias* (pp. 156–184). Boston, MA: College Hill.

Klein, M. D. (1982). *Pre-writing skills: Skill starters for motor development.* Tucson, AZ: Communication Skill Builders.

Kopp, C. B. (1982). Antecedents of self-regulation: A developmental perspective. *Developmental Psychology, 18,* 199–214.

Lawhon, G., & Melzar, A. (1988). Developmental care of the very low birth weight infant. *Journal of Perinatal and Neonatal Nursing, 2*(1), 56–65.

Linn, P. L., Horowitz, F. D., & Fox, H. A. (1985). Stimulation in the NICU: Is more necessarily better? *Clinics in Perinatology, 12,* 407–422.

MacGregor, S. N., Keith, L. G., Chasnoff, I. J., Rosner, M. A., Chisum, G. M., Shaw, P., & Minogue, J. P. (1987). Maternal cocaine use and genitourinary tract malformations. *Teratology, 37,* 201.

McCormack, G. L. (1990). The Rood approach to the treatment of neuromuscular dysfunction. In L. E. Pedretti & B. Zoltan, *Occupational therapy practice skills for physical dysfunctions* (pp. 311–333). St. Louis, MO: C. V. Mosby.

McWilliam, R. A., & Strain, P. S. (1993). Service delivery models. In *DEC Task Force on Recommended Practices: Indicators of quality in programs for infants and young children with special needs and their families* (pp. 39–48). Reston, VA: Council for Exceptional Children.

Masin, H. L. (1991). *Parental attitudes toward physical therapy services at the Debbie School Early Intervention Program.* Miami, FL: University of Miami, Department of Pediatrics. Unpublished manuscript.

Morris, S. (1982). *Pre-Speech Assessment Scale.* Clifton, NJ: J. A. Preston.

Morris, S. (1989). Development of oral-motor skills in the neurologically impaired child receiving non-oral feedings. *Dysphagia, 3,* 135–157.

Morris, S. E., & Klein, M. D. (1987). *Pre-feeding skills.* Tucson, AZ: Therapy Skill Builders.

Newald, J. (1986). Cocaine infants: A new arrival at hospitals' steps. *Hospitals, 60*(7), 96.

Oro, A. S., & Dixon, S. D. (1987). Perinatal cocaine and methamphetamine exposure: Maternal and neonatal correlates. *Journal of Pediatrics, 111,* 571–578.

Palisano, R. J. (1989). Comparison of two methods of service delivery for students with learning disabilities. *Physical and Occupational Therapy in Pediatrics, 9*(3), 79–100.

Poulsen, M. K. (1990, February). *Children prenatally exposed to drugs: Challenge of the nineties.* Paper presented at Operation PAR, Third Annual Regional Conference on Substance Abuse and Pregnancy, St. Petersburg, FL.

Rogers, S. J., D'Eugenio, D. B., Brown, S. L., Donovan, C. M., & Lynch, E. W. (1981). Early Intervention Developmental Profile. In D. S. Schafer & M. S. Moersch (Eds.), *Developmental programming for infants and young children* (Vol. 2). Ann Arbor, MI: University of Michigan Press.

Sameroff, A. (1982). The environmental context of developmental disabilities. In D. Bricker (Ed.), *Intervention with at risk and handicapped infants* (pp. 141–152). Baltimore, MD: University Park Press.

Saunders, L. (1954). *Cultural differences and medical care.* New York: Russell Sage Foundation.

Schafer, D. S., & Moersch, M. S. (1981). Stimulation activities. In D. S. Schafer & M. S. Moersch (Eds.), *Developmental programming for infants and young children* (Vol. 3). Ann Arbor, MI: University of Michigan Press.

Schneider, J. W. (1988). Motor assessment and parent education beyond the newborn period. In I. J. Chasnoff (Ed.), *Drugs, alcohol, pregnancy, and parenting* (pp. 115–126). Dordrecht, The Netherlands: Kluwer Academic.

Schneider, J. W. (1990). Infants exposed to cocaine in utero: Role of the pediatric physical therapist. *Topics in Pediatrics, Lesson 6.* Alexandria, VA: American Physical Therapy Association.

Schneider, J. W., Griffith, D. R., & Chasnoff, I. J. (1989). Infants exposed to cocaine in utero: Implications for developmental assessment and intervention. *Infants and Young Children, 2,* 25–36.

Semmler, C. (1989). Positioning and positioning-induced deformities. In C. Semmler (Ed.), *A guide to care and management of very low birth weight infants: A team approach* (pp. 99–123). Tucson, AZ: Therapy Skill Builders.

Sommerfield, D., Fraser, B., Hensinger, R., & Beresford, C. (1981). Evaluation of physical therapy service for severely mentally impaired students with cerebral palsy. *Physical Therapy, 61,* 338–344.

Strominger, A. Z., Winkler, M. R., & Cohen, L. T. (1984). Speech and language evaluation. In S. M. Pueschel (Ed.), *The young child with Down's syndrome* (pp. 253–261). New York: Human Sciences Press.

Stuberg, W. (1992). *Milani-Comparetti Motor Development Screening Test for Infants and Young Children—A manual.* Omaha, NE: Meyer Rehabilitation Institute, University of Nebraska Medical Center.

Sugden, D. A. (1990). Role of proprioception in eye–hand coordination. In C. Bard, M. Fleury, & L. Hay (Eds.), *Development of eye–hand coordination across the life span* (pp. 133–153). Columbia, SC: University of South Carolina Press.

Sweeney, J. K., & Swanson, M. W. (1990). At-risk neonates and infants: NICU management and follow-up. In D. A. Umphred (Ed.), *Neurological rehabilitation* (pp. 183–238). St. Louis, MO: C. V. Mosby.

Taeusch, H. W., & Ware, J. (1980). Mechanics of follow-up clinics. In H. W. Taeusch & M. W. Yogman (Eds.), *Follow-up management of the high risk infant* (pp. 83–97). Boston, MA: Little, Brown.

Tasker, M. (1992). Children and AIDS. In W. M. Marcil & K. N. Tigges (Eds.), *The person with AIDS* (pp. 53–62). Thorofare, NJ: Slack.

Vergara, E. R. (1993a). Overview of neonatal intervention. In E. R. Vergara (Ed.), *Foundations for practice in the neonatal intensive care unit and early intervention: A self-guided practice manual* (pp. 1–111). Rockville, MD: American Occupational Therapy Association.

Vergara, E. R. (1993b). Neonatal occupational therapy intervention. In E. R. Vergara (Ed.), *Foundations for practice in the neonatal intensive care unit and early intervention: A self-guided practice manual* (pp. 117–241). Rockville, MD: American Occupational Therapy Association.

Vinter, A. (1990). Manual imitations and reaching behaviors. In C. Bard, M. Fleury, & L. Hay, (Eds.), *Development of eye–hand coordination across the life span* (pp. 157–187). Columbia, SC: University of South Carolina Press.

Wiener, L., & Septimus, A. (1991). Psychosocial consideration and support for the child and family. In P. A. Pizzo & C. M. Wilfert (Eds.), *Pediatric AIDS: The challenge of HIV infection in infants, children, and adolescents* (pp. 577–594). Baltimore, MD: Williams & Wilkins.

Werder, J. K., & Bruininks, R. H. (1991). *BodySkills manual.* Circle Pines, MN: American Guidance.

Zlatin, M. A. (1967). Development of speech, language, auditory, and oral function in the presence of congenital sensory neuropathy. In J. Bosma (Ed.), *Symposium on oral sensation and perception* (pp. 381–388). Springfield, IL: Thomas.

CHAPTER 13

Predicting the Costs
of Early Intervention

JOHN C. HALL

LINDA STONE

MICHAEL WALSH

DOUGLAS W. WAGER

ANITA ZERVIGON HAKES

MIMI A. GRAHAM

During the past decade, strong patterns of fiscal retrenchment have been evident in all levels of government, much of the private sector, and even in our own personal households. Economic issues overshadow most other concerns of Americans these days. Finding ways to fund our traditional spending practices without cutting costs or securing new income is becoming increasingly difficult.

Because social services, health care, and education constitute close to three-quarters of the budget in state government, expenditures in these areas are subject to extreme scrutiny and review. Long-standing entitlement programs such as public schools, Medicaid, and Aid to Families with Dependent Children programs account for most of the public spending for social services, health care, and education. For example in the state of Florida during 1991–1992, the combined appropriations for the departments administering education, health, and social services represented 60% of the total Florida budget. Similar patterns exist in the other states. State spending in these areas has climbed dramatically over the past 10 years both in absolute dollars and as a proportion of the total state budget.

In state fiscal environments such as this, the task of forecasting the cost of a new statewide entitlement program such as Part H of the Individuals with Disabilities Education Act carries a unique challenge. Unlike categorically funded programs, insufficient revenue is not an acceptable reason to curtail or deny services in an entitlement program. Decisions to spend scarce revenue for an open-ended entitlement, regardless of the potential benefits of the services, requires that all interests have the utmost confidence in the cost estimate (and the stated benefits). Yet, the broad eligibility populations in Part H have significantly different needs and require significantly different services—and therefore costs—among the potential client population. For instance, there are major differences in the cost of services for children with complex medical conditions as compared to those who are low birth weight. In addition, early intervention and prevention services can be configured in a variety of ways ranging from the very costly, medically oriented and therapeutic interventions to the less expensive services that could be provided by paraprofessionals and parent support groups. Further, it must be recognized that typical parameters for budgetary flexibility are curtailed under collaborative interagency initiatives such as Part H. Spending the budgetary resources of more than one state agency complicates the ability of participating agencies to shift funds among service categories as the need arises. If one agency is expected to perform all infant and toddler evaluations, the cost estimate for that particular service needs to be accurately projected because other funds may not be available to offset deficits.

Early intervention policy and planning, and evaluation of governmental spending and funding practices are our areas of interest. In this chapter, we will draw upon our experience and work on cost/funding studies for infants and toddlers to help others understand a new approach to developing reliable cost estimates for early intervention and prevention services. The methods presented here have direct implication for developing cost estimates in other areas, such as education, health, and social services, as well.

TRADITIONAL COST ESTIMATION APPROACHES

Historical methods used for forecasting the cost of a new program in education, health, and social services usually followed one of two rather straightforward exercises, or a combination of both. One common approach involves determining the average cost per client in a state that already operates the desired program (often established through the estimate of some "informed" source). The "average cost per client" is then applied to a theoretically derived number of the potential clients in the jurisdiction under consideration. In contrast, the other approach might aptly be named the "back door" costing method. This method assumes that existing personnel and the related administrative and programmatic resources will simply take on an additional responsibility or entirely new function with the forecasted cost equal to the current budget parameters. Both approaches have serious limitations with potential for escalating the costs because of (1) inherent inefficiencies or understatement of the costs because of a poor understanding of the actual spending functions, or (2) costly antecedents linked to the consolidation of work functions and activities.

We confirmed the limitations of traditional cost estimation approaches in our recent work on Florida's Part H Cost/Funding Study. At an early point in the research, the cost experience of other states was examined as a guide for developing cost estimates. Differences in eligibility definitions and services among other states restricted direct inferences for cost comparisons. The average cost of Part H services per child and family varied from $2,400 to $6,090 among the seven states studied. No state was found to have identical eligibility definitions or offer the same array and intensity of services considered.

A search of the literature found that published information regarding the costs of early intervention was limited and focused upon accumulating the costs in a particular program or group of programs for cost–benefit analyses (Barnett & Escobar, 1990). We designed a new approach.

"TABULA RASA": THE CLEAN SLATE APPROACH

To determine reliable cost estimates for a system of early intervention and prevention services (including Part H or most other programs in the areas of health, education, and social services), a methodology is recommended that flows from an effort structured to answer some very basic but interrelated research questions. These questions form the foundation for a theoretical blank budgetary ledger that is, in effect, a clean slate or "tabula rasa." The development of the necessary research questions evolve from an effort to identify the basic cost functions to be measured. Four essential research questions must be answered to determine reliable cost estimates for a statewide system of prevention and early intervention services. These questions are stated and discussed in the following paragraphs.

1. *How many infants and toddlers are potentially eligible?* This question addresses the program's eligibility definition and the estimated *prevalence* of the target client population. Eligibility characteristics must be measurable among the general population and a methodology developed to estimate, with confidence, the size of the client target group (see Foster & Foster, Chapter 4, this volume). Public Law 99-457, Part H, requires states to serve children with handicaps and developmental delays and provides discretion for broadening the potential eligible population to children with biological or environmental risks that are likely to lead to developmental delays (see Benn, Chapter 2, this volume). At a very basic level, the state must decide if children at risk of developmental delay will be eligible for the statewide early intervention services system. Estimates of the prevalence of infants and toddlers with established conditions or developmental delays as well as those at risk of developmental delay should be determined. The Part H eligibility definition involves

a number of biological factors in children that can, but rarely do, occur in isolation and usually occur in clusters. Further, accurate measurement of developmental delay, biological risks, and environmental risks among a population under the age of 3 is very difficult.

Prevalence estimates indicate the occurrence of conditions within the general population. Therefore, the Part H prevalence estimate should indicate, within a reasonable degree of accuracy, the proportion and number of children who are likely to meet the eligibility definition among *all* children aged birth to 3. Depending on available resources, a single-point-in-time (or multiple points in time, if feasible), stratified, random sample survey can be conducted in representative counties or statewide. One must first decide where families are currently accessing services for their children in need of early intervention services. Consideration should be given to sampling children seen in private physicians' offices, public health units, children's medical services clinics, and other relevant service agencies to accomplish this goal. The survey responses can then be weighted and demographically controlled to project prevalence estimates on a statewide basis. Later in this chapter we will use data obtained in a prevalence study conducted in 1990 in Palm Beach County, Florida. (For a detailed methodology, see Foster & Foster, Chapter 4, this volume.)

2. *How many potentially eligible infants and toddlers are likely to utilize the services to which they are entitled?* The second factor influencing costs requires judgment concerning the level of utilization of the statewide early intervention services system by those children who are potentially eligible. Voluntary human services programs, even if an entitlement such as Part H, rarely serve 100% of the prevalence population. As in many health and social services, participation in Part H services by the potential eligibility population is voluntary in nature. Not every family with an eligible child will chose to enter the program or use all the services to which they are entitled. For example, all Medicaid recipients under the age of 21 are entitled to Early and Periodic Screening, Diagnosis, and Treatment (EPSDT) services. However, the EPSDT participation rates among the potential (prevalence) population vary considerably from state to state, with an average of 41% nationally in 1991. Therefore, the development of reliable forecasts of the cost of early intervention and prevention services must also determine an estimate for the program *utilization* population.

Development of an estimate regarding the proportion of the prevalence population that is likely to enter the early intervention system should be approached carefully. For instance, it must be acknowledged that program utilization rates will vary over time. If effective public awareness and service outreach campaigns are coupled with programs of high quality, the utilization rate increases. However, it is highly unlikely that even very effective public awareness initiatives and "child-find" activities will result in 100% of the prevalence population utilizing a statewide early intervention system. In addition, some children in the prevalence population may not require any services (or their families may not want their children to have any services), even though they have established conditions or risk factors that are generally associated with developmental delays.

Two potential methodological approaches to estimating utilization are described here. One approach to determining the number of infants and toddlers who will utilize the services involves an extrapolation from a single-point-in-time survey. The method basically involves statistically estimating a statewide utilization estimate from a 1-day survey in a representative county or a group of counties. This approach assumes that the proportion of potentially eligible Part H children receiving services in typical programs under current policy will remain fairly constant under a new statewide entitlement of services. However, it is important to determine if children detected in a single-day survey receive only minimally appropriate levels of service or all the types of services needed. Additional children not in the caseloads of accessible public agencies that are in early intervention programs, operating with private revenue or public subsidies or contracts (instead of service rate agreements linked directly to caseloads) should also be considered. Knowledgeable administrators at the state and local level should be asked if there are capacity deficits in the existing system of early intervention services that make the single-day survey an underestimation of the potential annual caseload that the state may need to serve under Part H. The demand for early intervention services, both in terms of those who currently receive some but not enough services, and those who need but go without services, may exceed the capacity of the current system to meet the real level of need. Adjustments to findings may be warranted.

A second (and recommended) method of estimating service utilization involves an investigation beyond a single day. A cost estimate incorporating a 12-month time frame provides a more highly accurate utilization estimate. New questions are posed under this approach: How many eligible children access applicable programs over the course of a year, at what age do they enter services, and how long do they stay in services? This method acknowledges that children and families will *not* access services evenly throughout a 12-month period. Some children and their families may not require services for a year in duration; others will move; some will die; some will turn 3 and no longer be eligible; and others will be born during the year and require early intervention services. This phenomenon is referred to as "turnover." Similar to methods employed by the public schools and child care programs, this method focuses on the need to determine the number of full-time service delivery "slots" from which to derive a more refined estimate of utilization. The concept of "slots" incorporates the turnover phenomenon through focusing on the development of a measure of the full-time demand for services and, at the same time, incorporates the actual absolute number of children that constitute that demand over a 12-month time period.

To determine the utilization estimate under this second method, the following research steps should be undertaken:

1. Extend the period of investigation to 12 months. By including all applicable sources to accessing services (e.g., pediatricians, neonatal care units, developmental services programs, exceptional student education programs, public health offices, etc.), acquire an unduplicated count of all potentially eligible infants and toddlers accessing services over a 12-month period.
2. Determine (for the population identified in Step 1) the average age of entry into services. Under Part H, children are eligible from birth until their third birthday.
3. Determine (for the population identified in Step 1) the average length of service received by those accessing services.
4. Derive the number of slots applicable to 12-month funding requirements by multiplying the absolute total number of children accessing services over the year by the ratio derived from Steps 2 and 3. For example, if 100,000 children are expected to access early intervention services in a year, the average age of entry into services is 10 months of age, and the average length of service is 16 months, the funding requirement for utilization is 62,500 slots (100,000 × 10/16 = 62,500).

3. What are the service needs among the population eligible to utilize them? Determining service needs is the third question and one that this chapter will address in more detail. This step in the process is concerned with determining the specific service needs (array of services) and the amount or intensity required by the utilization population. The research objective in this area is concerned with systematically determining answers to such questions as: How many children will need physical therapy, and of those children who need it, how many hours of therapy will they need over a year? Will a therapist need to provide home-based services (such as for a medically complex child) or center-based services? Can therapies be provided in group or is individual therapy needed? Can a therapy aide provide adequate intervention or is a professional needed or required by state law or by the funding source?

Measuring and quantifying service needs on a statewide basis for children in this young age group with a wide range of conditions potentially associated with developmental delays is a complex undertaking. For instance, even within the Part H-required eligibility group of handicapped infants and toddlers, the service needs (and the related cost requirement) differ markedly. Among children with Down syndrome, there may be significant variations in service needs. Also, when children with Down syndrome are compared with others who have different congenital or metabolic disorders, there may again be significant variations in need for service. Similarly, risk conditions, both environmental and biological factors, are simply predictors rather than precise indicators of a need for service. Family conditions and parent coparticipation in planning services for their child introduce other variables that influence the need for services. Not all children will need the same array of service, and the intensity and/or amount of the services needed will vary by child and family. We recommend a method in the next section to predict individualized service needs for children and families within a potentially broad range of eligibility conditions.

4. How much will the services cost? The final step in the process is estimating the costs of the services themselves. The cost estimate is also a function of the specific services, and their related costs, to which eligible children will be entitled. Most programs (Head Start, Even Start, and Part H) require basic services be provided as part of the early intervention system, but allow states the discretion to include other services, as deemed appropriate. A cost estimation methodology employing a unit of service cost analysis is recommended.

The goal of the cost methodology is to capture significant cost variations in the provision of services, so that on the average, the computed cost will represent the funding need. As discussed in more detail below, research activities and purposeful sampling techniques can be undertaken to determine potential differences in the service needs among children with similar conditions and risks, as well as any patterns or clusters of similar service needs among children with different characteristics.

DEVELOPMENT OF A MATRIX
FOR PREDICTING SERVICE NEEDS

What types and amounts of services are needed by the eligible infants and toddlers who will utilize them? Child and family service needs vary significantly among children who may be eligible for early intervention services. For instance, two children with Down syndrome may have very different family resources and needs. One may be from a two-parent home where both parents had a college education. Another may be living in poverty in a single-parent home as the child of a teenager. The developmental status of two children with similar diagnosed established conditions can vary significantly. One may have significant health problems and delays in speech, gross motor, and fine motor skills, whereas the other may only display minor delays in language development. Therefore, estimating need based on the child's diagnostic label and the usual methodology of per child cost averaging would not produce reliable estimates of service needs or costs.

We have found a matrix useful as a conceptual tool for integrating child and family risk factors and best intervention practices. The matrix provides an operational model to help predict need for service and the related costs. The first step in designing a matrix involves analysis of prevalence survey data coupled with in-depth case studies. This is done to detect the natural clustering of needs based on the interactive and cumulative effect of child and family risks. Risks can then be generalized into a hierarchy along two axes, the vertical axis displaying the child's biological risks and the horizontal axis representing the family's environmental risks. Using a series of decision rules, risks are clustered so there is more consistency in the types of children and families (and the needed services) found along each column, row, and cell with the understanding that there is some variability accounted for by individual uniqueness. The final matrix serves as the basis for recommending the array of early intervention services most likely needed for various child and family risk levels, the settings in which these services might be delivered, the estimated intensity of these services, and the predicted costs.

The matrix displayed in Figure 13.1 was used as an organizer to forecast child and family services based on needs rather than programmatic or categorical definitions. The matrix is a planning tool to conceptualize potential child and family need for services. It was not developed to exchange one form of categorical funding or labeling of children with another.

The methodological process to develop the matrix was based upon a series of decision rules for predicting the relationship between service needs and risks. Environmental and biological risks were distributed along two axes of the matrix to indicate a hierarchy of intensities of service needs. The vertical axis represents the predictions of the cumulative impact of established conditions and biological risks upon the child's needs for services. For example, children with certain neurological abnormalities such as cerebral palsy very often have sensory as well as motor impairments and developmental delay. The decision rules for the matrix incorporate these kinds of considerations. The horizontal axis represents the predictions of the family's needs for services based upon environmental risks. The intersection of the two axes represents the cumulative and interactive effect on the need for services when the child's established conditions, biological risks, and families' environmental risk factors are viewed as a whole or "gestalt."

Levels of Service

Both the child's biological and environmental risks are significant and must be fully considered to determine the level of service needed. The service needs

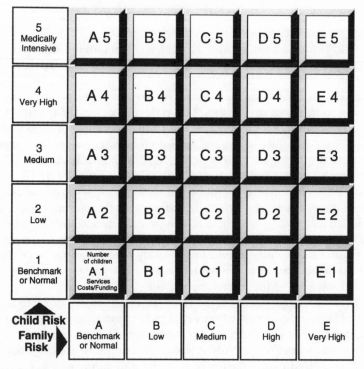

FIGURE 13.1.   Matrix for predicting early intervention service needs based on risks.

and the appropriate service delivery options for two children with an identical single biological risk may be quite different because one of the two lives with multiple environmental risks. Similarly, the types and levels of services needed by children with multiple biological risks as compared to those with a single biological risk factor may differ substantially.

The concept of an early intervention services matrix evolved from efforts aimed at configuring service need based on the interactive and cumulative impact of both biological and environmental risks. Toward this effort, a multidisciplinary group of eight experts was assembled to develop decision rules predictive of the relationship between risk-related characteristics and the level of service need for infants and toddlers. As a first step, the team considered every conceivable service configuration (e.g., types of services, intensities and duration of service, mode of delivery) appropriate for children with established conditions and developmental delay and their families. Five levels of service, defined in Table 13.1, were determined sufficient to capture the needs for both the children and families. In considering the children's services needs (the vertical axis), the levels of service range from low to medically intensive. A low level of service need was defined as tracking and monitoring the child's developmental status with a possible need for short-term service intervention. A high level of service need was characterized as high-intensity services with ongoing health, educational, therapeutic, and related psychosocial interventions. Benchmark children were defined as those with no early intervention service needs. Considering the families' services needs (the horizontal axis), the levels of service range from none (none being defined as just those family supports that are necessary because the child manifests a condition) to very high. Significant needs for service included intensive supports and potential out-of-home placement services for the child. Benchmark families were defined as those with minor need for services beyond those related to understanding the child's risk factors.

Child and Family Service Needs

As is shown in Table 13.2, 13 variables were available in the database from the survey to be considered for predicting the child's need for service. As a first step, each established condition and biological risk variable was separately ranked by each team member relative to its probable implication for one of the five levels of service needs. Interrater reliability was excellent allowing for the averaging of all rankings. Further evidence of reliability (and validity) was gained through a review of the literature and through representative case studies, which generally confirmed the predicted level of service needs established by the team of experts. Table 13.2 illustrates the decision rules that were established relative to single risk conditions. Children with atypical developmental disorders, sensory impairments, or illness and trauma associated with delay were predicted to have a high level of service need. In contrast, children with developmental delay or a neurological abnormality were considered to need a medium level of service, whereas, infants with a birth weight under 1,000 grams without overt signs of disability were predicted to need a low level of service.

The team of experts used 20 variables considered to be environmental risks or family stressors to predict the level of service needs for families of children with established conditions and developmental delay (see Table 13.2). When present as a single risk factor, 13 of these risks/stressors are considered to indicate a need for a low level of service. A few family conditions were expected to require medium, high, or very high levels of service. For example, migrant families are predicted to need a medium level of services (i.e., most are homeless, poor, and lacking basic health care). Parents who leave their children without supervision are predicted to need a high level of ser-

TABLE 13.1. Child and Family Risk Level Descriptors and Predicted Need for Services

Child

Intensity of child's needs	Child risk factors	Predicted need for intervention services
Low	One or two biological risk factors are present in the child's history such as very low birth weight.	Tracking and monitoring and/or short-term support or intervention. This might include health and developmental monitoring.
Medium	The child has congenital and/or neurological problems with a visible developmental delay.	Regular child-focused interventions and/or therapy(s) and periodic health checks.
High	The child has significant health and/or developmental problems including sensory impairments stemming from a physically or neurologically compromising illness or trauma.	High-intensity, on-going health, educational, therapeutic, and/or psychosocial interventions.
Very high	The child has two or more established conditions or multiple biological risks accompanied by emotional problems and developmental delays.	Very intensive behavior and other specialized therapies.
Medically intensive	The child has multiple medical problems and developmental delays that have often been environmentally induced and that require extensive technological and medical support.	Intensive and costly medical, developmental, and psychological services that last for an indefinite time period and that include specialized procedures and treatments.

298

Family

Intensity of family needs	Conditions and risks	Predicted need for intervention services
Benchmark or normal	The family is able to provide social, economic, emotional and health needs. Most families have two educated parents, who are not poor. Essential parenting functions are provided.	The family only needs services as they pertain to the risk factors in the child such as peer support and developmental guidance.
Low	Some environmental risk factors or stressors are present such as a single-parent family and/or poverty.	The family needs some intervention and/or preventative and support services such as child care and/or economic and educational services.
Medium	Several environmental risk factors or stressors are present such as low parent education, poverty, single-parent family, teen mother.	In addition to the above, the family may need drug treatment and/or crisis counseling.
High	There are significant chronic family problems. In addition to those named above, there are multiple stressors and risks that impact parenting such as child abuse, drug abuse, and/or family violence. Many children do not live with their biological family. Many homes have another incapacitated person.	The family needs intensive psychosocial supports such as family supervision, drug rehabilitation, or an out-of-the-home placement for the child.
Very high	There are multiple pervasive family risk factors including poverty, teen parent, drug abuse. Most of these children live out of the home.	The child needs residential services outside the family structure. Family needs extensive crisis management services, counseling, therapy/ rehabilitative supports and services.

TABLE 13.2.   Decision Rules to Predict Child and Family Service Needs[a,b]

Child Needs

Biological risks	Need for service				
	Low	Med.	High	Very high	Medically intensive
Medical complex/tech. dependent					✓
Atypical developmental disorders			✓		
Sensory impairments			✓		
Illness/trauma assoc. with delay			✓		
Genetic disorders		✓			
Neurological abnormalities		✓			
Congenital infectious diseases		✓			
Developmental delay		✓			
Drug exposure		✓			
Other factors impinging on developmental progress		✓			
Birth weight < 1,000 grams	✓				
Abuse/neglect	✓				
Exposure to poisons/toxins	✓				

Family Needs

Environmental risks	Need for service			
	Low	Med.	High	Very high
Foster/shelter care				✓
No legal guardian				✓
No legal guardian/relative or adoptive home			✓	
Children left without supervision			✓	
Parent unable to perform essential functions			✓	
Family member retarded, ill		✓		
Migrant/homeless		✓		
Relative/adoptive home	✓			
Teen mother [c]	✓			
No high school	✓			
Single mother [c]	✓			
Impoverished family [c]	✓			
Family immigrated in past year	✓			
Death in home in past year	✓			
Chronically ill mother	✓			
Family member < 18 pregnant	✓			
Separated/divorced in past year	✓			
Family moved more than twice	✓			
Family member serious crime victim	✓			
Violent home	✓			

[a] Level of service need for children is increased by one level when two or more conditions are present and the level of service is less than very high.
Exception:
[b] The level of service needs is not increased for children with conditions where factors cluster, that is, a child with neurological abnormalities will generally be developmentally delayed and have other impingements on developmental progress.
[c] Service need is increased by one level when any one or more of these three conditions is combined with some other family condition and the level of service is high or less.

vices. A very high need for service is predicted for situations were the child lives in an out-of-home placement or the natural parents have lost parental rights.

Decision Rules for Multiple Risk Factors

Extensive research has determined that children with established conditions and developmental delay typically have more than one biological risk present at a time. In one state, 87% of the children with established conditions and developmental delays had more than one type of biological risk. In addition, almost half of the children with established conditions were also developmentally delayed. Similarly, these families generally had more than one environmental risk and family stressor. Migrant families were poor, and teen mothers typically had less than a high school education. Therefore, services could not be predicted simply on the basis of a particular single condition or risk factor. The group of experts had to establish further decision rules to incorporate service need considerations for the typical clustering of risks.

Multiple Child Risks

The preliminary cell assignment of a hypothetical child with more than one risk condition was based on the risk condition with the highest level of service value. For example, if the child had a sensory impairment (high level of service) and a birth weight under 1,000 grams (low level of service), he/she was predicted to need a high level of service. As a general rule, it was decided to increase the predicted level of service need by one level if two or more conditions or biological risks were present and the child was not already in the very high service need level. Therefore, the child with sensory impairments and a very low birth weight was categorized in the very high level of services need as a way to take into account the interactive and cumulative nature of risks on a child's needs for service. The presence of each additional risk increased the level of service need by one level but did not exceed the very high level of service need. For example, if that same child with a sensory impairment and low birth weight was also drug-exposed, he/she was still predicted to need a very high level of services. In contrast, a child with congenital or genetic disorders (medium level of services), who was drug exposed (medium level of services) and also neglected (low level), was predicted to need a very high level of services—an increase of two levels of service.

The experts had to further qualify the decision rules. They believed it was important to maintain the integrity of the medically intensive category where costs tend to be extremely high. Furthermore, they wanted to provide for the clustering of factors found in certain established conditions and bio-logical risks. Therefore, exceptions to the general decision rules were estab-lished, as follows:

1. A child had to be medically involved or technologically dependent to be placed in the medically intensive level of service need category regardless of the number or type of other established conditions and biological risk factors.

2. The level of predicted service need would *not* be increased for chil-dren with neurological abnormalities (medium level of services) when "other factors impinging on their developmental progress" (medium level of services) were also present, because these two factors gener-ally go hand in hand. A third risk factor had to be present to increase the predicted level of service need under these conditions.

3. The predicted level of service need would *not* be increased for chil-dren with any single established condition when developmental delay is also present. For example, a neurological abnormality coupled with developmental delay would remain a medium level of service need prediction because most children with this condition do manifest this type of delay. However, a child with a neurological abnormality, developmental delay, and drug exposure would be increased to a high level of predicted service need.

The latter two exceptions were to account for the expected clustering of symp-toms with many conditions.

Multiple Family Risks or Stressors

The predictive decision rule for considering the interactive and cumulative impact of multiple environmental risks and family stressors called for increas-ing the level of service need beyond the level associated with single risks under one circumstance. The need for service was increased by one level if one or more of the following risks was also present—(1) teenage mother, and/or (2) single mother, and/or (3) poverty—and if the level of service need indi-cated from the single risk was not already high. These conditions exacerbate other environmental risk factors.

Later in this chapter, these decision rules for predicting the relationship between biological and environmental risks and need for services are applied to information about Florida's Part H-eligible population. Application of the predictive relationships is essential to the recommended approach for esti-mating the cost of an early intervention program. Others are encouraged to use the rankings discussed above; however, our main objective is to stress the importance of systematically differentiating the service needs for accurate cost estimation purposes.

SERVICE UNIT COSTS

How much do early intervention services cost? The method recommended to determine the relative cost of the services considered for inclusion in the statewide early intervention services system is a unit cost analysis. Instead of methods based on determining the average cost per child (derived from extrapolations of personnel requirements or the budgetary experience from other jurisdictions), a unit cost approach should be undertaken within early intervention programs for three primary reasons:

1. Unit cost budgeting facilitates the development of funding strategies.
2. Unit costs support the capability to implement and monitor appropriate levels of service intensity.
3. Unit costs allow for the establishment of a funding framework for model programs.

Development of Funding Strategies

Most revenue sources under consideration for funding early intervention are categorical, that is, funds that restrict eligibility to certain categories of children or prohibit the use of the revenue for funding particular services. Medicaid funds (Title XIX) in most states operate on a unit cost (fee-for-service) reimbursement basis or capitated rates developed from unit costing. Using a unit cost methodology compatible with the Medicaid reimbursement methodologies can set up access to a major potential federal revenue source for early intervention and Part H services.

Support Implementation and Monitoring

Existing early intervention programs vary in terms of the types of services offered and the intensity of the services delivered (e.g., the number of hours of physical therapy provided). A unit cost approach supports the development of a cost-estimating framework based on the actual cost experiences of representative programs, but independent of current, sometimes insufficient, cost reimbursement rates and levels of service intensity. Service needs including both types of services and their intensities should be factored into the statewide cost estimates and should be adjusted based on actual program experience.

Unit costs will also be useful for monitoring the efficiency patterns of future service delivery. Economies should be realized through decreasing unit costs instead of reducing the intensity or amount of service delivered.

Establishment of a Funding Framework

Unit costs provide discrete information on the basic components affecting the costs of early intervention programs. Accumulation of cost information at the unit of service level provides a method to estimate the potential costs of new program models with characteristics that differ from the current situation. Potential economies of function (i.e., consolidating work activities through role redefinition), such as integrating the case management function with home visits, is more readily determined with knowledge of the unit cost of each function individually. Also, understanding the related unit costs of services delivered in programs with primarily paraprofessional staff as compared to those in medical facilities with high levels of professionalization will support cost simulations for various combinations of staffing patterns in program models.

Estimation of Unit Costs

The first task required to estimate unit costs involves the development of mutually exclusive and quantified definitions of each type of service under consideration. For early intervention programs, it is important to consider both the child-focused services as well as the family support services. Recognition should also be given to the fact that some services can be delivered by various professional disciplines, which could affect unit costs. For example, case management services are in some situations most appropriately delivered by a health professional (e.g., nurse) and in other cases by a social worker. Salary requirements can vary substantially among professional disciplines. Therefore, the cost of a unit of case management service will vary by the required professional credentials of the service provider. To accommodate these situations, discipline-specific units of service cost should be developed.

In addition, two different types of cost units must be developed for early intervention services. The first involves a flat cost rate developed for services that generally are episodic or limited in use over a fixed period of time and include more than a portion of an employee's time. Examples of flat or fixed unit cost service are evaluations that are performed a limited number of times during a period, on a nonroutine, periodic basis and often involve other cost factors such as the cost of instrumentation and the interpretation and documentation of diagnostic assessment. Family assessments, intake/screening, service planning, and transportation are others that involve unit costs for each episode of service.

The second type of unit cost is the unit-of-service cost. Applying an hour- or day-of-time measure to the unit-of-service cost is used for those services that are primarily time sensitive and reoccur on a periodic basis. An example of this type of service is therapy. Therapies are performed on a scheduled, recurring basis (weekly, monthly, etc.) for a specific amount of time (30 minutes, 1 hour, etc.). Case management, counseling, health services, special intervention services, developmental child care, medical child care, and family support services are costed as hourly units of services. Therapeutic foster care and medical foster care are also costed as daily units of services.

A cost questionnaire should be developed for conducting unit cost analysis. The instrument should be designed to capture all of a program's direct and indirect expenses relative to the delivery of specific types of early intervention services. Questions must be specifically designed to determine a program's spending on administrative functions and program operations for the delivery of each type of early intervention service. Revenue from all sources, including in-kind contributions, must be considered in a program's expenditures. Specific categories of program expenses included in the unit cost analysis are:

- Salaries, wages, and benefits.
- Facility expenses.
- Utility expenses.
- Insurance and interest expenses.
- Maintenance expenses.
- Administrative and program equipment.
- Administrative and program supplies.
- General administrative expenses.
- Food purchases and services.
- All other direct and indirect administrative and program expenses.

Calculation of unit costs requires the allocation of both program and administrative costs over the most recent 12-month period to the applicable service categories. Additionally, the number of units of services (hours or days) or service units (episodes) provided (with the allocated costs) within each service category is obtained to determine the applicable unit costs within the program.

Agencies selected for unit cost analyses should operate programs with diverse characteristics including:

- Programs with varying levels of staff representing a range of different professional disciplines.
- Programs specializing in services solely to children with risks or only disabilities, as well as programs with integrated client populations.
- Programs operating with public revenue on a fee-for-service and fixed-grant-amount basis, some with only private sources of revenue, and some with a mix of revenue sources.
- Programs delivering only a single service and some offering an array of different services.
- Programs providing services through various contexts, including in-home and center-based, and some delivering the same service to some children on an individual basis in their homes and to others on a group basis at centers.
- Programs serving children only and programs serving both children and adults.

The administration of the unit cost questionnaire should be conducted on-site if possible. This is recommended because generally no agency will maintain its fiscal records in a manner that directly supports the interpolation of its expenditures into a unit cost structure. Generally, agency fiscal records will not record expenditures so they can be related directly to the object of cost nor will they define services in a manner comparable to a unit cost methodology. Considerable effort will be expended in attributing agency expenditure objects and assigning costs to those services that most resemble the applicable unit cost structure. The site visits typically will require interviews with administrative, fiscal, and senior program staff to complete the fiscal analysis. Although audit statements and fiscal year expenditure reports should serve as the basis for the fiscal analysis, informed judgments and estimates from the best information available can be considered as reliable indicators of service costs.

Estimation of Florida's Statewide Cost for Early Intervention Services

As an exercise to illustrate the application of the early intervention services cost methodology, summary statistical tables are provided below based upon our work on Florida's Part H Cost/Funding Study. The research information acquired through this study provides an actual framework for empirical data upon which the methodology can be applied.

The prevalence estimate for Florida's Part H eligibility definition was 8.6% of the applicable age cohort, or 48,493 children under the age of 3 years. Research undertaken to determine the service utilization estimate revealed that 30,504 infants and toddlers (62.9% of those eligible) were expected to participate in services throughout a year. The average age of admission to services was 11.8 months, and the average child stayed in services 13.9 months. Using the second utilization estimation method described earlier in this chapter, these results allowed us to calculate the need for an estimated 10,066 slots for full-time service demands.

Application of the matrix decision rules to the estimated utilization population (through the prevalence database) allowed us to distribute Florida's children and families into the applicable cells of the matrix. Using the 13 available child variables and 20 family variables, demographic profiles were constructed for each row (representing the children), column (representing families), and cell (representing the interaction of child and family risks). From these profiles, service needs were predicted for the hypothetical child and family in each cell of the matrix.

Here we will use cell C3 of Figure 13.1 as an example. Of the children and families expected to utilize services 14.2% are predicted to have characteristics as described for this cell—medium levels of child and family needs. Half of the 4,332 children expected to utilize services in this cell had delays or other factors that affect their development (56%). Many had infections associated with delay (42%), and over a third were drug-exposed (36%) or were in a neonatal intensive care unit. A few were low birth weight or abused (13%).

Of the families, 70% were single-parent and the majority had a very low educational level, with 82% having a high school education or less and 67% having only a junior high school education. About half the families lived in poverty (47%). A fifth were teen mothers. Most of the children lived with their biological family, but 30% lived with relatives or outside the family home. A fifth or more had additional family stressors that included a recent death in the family (20%), a separation or divorce (25%), or a teen pregnancy in the household (22%).

What kinds of services will such children and families need? Table 13.3 indicates for cell C3 the type of service need predictions made by our expert team. As Table 13.3 illustrates, half the children in this cell will most likely need physical, occupational, and speech therapies. Many will need psychological supports due to attachment problems resulting from either extended hospitalizations or drug exposure. Periodic health monitoring is needed for those with infections. Extensive parent training and support will be needed for the poor, uneducated single mothers whose children have problems. Financial counseling and job training are needed to help the family out of poverty. Drug rehabilitation is needed for families of the children who have been drug-exposed.

These recommended interventions are based upon the general cell demographic profile and are not the only array, intensity, or duration of services that may be provided to children and families within this cell. Each individual will have his/her own unique service configuration. Table 13.3 represents the average need for service, which is costed to determine the typical funding

TABLE 13.3.   Predicted Service Needs for Children and Families in Matrix Cell C3 (Figure 13.1)

Child-related services	Intensity	Duration	Method	Personnel	Percentage of cases in cell
Case management consultation	6 hours per month	12 months	1:1	Community resource mother, nurse, social worker, or teacher	all
Parent training	8 hours per month	12 months	1:10	Community resource mother, nurse, social worker, or teacher	all
Health services (includes nutrition)	6 hours per year	annually	1:1	Nurse or home health aide	all
Multi-disciplinary evaluation	9 initial in-depth[a]	1st yr	1:1	Speech therapist, physical therapist, occupational therapist, psychologist, nurse/nutritionist, audiologist	33%
	6 in-depth	2nd yr			33%
	5 in-depth	3rd yr			33%
Special intervention or developmental child care	30 hours per week	12 months	1:4	Early interventionist or early childhood educator	75%[b]
	15 hours per week				25%
Occupational therapy	4 hours per month	12 months	1:1	Occupational therapist or assistant with supervision	50%
Physical therapy	4 hours per month	12 months	1:1	Physical therapist or assistant with supervision	50%
Speech/language therapy	4 hours per month	12 months	1:1	Speech therapist or assistant with supervision	50%
Transportation	5 days per week for child 1 day per week for parent	12 months	NA	Driver	60%
Behavioral therapy	1 hour per week	6 months	1:1	Psychologist	50%
Service planning	Twice a year	Twice a year	NA	Team - 8 professionals - for initial Family Support Plan, 4 for next	all
Family-related services					
Financial counseling	4 hours per year	NA	NA	Financial counselor	82%
Job training for GED	NA	Until GED	NA	Adult educator	82%[c]
Drug rehabilitation	NA	NA	NA	Drug counselor	36%
Counseling for self-esteem building	2 hours per week	12 months	1:10	Therapist	81%[d]
Subsidized child care	NA	NA	NA	NA	82%[e]

a Quarterly OT, PT, speech, psychology, nutrition, and health services in lieu of regular therapy, includes 3 health evaluations (at 3, 6, and 12 months)
b Those in poverty and drug exposed are recommended for full-time intervention
c 82% have less than a high school education
d Counseling for the drug users (36%), divorcees (25%),those with a death in family(20%)
e Child care needed while pursuing education

need. Based on the average cost of each of these services (see Table 13.4), each slot in cell C3 would be allocated $10,079 for services, constituting 14.2% of the statewide slots.

Following the unit of service cost methodology discussed earlier, we conducted a cost survey of representative early intervention programs in Florida to answer the fourth pertinent research question—how much do the predicted service needs cost? Table 13.4 displays the results of this unit cost survey. Some categories of service cost could not be estimated based on actual

TABLE 13.4.   Early Intervention Services Unit Costs

Required Part H Services	Programs Providing Service	Low Cost	High Cost	Average Cost	Decision Rule	Unit of Service
Case Mgt - Medical (H=Hour)	2	$27	$52	$40		$40
Case Mgt - Social (H)	11	$16	$60	$28		$28
Case Mgt - Parapro (H)	1	$15	$15	$15		$15
Case Mgt - Other (H)	1	$21	$21	$21		$21
Counseling/ - W/Parent (H)	14	$11	$57	$29		$29
Counseling/ - W/Other (H)	0				$29	$29
Eval - Audiology (E = Episode)	1	$30	$30	$30		$30
Eval - Medical (E)	4	$59	$100	$76		$76
Eval - Health (Md/Nur)	1	$29	$29	$29		$29
Eval - Nutrition (E)	3	$25	$59	$44		$44
Eval - Occup Therapy (E)	6	$31	$123	$67		$67
Eval - Phys Therapy (E)	6	$44	$123	$76		$76
Eval - Speech/Lang (E)	6	$28	$160	$82		$82
Eval - Psych (E)	5	$37	$166	$100		$100
Eval - Social/Emot (E)	6	$22	$166	$72		$72
Eval - Lab Tests (E=Episode)	0				$100	$100
Family Assessment (Formal) (E)	8	$11	$207	$82		$82
Health Svcs - Med Consult (E)	1	$111	$111	$111	$38	$38
Health Svcs - Nursing Care (H)	2	$32	$37	$34		$34
Health Svcs - Home Aide (H)	0				$17	$17
Health Svcs - Med Eq (E)	0				$250	$250
Health Svcs - Med Supplies (E)	0				$250	$250
Intake and Screening (E)	5	$12	$55	$29		$29
Service Plan (2 per yr min) (E)	9	$14	$103	$38	$345	$345
Spec Intervention (Ed) Svcs (H)	7	$8	$55	$29		$29
Ther Svcs - Audiology (H)	1	$128	$128	$128		$128
Ther Svcs - Nutrition (H)	1	$24	$24	$24		$24
Ther Svcs - Occup (H)	6	$20	$80	$53		$53
Ther Svcs - Physical (H)	6	$14	$80	$52		$52
Ther Svcs - Speech/Lang (H)	5	$27	$80	$43		$43
Ther Svcs - Psych (H)	4	$14	$80	$54		$54
Trans - Indep/Support (TI=Trip)	2	$1	$4	$3		$3
Trans - Dependent (TD=Trip)	0				$3	$3
Other Services						
Childcare (H)	7	$2	$4	$3		$3
Medical Childcare (H)	1	$9	$9	$9		$9
Ther Foster/Shelter Care (D=Day)	1	$67	$67	$67		$67
Medical Foster Care (D)	0				$75	$75
Family Support - Respite Care (H)	1	$6	$6	$6		$6
Family Support - Homemaker (H)	0				$6	$6

costs because no programs were providing those services. The expert team estimated a cost for those 10 services (e.g., home-aide health services).

The next and final step was to apply the service unit costs to the predicted service needs in each cell to determine the average funding requirement to meet the needs for early intervention services for the estimated utilization population. Tables 13.5 and 13.6 illustrate a completed matrix and cost distribution for the Florida study summarizing prevalence, utilization, slots, and the predicted statewide costs for funding those slots.

SUMMARY AND CONCLUSIONS

Extensive and reliable research has demonstrated the cost effectiveness of early intervention services. Programs such as Part H make sense. However, our country's history of largely uncontrollable entitlement programs dictates caution when proposing new programs. Reliable cost estimates are imperative. Inadequacies of traditional cost estimation techniques necessitated a new methodology for generating reasonably accurate cost estimations for early intervention programs.

This method of cost estimation requires answers to four essential research questions. First, an estimate of the prevalence of the target client population is needed. We discussed the need for a precise eligibility definition and methods to conduct prevalence surveys. Next, an estimate of the proportion of the prevalence population expected to use the services is needed. We discussed two basic methods to derive estimates of the utilization population recommending application of a "slot" concept for funding purposes. The third question addresses the cost of the services to be included in the program.

TABLE 13.5. Matrix for Predicting Early Intervention Service Needs in Florida (Distribution and Annual Cost per Slot)

		FAMILY NEEDS						
C		A Benchmark	B Low	C Medium	D High	E Very High	Total	
H	5	0.4%	8.2%	6.1%	1.3%	3.5%	19.5%	Medically
I		$25,812	$22,648	$26,414	$27,623	$28,340		Intensive
L	4	4.5%	3.6%	1.0%	3.1%	8.4%	20.6%	Very High
D		$13,142	$13,813	$13,965	$14,067	$16,347		
	3	17.6%	2.8%	14.2%	6.0%	5.1%	45.7%	High
N		$5,032	$8,523	$10,079	$11,730	$12,042		
E	2	2.8%	3.1%	0.5%	0.2%		6.6%	Medium
E		$6,389	$9,061	$9,865	$9,759			
D	1	3.8%	3.8%				7.6%	Low
S		$1,446	$1,269					
	Total	29.1%	21.5%	21.8%	10.6%	17.0%	100%	

TABLE 13.6. Average Cost per Cell and Total Statewide Costs in Florida

Cell	0-36 Avg. Cost	Prevalence	Utiliza-tion	Slot # Full-Time-Equivalent Clients	TOTAL STATEWIDE COST with slot concept applied
A-1	1,446	1,843	1,159	382	552,287
A-2	6,389	1,358	854	282	1,801,698
A-3	5,032	8,535	5,369	1,772	8,916,704
A-4	13,142	2,183	1,373	453	5,953,326
A-5	25,812	194	122	40	1,032,480
B-1	1,269	1,843	1,159	382	484,758
B-2	9,061	1,504	946	312	2,827,032
B-3	8,523	1,358	854	282	2,403,486
B-4	13,813	1,746	1,098	362	5,000,306
B-5	22,648	3,976	2,501	825	18,684,600
C-2	9,865	243	153	50	493,250
C-3	10,079	6,887	4,332	1,430	14,412,970
C-4	13,965	485	305	101	1,410,465
C-5	26,414	2,958	1,861	614	16,218,196
D-2	9,759	97	61	20	195,180
D-3	11,730	2,909	1,830	604	7,084,920
D-4	14,067	1,504	946	312	4,388,904
D-5	27,623	631	397	131	3,618,613
E-3	12,042	2,474	1,556	513	6,177,546
E-4	16,347	4,073	2,562	845	13,813,215
E-5	28,340	1,698	1,068	352	9,975,680
Total		48,497	30,506	10,064	$125,445,616

Note. Totals may vary slightly due to rounding.

Advantages of a unit cost estimation methodology were articulated. Finally, the service needs of the utilization population must be determined. We proposed and discussed extensively a predictive typology or matrix for determining service needs.

Recommending the use of a matrix as a conceptual organizer for planning services, and more importantly, as a predictive typology to estimate costs is, we believe, an advance in the field of program cost analyses in health, education, and social services. The method we described is consistent with contemporary theory in early intervention because it considers the interaction of the child's biological and environmental risks. The method is consistent with current statistical approaches for developing program cost estimates (i.e., it recognizes cost variations among client populations). Other important aspects of the matrix as a tool in cost estimation are that the matrix:

1. Incorporates the potential number of children to be served based on best practices knowledge regarding the relationship between biological and environmental risk factors.

2. Proportionally represents children with high-level service needs and high costs, such as medically complex children.
3. Predicts the volume of service capacity needs for personnel and program development planning.
4. Provides a framework for the allocation of resources and lends itself to programmatic outcome evaluations.
5. Establishes a management information system framework for addressing federal, state, and local reporting requirements.
6. Allows for movement away from categorical funding mechanisms to a basis for collaborative funding mechanisms.

Others are encouraged to apply this cost estimation methodology to their own program development initiatives. We believe the recommended research methods add logic and structure to what is often an emotional and difficult process. Answers to the four research questions discussed in this chapter are pertinent to most program development exercises in the area of health, education, and social services. The approach is adaptable at any level of programmatic consideration (e.g., statewide, county, municipal, etc.) and the conceptual underpinnings for the matrix are directly transferable to different client target populations as well. In fact, the predictive typology for estimating service needs is relevant for any early intervention program seeking to serve children with established conditions, those with developmental delay, and those at risk of delay.

ACKNOWLEDGMENTS

This research was funded through Part H dollars in a grant from the Florida Department of Education, Bureau of Exceptional Students. This chapter is adapted from *Florida's Cost/Implementation Study: Vol. 10. Costs and Funding for Early Intervention Services to Infants and Toddlers in Florida* by Florida TaxWatch. The research work was a collaborative project, interdependent upon the conceptual direction and research methods of many individuals and groups that contributed their wisdom and guidance to this effort. We acknowledge the special contributions of Ray Foster, PhD, and his staff at Therapeutic Concepts, Inc., and the support of Dominic M. Calabro and Neil S. Crispo, EdD, of Florida TaxWatch, Inc.

REFERENCE

Barnett, W. S., & Escobar, C. M. (1990). Economic costs and benefits of early intervention. In S. J. Meisels & J. P. Shonkoff (Eds.), *Handbook of early childhood intervention: Theory, practice, and analysis* (pp. 560–582). Cambridge: Cambridge University Press.

CHAPTER 14

Systems of Financing
Early Intervention

RICHARD M. CLIFFORD
KATHLEEN Y. BERNIER

The directive contained in Part H of the Individuals with Disabilities Education Act (IDEA) (now Subchapter VIII of Public Law 102-119, formerly Public Law 99-457) established policy requiring participating states to provide early intervention services for infants and toddlers with disabilities (birth to age 3) and their families and to finance this system through a combination of existing governmental and nongovernmental sources.

Financing the Part H service system is a complex process requiring coordination or, at least, use of several different sources of funds, including federal, state, local, and nongovernmental sources. In general, state leaders have experienced difficulty in developing and implementing a complete system for financing Part H services. Of the 14 components of the IDEA legislation, the Part H finance system has been the slowest to progress (Harbin, Gallagher, & Batista, 1992; Harbin, Gallagher, & Lillie, 1989, 1991; Harbin, Gallagher, Lillie, & Eckland, 1990). The development and approval of early intervention plans has been under way for 5 years, and the application of finance plans is only now occurring in some states. Although progress is being made in states in the ability to access various funding sources, multiple "barriers" to developing a coordinated system of financing, such as regulations, lack of resources, and "turf" issues, are still reported (Clifford, Bernier, & Harbin, 1993).

This chapter begins with a review of the financial requirements of Part H and an overview of the current status of implementation of the Part H financing system. A summary of the literature on financing Part H early intervention services, including research and technical assistance information, follows. Details regarding potential sources for financing Part H services are presented, including information on the current status of states' use of sources and future prospects for financing services at the state level. The chapter concludes with a series of recommendations for state and federal policy makers.

FINANCE ISSUES IN THE PART H LEGISLATION

The requirements for the statewide, comprehensive, coordinated, multidisciplinary, interagency early intervention program outlined in Section 1476 of Part H of IDEA include the designation of a lead agency to, in part, identify and coordinate all available resources within the state including public and private insurance coverage (Section 1476[b][9]). The state may designate an individual or an entity to be responsible for assigning financial responsibility among appropriate agencies (Section 1478[a][2]).

Yearly appropriations under Part H from the federal government to the states are tied to specific requirements of progress outlined in the legislation (Section 1478). Funds provided under Part H itself are to be used to plan, develop, and implement the statewide system, and may also be used to provide direct services that are not otherwise provided and to expand and improve services that are otherwise available (Section 1479). Part H funds may not be used to pay for services that would have been paid for from other public or private sources, except to prevent a delay in the receipt of services pending reimbursement, nor may states reduce other assistance to infants and toddlers with disabilities or alter eligibility for other programs (Section 1481).

Types of sources that provide funding for services for young children with disabilities include federal monies from programs such as Chapter I and Medicaid; state funds, such as dollars designated for special education and matching federal program allocations; and nongovernmental sources, such as private health insurance and voluntary service agencies. The sources and amounts of funds available to a state are, of course, related to the particular type of early intervention service being provided to an eligible child and to characteristics of the child and family. According to the law, services that are to be provided include family counseling, training, or home visits; special instruction; speech and language therapy; occupational therapy; physical therapy; psychological services; service coordination; diagnostic medical services; screening and evaluation services; health services necessary to enable the child to benefit from other services; social work services; transportation; vision services; audiology; and assistive communication, (Section 1472[2][E]). Of these, the four core services (screening, multidisciplinary evaluations, family service plans, and service coordination) must be provided to a family at no cost and are to be financed by various federal, state, local, and nongovernmental sources. Other services, such as therapies and medical treatments, have been and may continue to be paid for by the family or some third-party source.

Sources of Funds for Early Intervention Services

The *NEC*TAS Financing Workbook* (Williams & Kates, 1991) is perhaps the most comprehensive work on identifying and describing types of potential sources for Part H services. Out of the National Early Childhood Technical Assistance System (NEC*TAS), it provides a comprehensive picture of the many different sources and outlines approaches to accessing the various types of financing. The workbook was written in response to a survey regarding states' needs for technical assistance that revealed that the issue of financing was a major priority. Experts on special education and health financing met to help develop materials for states to use in defining and applying states' financing systems for early intervention. An assumption underlying the workbook is that "in any financing plan all existing financing resources ought to be identified, understood, and fully utilized as a prerequisite and context for seeking new resources" (p. 3). This position is fully congruent with the intentions of the requirements in Part H for financing the service system, as described above.

Seven steps have been detailed to help guide planning and implementation of a financing system for early intervention, including involving key players, developing a vision of the system, defining the desired system, identifying the existing system, identifying existing problems, developing change strategies, and implementing changes. A financing matrix has been developed to help understand the existing structure of services and financing. NEC*TAS identified, in the list of potential sources, 44 funding resources or categories of resources that may be used to support early intervention services (see Table 14.1). Of these, 30 sources are from federal funds, 8 from state and local funds, and 6 from nongovernmental funds. Of the federal, state, and local government sources, 14 are education funds, 14 are health funds, and 10 are social welfare funds. The wide variety of levels and types of funding sources would seem to indicate that accessing and coordinating funding for the Part H service system is a major task requiring a substantial input of resources—both monetary and human—from both the state and local programs. In addition, gaps and overlaps in financing particular services for particular children must be identified and resolved.

Other work in the area of identifying and accessing types of resources has focused on particular sources of financing early intervention services, such as Medicaid (Fox & Wicks, 1990; Fox, Wicks, McManus, & Newacheck, 1992; Kastorf, 1991; NEC*TAS, 1990; White & Immel, 1990) or private insurance (Fox, Freedman, & Klepper, 1989; NEC*TAS, 1990; Van Dyck, 1991). Private health insurance and Medicaid (public health insurance) are both potential sources of major financial support for the Part H system and are being used by a majority of states (Clifford et al., 1993). Each currently presents problems, including lack of full early intervention benefits and difficulty of access, which limit usability. Eligibility is an issue in the use of Medicaid. Families with private health insurance coverage face problems including premium costs, copayments, deductibles, and fewer early intervention benefits than Medicaid. These different sources of funding are discussed in the following sections.

Public and Private Expenditures

The roles and relationship of private enterprise and the public sector are constantly debated. The goals of efficient and equitable delivery of health services are given different priority under public and private systems. Passell and Ross (1978) assert, for example, that the Medicaid program cannot resolve the conflict between attempting to provide services to all eligible persons and providing quality services. Private health insurance companies would seem to have motivation for efficient delivery of services, but in fact have little experience in monitoring health care quality and exist in a state of constant conflict over client protection and company profit goals.

Allocation of resources among programs is a value-laden process. In a rather sentimental essay on standards and values in a rich society, Hansen (1965) directs that qualitative goals for fiscal growth and progress be set in accordance with the type of country we wish to build:

> We have reached a point in our economic and social evolution where social-value judgments, not the market, must control the uses to which we put ... our productive resources. ... Civilized countries mold their people into civilized ways of thinking, guided by values that experience and knowledge have laid down. We don't leave it to the market. We educate. (pp. 8–9)

Even theoretical frameworks of fiscal functions may be seen to involve value choices. Musgrave and Musgrave's (1990) theory of public finance includes the notion that the role of government is threefold: allocation of resource use to private and social goods, adjustment of the distribution of income and wealth to assure societal "fairness," and stabilizing prices and economic growth while maintaining high employment. The scope of the government's role in these functions is debated, and the policy resolutions reflect prevailing values.

Public Health Insurance: Medicaid

Medicaid, or the Medical Assistance Program under Title XIX of the Social Security Act of 1965, provides federal financial assistance to states for medical services for public assistance recipients and other medically needy low-income people. The federal government provides a match for state dollars that ranges from 50 to 80% and is determined by a complex formula based on state per capita personal income. Reimbursement is based on actual expenditures for covered services provided to Medicaid-eligible individuals, and there is no limit on federal funds available. The Medicaid program is administered by a state agency that must operate under a state plan approved by the Secretary of the Department of Health and Human Services and comply with the many federal program regulations. The Medical Assistance Program is a payor of last resort, in that service providers are required to pursue reimbursement from other sources before seeking Medicaid reimbursement.

Eligibility for the Medicaid program and the range of benefits provided to those eligible vary greatly from state to state. The Omnibus Budget Reconciliation Act of 1989 (OBRA '89 or Public Law 101-239) recently extended eligibility and benefits. Presently, one group of people whose eligibility is federally mandatory is the categorically needy: recipients of Aid to Families with Dependent Children (AFDC) (usually children under 18 years of age living in low-income, one-parent homes); pregnant women and their children under age 7 who meet financial but not other criteria for AFDC and do not receive AFDC benefits; pregnant women and their children under age 1 who live in families with incomes up to 133% of the federal poverty figure; children under age 6 in families with incomes up to 133% of federal poverty; and, in some states, those eligible under the Supplemental Social Security Income program. At a state's option, the medically needy (individuals who lack the resources to pay medical expenses); foster and adopted children; pregnant women and their children up to age 1 whose families have income up to 185% of federal poverty; and some recipients of model programs may also be covered.

Mandatory benefits that must be provided for Medicaid-eligible children include inpatient and outpatient hospitalization, laboratory and X-ray services, rural health clinic services, federally qualified health clinic services, physician services, pediatric and nurse-practitioner services, and Early and Periodic Screening, Diagnosis, and Treatment (EPSDT). The EPSDT screening schedules now include interperiodic and partial examinations, and if a condition is discovered during a screening, treatment services that are medically necessary, whether available to all Medicaid-eligible persons or not, must be provided. Optional service categories that a state may provide include preventative and rehabilitative services, home or nursing care, home- and community-based model programs, medical equipment and appliances, private duty nursing, home respiratory care services, and case management.

States have much latitude to set limits on the frequency, scope, and duration of services, to set service standards, and determine payment rates. Thus, among states there is much variation in the types of people served and the types and quantity of services covered. In fact, Medicaid expenditures per capita may vary nationally by a factor of 15, and between the South and the Northeast by a factor of 6 (Davis, 1974, cited in Passell & Ross, 1978).

Services provided under Medicaid must meet the criteria of "statewideness and comparability"; that is, services must be equally available in all parts of the state and for all persons who are Medicaid-eligible, with the previously stated EPSDT exception included in OBRA '89. In the Medicare Catastrophic Coverage Act of 1987 (Public Law 100-360), the original Medicaid legislation was amended to require reimbursement for covered medical services for a child with disabilities if the service is included in an Individualized Education Plan (IEP) or Individualized Family Service Plan (IFSP). This is not to say that education services may be paid for with Medicaid funds, but that related services, such as speech and language therapy, psychological services, physical and occupational therapy, are eligible for Medicaid reimbursement.

The cost of the Medicaid program to the federal and state governments has rapidly increased. Both Congress and the states have at times implemented various fiscal restraints, such as restricting eligibility, requiring prior authorization for services beyond a given limit, requiring copayments, and strictly limiting participating provider rates (Passell & Ross, 1978).

The consensus among those who have investigated Medicaid as a possible source of payment for Part H services is that the Medicaid system is complex, in part because of the tremendous variability among states in details of the Medicaid plan regarding such issues as defining eligible populations and covered services. Many consider Medicaid to be a major source for funding Part H services. One option for financing states' early intervention systems would be to fund all Part H services under Medicaid for all children regardless of family income (Clifford, Kates, Black, Eckland, & Bernier, 1991). Although the benefits of such a method would include use of existing bureaucratic structures, ability to take advantage of the work that states have already done to move to a fee-for-service system, and simplification of the funding system, a major disadvantage would be the continuing difficulty of accessing reimbursement.

In a recent report of the results of two national surveys on private and public health insurance reimbursements for health-related services for infants and toddlers with developmental delays, Fox et al. (1992) conclude that "health insurance, especially Medicaid, can provide reimbursement for many, if not all, health-related early intervention services furnished under the Part H program" (p. 119). Their secondary data analysis of the 1988 National Health Interview Survey results suggested that a majority of children (59%) who were eligible for early intervention services were covered by private health insurance only, 16% had Medicaid coverage only, 12% had both Medicaid and private health insurance coverage, and 12% had no coverage. With the recent broadening of eligibility for Medicaid and concurrent expansion of services covered in the various state plans, current levels of Medicaid coverage should be substantially higher than in 1988.

In the 1988 study (Fox et al., 1992), private health insurance plans were found to more often offer coverage for ancillary therapists (physical, occupational, and speech therapists), whereas Medicaid tended to use less strict criteria for providing these services. Medicaid also tended to reimburse services in more types of settings than private insurance, including clinics that could provide early intervention services. Home health service coverage was greatly restricted under both Medicaid and private plans, but case management services, or service coordination, were more commonly provided under Medicaid than private insurance.

Medicaid is likely to present a better financing option for Part H services than private insurance (Fox et al., 1992). Unlike most private health insurance plans, Medicaid requires no or only a minimal copayment from the beneficiary. Because state dollars are supplemented by a federal match, states have a strong incentive to use Medicaid dollars for service reimbursement. Medicaid has no dollar caps on service costs; private insurance often caps costs. States have much more flexibility in structuring a Medicaid plan to meet the needs of children requiring early intervention than in directing the private health insurance industry in benefit provision. In addition, the recent (1989) mandatory EPSDT benefit allowing EPSDT coverage of any "medically necessary" service need discovered during an EPSDT screening provides a ready-made method to provide early intervention services, unlike set benefits offered under private plans. Although Medicaid seems to be a better financing option, Fox and colleagues cited problems including restricted reimbursement rates and lack of funds within states to expand services.

Basic information about the legislation and regulations regarding Medicaid and the EPSDT program of preventative screening and follow-up services for Medicaid-eligible children is available through several sources. The NEC*TAS Information Packet (1990) chapter on Medicaid is a collection of memoranda and short publications, from such organizations as the Children's Defense Fund and the National Governors' Association, detailing 1990 Medicaid and EPSDT federal mandates for coverage, changes in coverage, and status of coverage in each state. General information about Medicaid mandates and options, state-specific variations in benefits, and implementation issues for Medicaid financing of health-related early intervention services is also available (Fox & Wicks, 1990). White and Immel (1990) summarized the basic elements of Medicaid and detailed a plan to access Medicaid funds based on the successful experiences of several states.

In addition, Fox and Wicks (1990) argue that Medicaid is an appropriate source of financing health-related early intervention. Kastorf (1991) also states that the "authority of states to use Medicaid funds for the provision of early intervention has been well established by federal legislation, regulation, and court decisions" (p. 2), although he reminds us that states must make the choice to design and implement a system to do so. Kastorf further presents the experience of Massachusetts in implementing Medicaid funding for early intervention and details the benefits that Massachusetts has enjoyed. He suggests that one barrier states may face in applying the process is the requirement of a substantial commitment of state funds, staff, and time for start-up.

In summary, recent changes in the Medicaid legislation, regarding eligible income levels, ages of children covered, expansion of benefits, and service provision for medical treatment of conditions discovered during EPSDT screening, have prompted suggestions that Medicaid is the most likely source for major funding and coordination of the Part H service system.

Private Health Insurance

Although the Part H legislation directs states to include private health insurance as a source of financing services to eligible children, access to these funds has not been straightforward. Issues regarding the use of private health insurance for Part H services include who is covered, scope of services covered, quality of coverage, limitations on services or dollar amounts, and family financial responsibilities including premium costs, deductibles, and copayments.

States are beginning to develop plans and strategies to access private health insurance to cover early intervention services, as directed under Part H. Information on mandated insurance benefits by state that may be used to cover early intervention services, methods for estimating costs of the benefits, and options for implementing payment-for-services plans are available (McManus, 1989; NEC*TAS, 1990; Van Dyck, 1991).

The Children's Defense Fund reported that in 1990 more than 25 million children in the United States, or approximately 40% of all children, lacked employer-provided health insurance coverage (Rosenbaum, Hughes, Harris, & Liu, 1992), even though 85% of all American children live in employed families. Some form of non-employment-based private insurance covers 10%; 18% are covered by Medicaid; and 13% are completely uninsured. The trend in numbers of covered children is one of decline, especially among minority, low- and middle-income, and rural children.

Private health insurance coverage varies state to state, as well as by plan. Early intervention services that are most likely to be covered by private plans include evaluation/diagnosis, physical therapy, occupational therapy, speech therapy, outpatient mental health counseling, nutrition services, case management, therapeutic nursery, and medical equipment and supplies (McManus, 1989). Private health insurance plans tend not to offer any clinic services coverage, which are often needed by infants and toddlers with disabilities (Fox et al., 1992). Also, case management services, common among state Medicaid plans, are infrequently part of private insurance coverage.

Services often required by children with disabilities have traditionally been excluded from insurance coverage when children are school aged, because special education and related services have been viewed strictly as being provided at public expense. However, Fox et al. (1992) found that speech therapy, occupational therapy, physical therapy, and social work services were more likely to be covered under private health plans than under Medicaid. Private plans tended to limit provision of these services through criteria requiring therapy to restore a lost function, rather than improve or correct a congenital condition. Criteria such as these may prevent children needing early intervention services from obtaining coverage under private insurance.

Types of private health plans include traditional, self-insured, health maintenance organizations, and prepaid health plans. The possibility of and need for a national health insurance plan is a current topic of discussion in the current federal administration, the media, and published reports. The Children's Defense Fund, for example, recommends three basic elements for an acceptable national health plan: universal and accessible coverage, sufficient funds for the development of health services in areas suffering a shortage of primary care, and a strong basic public health infrastructure (Rosenbaum et al., 1992).

Because of escalating health care costs, there is political pressure to expand the role of the federal government in provision of health insurance. One method that has been suggested to address the health care problems of efficiency, equity, and their interrelationship is government regulation of insurance (Passell & Ross, 1978). Federal or state government could standardize insurance options available or some options could be prohibited or required. Involvement of the federal government could produce more uniformity among states and provide greater fiscal capacity.

Private health insurance companies face issues that differ from those discussed in regard to the government and Medicaid. For example, there is the basic "inescapable conflict between the beneficiary's motive for buying insurance—protection against risk—and the insurance company's means for deterring overutilization—coinsurance and deductibles" (Passell & Ross, 1978, p. 109). Private health insurance companies do not have the power to control provider rates or set standards, as the Medicaid program directs. Annual or lifetime caps on amounts paid to the insured and supplemental fees for clients with serious health problems are examples of policies that negatively affect families with children with disabilities.

Cost of Part H Services

Examining the cost of providing Part H services is clearly of importance to states. Overall, the information regarding early intervention costs is quite limited (Barnett & Escobar, 1990). However a recent guide has been produced to assist states in estimating the costs of providing early intervention services (Bowden, Black, & Daulton, 1990). Accurately determining fund availability and estimating the additional funds needed to implement a statewide system is important because Part H directs the maximization and coordination of existing and potential resources. Accurate cost estimates also offer a realistic perspective for those who make and seek increases in allocations. The guide suggests and illustrates a framework for planning and conducting a statewide cost analysis, with examples from several states, including results.

Cost analyses of Part H early intervention services have been conducted within several states. Hall, Stone, Walsh, Wager, Hakes, and Graham described the Florida cost and implementation study in the preceding chapter of this volume. As they pointed out, "the current discipline-specific, single-focused, program-bound delivery system of early intervention tends to be more expensive [than inclusive programs] when it tries to meet the holistic needs of families and children" (Florida State University Policy Studies Clinic, 1991, p. 14). The work of the Florida study has so far indicated a variation of costs depending on the nature of the child's and family's risk factors, the age of the child, the age of identification and intervention, the nature of the services provided, the intensity of the services, and the setting in which the services are delivered. Factors used by Florida to estimate the cost of this "multi-faceted entitlement system" include eligibility definitions and prevalence, client utilization levels, service unit costs, service needs, and service delivery models. Average per-child costs in the Florida study varied greatly, depending on differences in needs for anticipated Part H services. The large variation in costs of serving Part H children with different characteristics is a reminder of the importance of the consideration of this issue in determining costs of the Part H service system.

In contrast to Florida's conceptual matrix of service needs and costs, Rhode Island has conducted a study, following particular children through their service programs to gain an understanding of fluctuations of service usage costs and continuity of funding Part H services over time (Kochanek, 1991). Age of child, level of functioning, and eligibility condition were considered, as well as service setting and type of provider.

Several other states, including Massachusetts and Maryland, have collected early intervention service cost data that have been applied as the Part H requirements are being phased in. Massachusetts conducted an extensive unit cost study that resulted in their fee-for-service contracting system with a uniform service-unit cost structure. Maryland estimated average costs per child by service and percentage of children expected to receive each service. Costs were high, compared with other states, because transportation costs were assumed for all children and salaries of Maryland professionals providing early intervention services are higher than average.

States' Progress in Implementing the Financing of the Part H System

The least studied area of financing is that of the progress of states in actually developing and implementing plans for making use of the various sources of funds for service provision. Fox et al. (1989) maintain that the Part H program "undoubtedly will enhance the contact that agencies have with one another," but admit that the "interdigitation of agencies and the coordination of required resources . . . will not be accomplished without stress" (p. 172). They further assert that the "identification and use of appropriate public and private funds is particularly vital to the success of a state's Part H program" (p. 172), and that the financing of the system is the responsibility of the states, with the federal monetary role being minor. This system has been a major deterrent to the implementation of a coordinated system of financing Part H services within the states.

Fox and Wicks (1990) report on strategies that states are using to access Medicaid coverage for early intervention and preschool services. The diversity of approaches is striking. Four states are reported to allow school districts to be Medicaid providers of certain services. Five states are adding a new benefit to the state Medicaid plan specifically for IFSP- or IEP-related services for infants, toddlers, and preschoolers with disabilities. Two states are using the EPSDT discretionary service option to provide Medicaid coverage for certain services only to the population of young children with disabilities. It should be noted that these examples were cited in 1990 when many states were not committed to the Part H program or were in the nascent stages of planning. Much has changed since then, in as far as the extent to which Medicaid is being used within and among states.

Numerous states have conducted studies examining the status and prospects for financing services within their own state. The most ambitious of these efforts has been the work in California. Under a contract with the Part H lead agency in the state of California, the American Institutes for Research (AIR) conducted a major examination of the costs and benefits of an early intervention program and of existing and potential funding sources. The first report from this study (McDonald et al., 1990) describes features of state departments and programs that currently fund early intervention such as the service system structure, services provided, children and families served, and funding issues raised by different programs. Conclusions of this investigation of the funding of California's early intervention system are threefold: (1) The current system of early intervention program services in California is neither coordinated nor comprehensive, but rather is a series of separate programs; (2) California currently invests substantial state resources in early intervention services through the separate programs; and (3) a state tobacco tax and federal Part H funds are seen as two new major sources for funding early intervention services, with the existing sources of Medicaid and Chapter I expected to be expanded.

Another AIR report examined Nebraska's early intervention system (Parrish, 1990). Similar to the project in California, the purpose of this study was to analyze existing and potential funding sources, design service delivery models, and develop a detailed financing plan for early intervention services in Nebraska. Low-, medium-, and high-level cost estimates were made, based on different models of service delivery. Additional costs to the existing early intervention system needed to implement the Part H system and supplemental resources predicted to be available were compared to estimate additional funding needs and the impact on the state's general fund. Nebraska revenue projections were stated to be dependent on the development and implementation of a statewide billing system to Medicaid for related services.

The analysis of existing, underutilized, and potential funding resources for Part H services from federal, state, and local sources outlined common difficulties states encounter when trying to determine Part H expenditures. For example, it was reported that in Nebraska, as in most states, "certain services will be found in their entirety in some agencies and only bits and pieces of other services may be found across agencies" and "it is sometimes difficult to discern exactly what elements of a given service fall under Part H and which do not" (Parrish, 1990, p. 18). Thus, although specific figures for fiscal year 1990 expenditures are reported by agency, and federal, state, and local share of funding services are detailed, further estimates had to be made as to the extent a given service qualified under Part H and of the number of Part H-eligible children using the service. If Nebraska were to implement the Part H system, the only "new" funds for Part H services would be Part H dollars themselves. At present, all children birth to age 3 years and eligible for Part H can be served under Chapter I/Handicapped programs in Nebraska.

Florida, in developing funding strategies to implement the "fourth year" of Part H, investigated the current use of funds by state departments for early intervention services and potential sources of revenue. Estimates were made of costs for case management, multidisciplinary evaluations, intake and screening, and service planning for infants and toddlers with established conditions and their families. Potential revenue was detailed for each service and possibilities for new funds were suggested, such as maximizing the use of Medicaid, accessing additional resources, developing more efficient use of available dollars, and coordinating financing strategies with local and private revenue.

No recent reports have been prepared for Congress on the topic of states' progress in the financing of Part H. A report entitled "Meeting the Needs of Infants and Toddlers with Handicaps" was produced by the U.S. Department of Education and Department of Health and Human Services (1989). The report identified and described federal funding sources and services in the two departments and outlined interagency actions to coordinate services and resources, based on a Congressionally mandated study. Several sources (e.g., Gallagher, Harbin, Thomas, Wenger, & Clifford, 1988; Trohanis et al., 1988) were used to identify federal funding sources and services. Sixteen programs with "significant potential to contribute resources toward the successful implementation of a statewide system of comprehensive, coordinated, multidisciplinary, interagency programs of early intervention services" were specified for use in providing direct services:

1. Part H of Public Law 99-457
2. Chapter I/Handicapped
3. Part B of Public Law 99-457
4. Services for Deaf–Blind Children and Youth
5. Head Start Program
6. Medicaid
7. Maternal and Child Health Block Grants
8. Child Welfare Services Program
9. Developmental Disabilities Basic State Grants Program
10. Alcohol, Drug Abuse and Mental Health Administration Block Grant Program
11. Community Health Service Program
12. Indian Health Service Program
13. Migrant Health Services Program
14. Preventative Health and Health Service Block Grant
15. Health Care for the Homeless Program
16. Social Service Block Grant

These programs differed in eligibility criteria, such as ages served or income status, flexibility at the state level of discretion in providing early intervention services, and funding approach (e.g., single-focus grants, multipurpose block grants, and entitlement programs). Only one source of funds, Part H dollars themselves, was specifically targeted to the Part H population; infants and toddlers with special needs must "compete" with other populations for dollars from other programs. Coordination of these funds was described in this report as a difficult task, given the differences in the programs previously cited and the task of coordinating federal funds at the state and local levels. Tracing funding of early intervention services through the various programs is nearly impossible, because the fiscal reporting procedures of the programs are not now designed to do so.

In work done through the Carolina Policy Studies Program (CPSP) at the Frank Porter Graham Child Development Center, University of North Carolina at Chapel Hill, staff have conducted surveys of 50 states and the District of Columbia and case studies of six states regarding their efforts to implement Part H of IDEA. CPSP surveys of early state progress indicated that states are slower in implementing the major financial provisions of the law than other requirements (Harbin et al., 1989, 1990, 1991, 1992). Two reports have been issued that point to the difficulties that states have been having with actually accessing the funding sources originally envisioned by the authors of the legislation (Clifford, 1991; Clifford et al., 1991). Clifford (1991), in the first round of case studies in 1989–1990, collected information from six states on details of the processes involved in accessing and coordinating various financial resources. Clifford noted that, "in general, state agency personnel did not have detailed information on exact expenditures for Part H services" (p. 4). There were two factors contributing to this lack of information: (1) states had only begun the implementation and had not had sufficient time to gather all necessary data; and (2) program reporting systems across agencies and programs were not designed to provide subset expenditures for the birth to age 3 group of children and families.

Knowledgeable personnel in each of the six states were asked to rate the use of seven sources of funds: Medicaid, state or interagency health, Chapter I/ Handicapped, state education, private insurance, parent fee, and local funds. On the average, only one or two funding sources were described by states as major, or essential to and substantial in the state's financial plan. The funding source most frequently cited as major was state or interagency health, which included both specific financing through a state health agency and financing through an independent interagency group in state government.

Clifford (1991) also asked state personnel to indicate which of the following approaches to financing services were evident: unit rate financing, contracting for services, state core financing, local funding initiatives, formal agreements, informal agreements, local coordination, and state level coordination. A variety of packages of approaches was reported. All of the states that had relatively advanced financing plans used some state core financing, implying not only that states were committed to early intervention, but also that state funds allowed access to other funds.

A recommendation based on the results of this first round of case studies of states implementing Part H is that states should concentrate financing efforts on a small number of sources and access state government funds to match federal dollars, "fill the gaps" in financial assistance, and initiate or expand local programs (Clifford, 1991). Staff time and expertise must be committed to bring about a successful financing plan.

Reconceptualized alternative approaches to Part H financing are necessary to achieve the goals of the legislation, as data from CPSP case studies and other sources indicate that states are having great difficulty implementing the concept of developing a coordinated system of funding (Clifford et al., 1991). Several alternatives were suggested for the short term and the long term. In the short term, a two-tiered system of financing, or extended time of phase-in of federal requirements, will help to keep all states participating in Part H. This change was in fact accomplished with the passage of the Americans with Disabilities Act in 1991. In the long run, however, changes will be needed in the methods and sources of financing Part H services that will help overcome the difficulties inherent in trying to fund services within available categorical sources.

Clifford et al. (1991) suggested that all Part H services could be funded under Medicaid; that portions of each major piece of federal legislation affecting children could be earmarked for Part H financing; or that Part H could be transformed into a new funding entitlement program. Each option has its advantages and disadvantages, which are detailed in the report, but all address the long-term need for financial stability for the Part H program.

In a report of a CPSP finance survey (Clifford et al., 1993), hypotheses suggested by previously collected CPSP data and other studies regarding the status of the Part H financing system in states were investigated. Mechanisms used to develop and implement plans for financing and coordinating financing across the various state agencies involved were examined, as well as the extent to which states responding to the survey were accessing the various sources that had been identified as viable for funding Part H services.

Part H coordinators in the 50 states and the District of Columbia were asked to indicate the percentage of their state's total funding for financing the implementation of Part H for each of 44 potential sources (see Table 14.1). The sources ranged from federal education and health and human services to state and local sources and nongovernmental sources, such as private insurance and voluntary health or service agencies. Every one of the 44 sources was used by at least one state for at least 1% of its Part H system costs. States reported using, on the average, about 21 different sources of funding. Most sources named were federal, as might be expected because 30 of the 44 sources listed were federal. About half of these were federal education programs and half federal health and human services funds.

States most frequently reported using three sources moderately to heavily (at least 5% of the total funding). When use was weighted by the amount that state Part H coordinators reported for each of the sources, over half of the dollars used to fund the Part H system were federal (56.7%), about one-

TABLE 14.1.   Funding Sources Used to Support Early Intervention Services

Federal Department of Education
1. Education of the Handicapped Act, Part H; Handicapped Infants and Toddlers
2. Education of the Handicapped Act, Part B; State Grants, Assistance for Education of All Handicapped Children
3. Education of the Handicapped Act, Part B; Section 619, Preschool Grants
4. Education of the Handicapped Act, Part C; Services for Deaf–Blind Children and Youth
5. Chapter I, Programs for Handicapped Children
6. Chapter I, Even Start Programs
7. Chapter I, Disadvantaged Children
8. Bilingual Education Act
9. Chapter I, Programs for Migratory Children
10. Technology-Related Assistance for Individuals with Disabilities Act

Federal Department of Health and Human Services
11. Medicaid, Social Security Act, Title XIX (federal share only)
12. Early and Periodic Screening, Diagnosis and Treatment Program
13. Maternal and Child Health Block Grant, Social Security Act, Title V (federal share only)
14. Developmental Disabilities; Basic Grants to States
15. Developmental Disabilities; Grants to University Affiliated Programs
16. Head Start Act
17. Child Welfare Services, Social Security Act, Title IV-B
18. Social Services Block Grant, Social Security Act, Title XX
19. Public Health Service Act; Alcohol, Drug Abuse and Mental Health Administration Services Block Grant
20. Public Health Service Act; Community Health Centers
21. Indian Health Care Improvement Act
22. Public Health Service Act; Migrant Health Centers
23. McKinney Homeless Assistance Act; Categorical Grants for Primary Health Services and Substance Abuse Services
24. McKinney Homeless Assistance Act; Block Grant for Community Mental Health Services
25. Comprehensive Child Development Act
26. Developmental Disabilities; Grants to Protection and Advocacy Systems

Other Federal Programs
27. Civilian Health and Medical Program of the Uniformed Services (CHAMPUS)
28. Special Supplemental Food Program for Women, Infants, and Children (WIC)
29. Community Development Block Grants, Housing and Urban Development
30. Bureau of Indian Affairs

State and Local Sources
31. State matching portion for Medicaid
32. State matching portion for Maternal and Child Health Block Grants
33. Special Education Funds
34. Other Education Funds
35. Public Health/Mental Health Funds

(*continued*)

TABLE 14.1. *(continued)*

36. Targeted appropriations for children (e.g., for high-risk children)
37. Foster Care/Protective Services/Child Welfare Funds
38. Mental Retardation/Developmental Disability Funds

Nongovernmental Resources
39. Private insurance—individual and group policies and self-insurers
40. Health maintenance organizations, preferred provider organizations, and other managed care systems
41. Voluntary health agencies (e.g., United Cerebral Palsy, Easter Seals, Association for Retarded Citizens)
42. Foundations and corporate giving programs
43. Families—sliding fee scale (e.g., tuition, fees, insurance deductibles, copayments)
44. Voluntary service programs (e.g., churches, Lions Clubs, Shriners)

Note. Adapted, by permission, from Williams and Kates (1991).

third were state/local (31.8%), and the remaining dollars were nongovernmental (11.5%). This finding was reiterated in examination of the top 15 sources, compiled through weighting by amount of use (see Table 14.2). Of the top 15 sources, 7 were federal, 6 were state/local, and 2 were private. Besides Part H funds themselves, states most frequently reported moderate to heavy use of funds from the following sources: state mental retardation/developmental disabilities, federal Chapter I/Handicapped, federal and state Medicaid, federal and state Maternal and Child Health Block Grants, and federal EPSDT.

A trend that seemed to hold across the states responding to the survey indicated that as the number of people involved in the development and implementation of the Part H finance system increased, the total number of sources used increased and the number of sources used moderately to heavily decreased. This may reflect a recognition by state personnel of the need to concentrate efforts on a contained group of funding sources, rather than attempting to coordinate all available monies.

States reported improvements in efficiency and effectiveness in accessing Medicaid and EPSDT funds, and they had expectations that these sources of funds for the Part H system would increase over the next 3 years. An additional source of funds expected to increase was Chapter I/Handicapped. States also seemed to expect more use of private insurance and sliding fee scales for families to pay for Part H services, in that intentions to continue or institute new formal state plans or state requirements to include these funding sources by 1995 were indicated.

Most states have centered responsibility for coordination of financing services at the state, rather than regional or local, level and rely on formally signed interagency agreements to facilitate the process. States continue to report multiple barriers to developing a coordinated system of financing, and

TABLE 14.2.   Top 15 Sources of Financing Part H Early Intervention Services Reported by Part H Coordinators (n = 30)

Rank	Source	Type of $	No. states using	No. states using at least 5%
1	Part H	Federal Education	29	19
2	Mental Retardation/ Developmental Disabilities	State	24	14
3	Chapter I/Handicapped Children	Federal Education	27	15
4	Medicaid	Federal Health and Human Services	23	17
5	Medicaid match	State	23	10
6	Public Health/Mental Health	State	18	10
7	Maternal and /Child Health Block Grant	Federal Health and Human Services	25	7
8	Maternal and Child Health match	State	17	7
9	WIC Supplement Food Program	Federal other	19	6
10[a]	Special Education	State	15	5
10[a]	EPSDT	Federal Health and Human Services	24	4
12	Social Services Block Grant	Federal Health and Human Services	15	5
13	Private health insurance	Nongovernmental	22	4
14[a]	Targeted appropriations for children	State	15	5
14[a]	Voluntary health agencies	Nongovernmental	20	4

[a] Weighting by amount of use resulted in two pairs of tied sources.

relationships regarding use of formal workgroups and number of interagency agreements indicate that barriers are perceived to be reduced with formal participation and definition. The Part H coordinator and agency-level decision makers were named as the most important participants in developing a vision of the Part H finance system.

CONCLUSIONS AND RECOMMENDATIONS

The review of literature, survey results, and states' reports attest to the huge efforts of state personnel to implement Part H of IDEA. The legislation envisioned states accessing a broad array of funding sources to support a system of services for infants and toddlers with disabilities and for their families. In fact, each of the 44 different sources of financing is being used by at least one state for at least 1% of the financing package for Part H services. On average, states report using some 21 different sources to support the service delivery system. The states have put forth incredible energy to make the most of the opportunities and challenges to identify and coordinate funding sources.

In implementing the law, states have found that financing the system was not simply a matter of gaining access to federal sources of funds to pay the full cost of the services needed, but that a substantial investment of state resources was required as well to take full advantage of the array of federal sources. It is clear from both the recent survey (Clifford et al., 1993) and previous interactions with a small number of case study states (Clifford, 1991) that gaining access to Medicaid, in particular, is a process consuming time and human resources. Still, some 25% of states reported that Medicaid was not used at all and another 20% reported that the federal portion of Medicaid accounted for less than 5% of their program costs—and these figures reflect the situation some 5 years after the Part H legislation was enacted.

Of course, part of the difficulty in accessing Medicaid is tied to the fact that it is jointly funded by the federal and state governments. State governments have seen dramatic increases in the proportion of their budgets required to finance the rapidly expanding budget needs of Medicaid in general, and they have been reluctant to support adding new cost items to the program. In spite of these difficulties, most states are making the commitments necessary to make Medicaid a key element in financing Part H services.

Other federal programs have also played an important role in financing the needed services—the Part H program itself, the Chapter I/Handicapped program, Maternal and Child Health Block Grant program, WIC, the EPSDT portion of Medicaid, and the Social Services Block Grant. Of the 15 most heavily used funding sources, 7 are federal. We estimate that more than half of the total financing for Part H activities has been borne by the federal government.

As mentioned above, state funding has played a critical role in financing services. State mental retardation/developmental disabilities programs have been used most heavily. The state portion of the Medicaid program has been the next most heavily used source, with public health/mental health programs a close third. The state has also had to match the Maternal and Child Health Block Grant program of the federal government. State special education funds also have been a major source of financing of services, with targeted state appropriations playing a less significant but still important role. State resources have contributed an estimated one-third of the total revenues of operating the program.

In addition, nongovernmental sources have played a much smaller, but still important role in the financial picture. Private health insurance and voluntary health agencies have been at the bottom of the 15 most used sources of support for Part H services. Overall, we estimated that the nongovernmental sources have supported only about one-tenth of the total cost of Part H services.

Although states have made major efforts to obtain financing for Part H services, they are still short of obtaining the total amount necessary to move to full financing of the system. Thus we have seen the vast majority of states electing to postpone "full implementation" of participation in the Part H program. Below we present several recommendations regarding future efforts at both the state and federal level to improve the current situation.

1. *States should continue to focus on Medicaid as a source of financing Part H services.* Most states have found ways to access Medicaid and are doing so substantially. Several states, in fact, have moved from no utilization of Medicaid to implementation of regulations allowing educational agencies to bill Medicaid directly, since the beginning of Part H. However, there is much more that needs to be done in states to fully utilize the Medicaid options. There are questions about how a proposed "cap" on Medicaid would affect the ability of states to maximize the potential use of Medicaid as a source of financing for Part H services.

2. *States should also focus on state sources.* The particular sources used most within a state—education, developmental disabilities, or health—seem to be dependent on the situation in a given state. A state core of funding for the Part H early intervention program has previously been found to be necessary to initiate and maintain a state's system (Clifford, 1991). Broadening the network of formal state agency involvement in the planning appears to facilitate access to sources of financing.

3. *States should broaden their focus to include more sources.* Findings from previous examinations of Part H financing indicated that successful states were targeting a few major sources of funding in the early stages of implementation. This seemed to, in part, be the result of scant available staff and the lack of time to do more than focus on a few key sources. The survey results indicate that states have now been able to broaden their efforts to access multiple sources. As states increase the capability to successfully obtain funds from multiple sources, the total amount available for the early intervention program should increase.

4. *States should work with federal agency personnel and Congress to develop a more coherent, simplified approach to financing Part H Services.* Although we recommend efforts to maximize use of a broader range of sources of funds for Part H services (3, above), we are convinced that major reform is needed to sharply reduce the number of sources and simultaneously greatly increase the amount of funding from this small number of sources of financing. The process of accessing many different sources of funds is inherently expensive

to carry out. With tax dollars in short supply, it is inappropriate to spend large sums in the pursuit of new dollars. Neither do we want to follow the example of the health insurance industry in which much of the money is spent on administration of the system.

5. *A new federal approach to financing Part H should be developed and implemented.* The federal government should reform the system to provide a greatly simplified and focused approach to financing appropriate services to infants and toddlers with disabilities and to their families, beginning at the earliest possible time in the lives of these young children. Several reasonable alternatives exist for reducing the current excessive costs of attempting to coordinate the large number of funding streams required to adequately finance services. Some suggested options are funding all Part H services under Medicaid, earmarking portions of each major piece of federal legislation affecting children to fund Part H services, and increasing Part H funds themselves to cover financing of services (Clifford et al., 1991).

Although substantial cost savings are possible by simplifying the financing of Part H services, these savings are not likely to be sufficient to cover the additional funds needed to support the cost of fully implementing the Part H program nationwide. Thus, it is imperative that the total funding levels be increased substantially, at the same time that the number of funding streams are reduced and simplified.

REFERENCES

Barnett, W. S., & Escobar, C. M. (1990). Economic costs and benefits of early intervention. In S. J. Meisels & J. P. Shonkoff (Eds.), *Handbook of early childhood intervention: Theory, practice, and analysis* (pp. 560–582). Cambridge, MA: Cambridge University Press.

Bowden, J. D., Black, T., & Daulton, D. (1990). *Estimating the costs of providing early intervention and preschool special services.* Chapel Hill, NC: NEC*TAS.

Clifford, R. M. (1991). *State financing of services under P.L. 99-457, Part H.* Chapel Hill, NC: Carolina Policy Studies Program, Frank Porter Graham Child Development Center, University of North Carolina at Chapel Hill.

Clifford, R. M., Bernier, K. Y., & Harbin, G. L. (1993). *Financing Part H services: A state level view.* Chapel Hill, NC: Carolina Policy Studies Program, Frank Porter Graham Child Development Center, University of North Carolina at Chapel Hill.

Clifford, R. M., Kates, D. A., Black, T., Eckland, J. D., & Bernier, K. (1991). *Reconceptualization of financing under P.L. 99-457, Part H.* Chapel Hill, NC: Carolina Policy Studies Program, Frank Porter Graham Child Development Center, University of North Carolina at Chapel Hill.

Florida State University Policy Studies Clinic (Florida Tax Watch). (1991). *Florida's cost/implementation study for Public Law 99-457, Part H, infants and toddlers, phase II findings: Costs and funding for early intervention services to infants and toddlers in Florida, preliminary findings.* Tallahassee, FL: Author.

Fox, H. B., Freedman, S. A., & Klepper, B. R. (1989). Financing programs for young children. In J. J. Gallagher, P. L. Trohanis, & R. M. Clifford (Eds.), *Policy implementation and P.L. 99-457: Planning for young children with special needs* (pp. 169–182). Baltimore, MD: Paul H. Brookes.

Fox, H. B., & Wicks, L. B. (1990). *The role of Medicaid and EPSDT in financing early intervention and preschool special education services.* Washington, DC: Fox Health Policy Consultants.

Fox, H. B., Wicks, L. B., McManus, M. A., & Newacheck, P. W. (1992). Private and public health insurance for early intervention services. *Journal of Early Intervention, 16,* 109–122.

Gallagher, J. J., Harbin, G., Thomas, D., Wenger, M., & Clifford, R. (1988). *A survey of current status on implementation of infants and toddlers' legislation* (Report for Cooperative Agreement No. G0087C3065) Washington, DC: U.S. Department of Education, Office of Special Education Programs.

Hansen, A. H. (1965). Standards and values in a rich society. In E. S. Phelps (Ed.), *Private wants and public needs* (pp. 1–15). New York: W. W. Norton.

Harbin, G. L., Gallagher, J., & Batista, L. (1992). *Status of states' progress in implementing Part H of IDEA: Report #4.* Chapel Hill, NC: Carolina Policy Studies Program, Frank Porter Graham Child Development Center, University of North Carolina at Chapel Hill.

Harbin, G. L., Gallagher, J., & Lillie, T. (1989). *States' progress related to fourteen components of P.L. 99-457, Part H.* Chapel Hill, NC: Carolina Policy Studies Program, Frank Porter Graham Child Development Center, University of North Carolina at Chapel Hill.

Harbin, G. L., Gallagher, J., & Lillie, T. (1991). *Status of states' progress in implementing Part H of IDEA: Report #3.* Chapel Hill, NC: Carolina Policy Studies Program, Frank Porter Graham Child Development Center, University of North Carolina at Chapel Hill.

Harbin, G. L., Gallagher, J. J., Lillie, T., & Eckland, J. (1990). *Status of states' progress in implementing Part H of P.L. 99-457: Report #2.* Chapel Hill, NC: Carolina Policy Studies Program, Frank Porter Graham Child Development Center, University of North Carolina at Chapel Hill.

Kastorf, K. (1991). *The Massachusetts experience with Medicaid support of early intervention services.* Chapel Hill, NC: Carolina Policy Studies Program, Frank Porter Graham Child Development Center, University of North Carolina at Chapel Hill.

Kochanek, T. (1991, December). *Impact studies on child and family needs, service utilization, and cost in early intervention programs.* Paper presented at the meeting of NCCIP, 7th Biennial National Training Institute, Washington, DC.

McDonald, W. R., Minicucci, C., Marquart, D. J., Hamilton, R. L., Block, A. H., & Yuan, Y. T. (1990). *Early intervention program (P.L. 99-457) cost evaluation study: Report A—Analysis of existing and potential funding sources* (Contract No. HD990070). Sacramento, CA: American Institutes for Research/California Department of Developmental Services.

McManus, P. (1989, June). *Special topics in private insurance.* Presentation at the

NEC*TAS Workshop on Collaborative Financing of Early Intervention and Preschool Services, Washington, DC.

Musgrave, R. A., & Musgrave, P. (1990). Fiscal functions: An overview. In P. Peretz (Ed.), *The politics of American economic policy making.* New York: M. E. Sharpe.

National Early Childhood Technical Assistance System (NEC*TAS). (1990). *Information packet on the financing of early intervention and preschool services.* Chapel Hill, NC: Author.

Parrish, T. B. (1990). *Nebraska financing study, P.L. 99-457: Part H, EHA.* Lincoln, NE: American Institutes for Research/Nebraska Department of Education.

Passell, P. & Ross, L. (1978). *State policies and federal programs: Priorities and constraints* (Twentieth Century Fund Report). New York: Praeger.

Rosenbaum, S., Hughes, D., Harris, P., & Liu, J. (1992). *Children and health insurance.* Washington, DC: Children's Defense Fund.

Trohanis, P., Kahn, L., Hurth, J., Danaher, J., Black, T., & Heekin, S. (1988). *The National Early Childhood Technical Assistance System national TA plan* (Report for Contract No. 300-87-0163). Washington, DC: U.S. Department of Education, Division of Educational Services, Office of Special Education Programs.

U.S. Department of Education and Department of Health and Human Services. (1989). *Meeting the needs of infants and toddlers with handicaps.* Washington, DC: Author.

Van Dyck, P. C. (1991). *Use of parental fees in P.L. 99-457, Part H.* Chapel Hill, NC: Carolina Policy Studies Program, Frank Porter Graham Child Development Center, University of North Carolina at Chapel Hill.

White, K. R., & Immel, N. (1990). *Medicaid and other third-party payments: One piece of the early intervention financing puzzle.* Bethesda, MD: Association for the Care of Children's Health.

Williams, S., & Kates, D. A. (1991). *NEC*TAS financing workbook: An interagency process for planning and implementing a financing system for early intervention and preschool services.* Chapel Hill, NC: NEC*TAS.

Note: Publications from the Carolina Policy Studies Program may be ordered by calling the Frank Porter Graham Child Development Center in Chapel Hill, NC, at (919) 962-7321. Publications from the National Early Childhood Technical Assistance Program (NEC*TAS) may be ordered by calling the Frank Porter Graham Child Development Center in Chapel Hill, NC, at (919) 962-2001.

CHAPTER 15

Policy Designed for Diversity
New Initiatives for Children
with Disabilities

JAMES J. GALLAGHER

The design of policy for children and families through federal legislation that then becomes implemented at the local level has had uncertain success (Goggin, 1987). The intent of Congress has often been modified or canceled out by local and state agendas. This has been the case particularly when the policy does not seem to take into account the diversity of the populations or settings that are affected by the policy.

Some examples of how the federal government has tried, through legislation, to cope with some of the more serious social and educational problems in the United States illustrate this point. In 1967, the Elementary and Secondary Education Act (Public Law 89-10) attempted to provide resources to deal with children from families at an economic disadvantage. In 1975, the Education for All Handicapped Children Act (Public Law 94-142) attempted to provide resources to help children with disabilities perform effectively in educational settings. In both of these instances, there have been concerns as to how the legislation was finally realized at the local level (Martin, 1989).

PART H—WHAT IS IT?

In 1986, Part H of Public Law 99-457, now referred to as the Individuals with Disabilities Education Act (IDEA), attempted to provide planning and development funds to the states to design a comprehensive service system for infants and toddlers with disabilities and their families. This system was to be set up to help such children at the beginning of their life cycle. Part H of IDEA is, on one level, the culmination of a 20-year dream of many special educators. By providing federal resources to aid the states in planning and developing programs for infants and toddlers with disabilities and their families, it completes a federal legislative program to provide educational and related services for children with disabilities from birth to 21 (Gallagher, Trohanis, & Clifford, 1989).

There are several significant differences between the current law (IDEA) and past programs for children with disabilities. First, there is the expectation that the lion's share of the costs of the program would be provided by the states from a variety of funds available (e.g., Medicaid, Title V of the Social Security Act), as described by Clifford and Bernier (Chapter 14, this volume). Second, there was a genuine effort to use this law to reform a variety of professional practices that have been observed to be, in one way or another, less than optimal. Such reforms include the empowerment of the family, marked by such provisions as the requirement that three parents participate in policy development by serving on the Interagency Coordinating Council, and that an Individualized Family Service Plan (IFSP) be developed with the active participation of family members in the design of treatment goals.

Another requirement is that the services to be delivered would be multidisciplinary in nature. Ten separate disciplines (medicine, social work, nursing, nutrition, occupational therapy, physical therapy, psychology, special education, speech/language pathology, and audiology) are specifically mentioned as expected to participate in these programs as appropriate.

The state is required by this law to establish personnel preparation programs and standards, a child-find system, a data system, a plan for financing the services, and a directory of services. In short, there is the expectation that many changes will be required in how services are delivered in the implementation of this law.

WHAT IS SOCIAL POLICY?

These social policy initiatives in Part H provide a working laboratory for the study of policy design and implementation. Social policy can be defined as follows: *Social policies are the rules and standards by which scarce public resources are allocated to almost unlimited social needs.* Written social policy should provide the answer to four major questions (Gallagher, 1992):

1. Who shall receive the resources (services)?
2. Who shall deliver the services?
3. What is the nature of the services to be delivered?
4. What are the conditions under which the services will be delivered?

There is little question that the design of policy and the production of policy statements are easier to formulate when the target group for the policy is relatively homogeneous. The challenge for the designers of social policy is how to shape it for diversity. In Part H of IDEA, we have an outstanding challenge for policy makers. In this instance, we have a diverse clientele (children with a variety of disabilities), from diverse families, treated by diverse sets of professionals, in diverse settings.

The extraordinary diversity of clients, professionals, and settings associated with early intervention calls for policies that are responsive to such diversity. This is a much easier principle to *state* than to apply, however, because of the natural consequences of the sequence of events by which policy is usually implemented. Once a law has been passed, there is a requirement that the federal government spell out, in considerable detail, what the various aspects of the statute mean, so that those service providers who must operate within the law can be assured that they are performing appropriately. A relevant federal agency is identified as the responsible agency to develop the rule making and regulations that will spell out the full intent of the law.

Because this is a critical stage in the implementation of legislation, the federal government is required to give public notice of such rule making and to encourage public comment on a draft set of regulations. Furthermore, the federal government is required to report the comments or concerns raised by the public and provide agency responses to those concerns. Sometimes these outside comments result in various regulations being modified or changed; sometimes the critiques are rejected, but with an extended justification as to why the suggestions have not been accepted.

Once the regulations have been finally approved, they assume the force of law. Thereafter, states, local communities, or citizens interested in the law will consult these regulations if they have concerns about how the law should be interpreted. Even after the regulations are in place, the problems of interpretation can be significant. If the 50 states are involved in such a law, it is always possible for one of the states to raise a particular issue and ask if their interpretation is correct. The federal government's answer to that one state, then, impacts upon all the states.

The important point about this entire sequence of events is how it gradually narrows and sharpens the acceptable area of performance. The more precise the answers become to questions about who is eligible, what services can be applied, under what conditions services may be provided, and so on, the clearer the territory becomes that falls outside acceptable boundaries. The history of such legislation has been to gradually constrain the acceptable behaviors through the regulation and review process. When this rigid bureaucratic process is applied to children, families, professionals, and settings as diverse as those in the Part H program, it runs the risk of inappropriately dealing with individual clients and situations.

Diverse Target Populations

The traditional thrust of policy statements has been to attempt to standardize, through clear rules and regulations, the parameters around which the policy will be implemented. For example, when there is an attempt to deliver resources to a distinct target population (e.g., children with disabilities ages birth to 3), a clear attempt would be made to carefully define who we mean by "children with disabilities."

The diversity of the target population for this Part H legislation for infants and toddlers was a direct challenge to policy makers. Not only do the children differ in the type of handicapping condition, from vision and auditory problems to orthopedic difficulties and mental retardation, but they also vary in degree from moderate to severe. (Mild problems such as articulation disorders or mild learning disabilities or behavioral problems are probably not easily identified in the age group of birth to 3.) Also, because development often appears in spurts in infancy, it is not always easy to determine who is developmentally delayed.

The irony of the rule making is that the more precision we achieve in definition, the more likely we as professionals will be unhappy with some of the results because our current knowledge of disabilities and our tools for identification are not as precise as the language of the rule maker. This is particularly true with infants. We need flexibility in defining eligibility rather than a set of rules from which we cannot dèpart (Harbin & Terry, 1990). This point is also made in Chapter 2 of this volume by Benn, who supports the use of clinical judgment in defining the condition.

Family Diversity

One of the areas of diversity that would seem to require some special planning is the range of needs and backgrounds that one would expect to find in a family with children eligible for these services. The multitude of genetic and neurological insults that can result in disabilities are not strictly related to social or economic classes. Anyone from the President of the United States to a homeless teenage mother can suffer these accidents, so the service programs have to plan for this level of diversity.

Arcia, Serling, and Gallagher (1992) have pointed out that there are relatively few (less than 10%) traditional two-parent families where the father earns an income above the poverty line, the mother stays home to care for the young children, and the mother did not have her child until she was 20 years or older. Yet Part H seems to be written with the expectation that interventionists will be dealing with an upper middle-class family where the problem of getting the child to appropriate services is not a large one. In addition, the family is expected to take on a variety of responsibilities that the law intends them to adopt for their children. Contrary to those expectations, many of the families who have become a part of this program will come from economically disadvantaged circumstances and may not speak English as their primary language. They may have very different cultural backgrounds and values that create barriers between them and the professionals who would be working with them.

For example, Hispanic families have a tradition of respect and deference to professionals that would substantially inhibit them from taking a dominant role in decisions concerning their child, as the "parent empowerment" initiative outlines for them. Although the legislation itself is quite clear in preserving parental decision making over the fate of their own children, during policy implementation there may arise situations where professionals will be coping with dysfunctional families, drug-dependent parents, or teenage single parents with limited educational backgrounds. These families also must be folded into the reality of policy implementation (Arcia, Keyes, Gallagher, & Herrick, 1992).

Professional Diversity

As noted above, there are many different professions involved in early intervention, each with its own traditions and practices that often differ from one another. For example, the case manager (service coordinator) in many health settings is supposed to be a nurse or social worker who carries out the wishes of the captain of the team, the physician (Fullagar, Crotser, Gallagher, Loda, & Shea, 1991). But in other educational settings, the case manager may play a very different role, combining the role of the physician and social worker in the health setting.

Family empowerment tends to be interpreted quite differently by various professions, and professional standards differ between disciplines. In one instance, a number of special educators wish to create a new specialty, early childhood interventionist, but few of the other professions have shown much interest in preparing specialists for a significantly new role (Gallagher & Coleman, 1990).

Interagency Coordination and Diversity

One of the sources of diversity involves the policies already established for children and families from at least three different sources: health, social services, and education. Such policies, created at different times and for different purposes, have been given to various administrative entities to carry out.

Separate agencies have been established at state and local levels of government for that purpose.

In order to fit Part H into this existing collection of programs, there has to be a considerable effort to establish interagency coordination and cooperation (Beder, 1984; Kaluzny, Morrisey, & McKinney, 1990). There is a growing history of experience that would suggest that such coordination will not be easy, given the diversity of authorities, purposes, and self-interests involved (DiStefano, 1984; Galaskiewicz, 1985; Milner, 1980; Oliver, 1990).

Service Setting Diversity

What are the settings where the services that are to be provided are delivered? The range here is even more impressive, as described by Graham and Bryant (Chapter 11, this volume), stretching from neonatal intensive care units, to private clinics, to individual clinicians, to home-based services delivered by a team of educator–family service personnel. To write rules that would fit each of these settings or would be adaptable to the institutional requirements of a hospital, but that still relate to the family day care provider, is a formidable task. But although diversity exists in all elements of this law, one of the predictable results of current legislative process is to narrow, or make more prescriptive, the rules.

THE REGULATIONS THAT BIND

One of the aspects of implementing a new law is the development of regulations that are designed to extend, expand, and interpret the legislation that was passed. There is an inevitable flow of questions from the field calling for interpretations. Each decision that is made that further interprets the legislation tends to function in a similar way to how a "class action" suit would in the courts. In a class action legal suit, the decision affects not only the particular case and people involved in the suit; it also applies to all persons in a similar class (Turnbull, 1986). Thus, in a suit brought as a class action to achieve rights for a child with mental retardation, the final judgment would affect all children with mental retardation, in addition to the one child on whose behalf the original suit was brought.

In a similar fashion, we can see that the decisions made by the executive branch in interpreting a law parallel the effects of a class action court suit. For example, a parent or professional could write to the federal government asking if the regulations under Part H would allow for the payment of a cleft palate operation on a child, on the grounds that it is a medical cost that is essential to effective speech and language development on the part of the child which, in turn, is essential to his/her education. Would this be an allowable expense?

The federal government has actually answered this question by issuing a clear statement in the regulations that cleft palate operations are not an allowable expense under Part H. Although that decision may have been reached based upon an individual case, it would also apply to any other child in the United States seeking help for a cleft palate operation. Although the child who originally asked for this help may have been from Florida, children with cleft palates in Colorado, California, and Michigan would all be affected by this decision.

The cumulative effect of these "class action executive branch" decisions sometimes creates a law that, in actuality, may differ considerably from the original intent of the lawmakers. It is important to note that all of this progressive tightening can happen without any single individual wishing it to happen, and the final result may not be pleasant for or acceptable to anyone. It is the consequence of a system and a set of procedures that need to be re-examined. The fundamental question is, "If we understand that the normal process of refining the meaning of the legislation leads to sharper and sharper distinctions—distinctions that may do a disservice to youngsters or families far from the norm of the legislation's target group, families, or settings—then should we consider alternative strategies for protecting and honoring the diversity that we have every right to expect from families when implementing this law?"

PROTECTING DIVERSITY

Skrtic (1991) proposes a different approach to policy implementation, calling for the design of an *adhocracy*, rather than a *bureaucracy*. He defines an adhocracy as "a problem solving organization configured to invent new programs." It deals with work that is so ambiguous and uncertain that neither the programs nor the knowledge and skills necessary for accomplishing it are known.

One of the purposes of Part H of IDEA—to serve infants and toddlers with disabilities and their families—was to create *flexibility* in the delivery of services. Although it demanded of the states who participated that they develop standards for personnel preparation, eligibility, family empowerment, and other areas, it left the specific design of such standards to the participating states (Gallagher et al., 1989). The federal statute implicitly recognized the great diversity of states, from Texas to South Carolina to Illinois to Vermont, and realized the futility of trying to write a set of precise standards or regulations that would match such diverse state situations. Passing the responsibility to the states, however, does not cope with the problem of diversity; it merely transfers it from the federal to the state level. Now, states like Illinois, for example, must provide rules that fit Chicago, Mattoon, Carbondale, Kankakee, and Peoria.

One other major effort at encouraging diversity in the federal statute was the provision in Part H that states, at their option, could include children "at risk" as a category of infants and toddlers eligible for services. This was designed to include a group of children who would be at risk for developing handicapping conditions unless appropriate intervention were made during the period from birth through 3 years. States interested in including the at-risk category among their eligibility requirements would have the responsibility of defining who would be considered an at-risk child (Harbin, Gallagher, & Terry, 1991). As an illustration of how sequential rule making can successively reduce flexibility, early in the implementation of this law an inquiry was made from a state to the federal government as to whether at-risk children would be deemed eligible for the entire range of services that other children, clearly identified as children with disabilities, would receive. The answer provided by the Office of Special Education Programs, in a rule-making letter interpreting the law, was that at-risk children would be eligible for all of the appropriate services for which other children with clearly defined disabilities were eligible.

Such an interpretation of the rights of at-risk children was a dash of cold water in the faces of many interested professionals, who saw the consequences of such a decision—an enormous expansion of needed services and the attendant costs—as being beyond the range of support they could hope to obtain from the legislative and executive branches in their states. This interpretation ultimately resulted in only a handful of small states (10 or 11) taking advantage of the presumed flexibility offered through the federal statute to include at-risk children—despite clear indications that the professional field was in substantial agreement with the at-risk initiative. See Chapter 13 by Hall, Stone, Walsh, Wager, Hakes, and Graham in this volume for a further discussion of needs for, and costs of, early intervention.

DIVERSITY AND KEY POLICY ELEMENTS

This section reviews the four key elements in the policy domain—who receives the resources, who provides the resources, the nature of services to be provided, and the conditions under which the services are provided—to observe potential problems with the implementation of legislation focusing upon young children with disabilities.

Who Receives the Resources?

One of the fundamental policy decisions in the allocation of resources is the definition of the recipient of these scarce resources. The American public has largely accepted the value position of vertical equity: "the unequal treatment of unequals in order to make them more equal." Vertical equity calls for persons with special needs to receive special resources. This value position has opened the door for special legislation aimed at improving the lives of children from economically disadvantaged families and children with disabilities, as Chapter 1 in this volume by Richmond and Ayoub describes. One of the clear consequences of such legislation is the necessity for drawing the boundary line between those who are eligible to receive resources and those who are not. The issue of how economically disadvantaged one needs to be, or how disabled one must be, becomes of central concern. It is also not unusual that the line separating children who should be served and those who should remain unserved moves around from time to time.

Over the years, the "poverty line" has often been redefined. If we say that all children below the poverty line are eligible for certain services, then moving the poverty line can obviously change the number of children receiving services. Recently, eligibility for some programs, such as Early and Periodic Screening, Diagnosis, and Treatment (EPSDT), has been opened to youngsters and families whose incomes are 133% of the poverty line or less, illustrating Wildavsky's (1979) position that it is inevitable that, for any social program, the eligibility requirements will be expanded to include more and more clients. A similar consequence can be seen in the field of children with disabilities in the rapidly growing number of children identified as learning disabled in the educational system (Kirk, Gallagher, & Anastasiow, 1993).

Another important part of the general public belief system is that it is better to intervene early developmentally to aid children with special needs. Such beliefs have been at the heart of the Head Start program (Zigler & Hodapp, 1981) and also the programs for infants and toddlers with disabilities and their families—programs that actually start intervention at birth, in many instances.

Maroney (1986) has suggested that the strategy of providing extra services for some targeted groups, such as "children with disabilities," has had unfortunate consequences. It tends to keep resources away from a large body of children, many of whom could use special services, and directs those resources to a limited number of children with special needs. By establishing a policy that all children would be eligible for all services, the need to spend an enormous amount of professional time on "eligibility" would, obviously, disappear. Maroney's suggestion would, of course, substantially increase the cost of the services, and that may be the most eloquent argument against full services for everyone.

The basic strategy for the past three or four decades has been to provide special services for those who demonstrably need such services and, in fact, cannot flourish without them. Over time, then, such services are made available to others whose problems are less severe. This has been known in legislative halls as the "salami" approach—taking thin slices off the public salami one at a time until, finally, one has the entire salami. Trying to convince the public that they should buy the whole salami at once (that is, provide services for *all* children) is generally assumed to make such a policy totally indigestible to the tax-paying public. The salami approach, with all of its attendant problems, would appear to be the preferred strategy for the near future, where economics will continue to drive policy development.

Who Provides the Services?

One of the key policy questions in the implementation of any particular program involves the qualifications of persons who provide the services necessary for the target population. Each professional group has found it necessary to establish some type of credential to certify the qualifications of the individuals who are service providers, whether it be certification, a license, or a particular degree from higher education.

The ten professions expected to play a role in Part H of IDEA, by providing services for infants and toddlers and their families, have each established some form of credentialing. The credential may be a medical license, certification as a special education teacher, a nursing degree, or some other professional measure of qualification, but such general credentials may not be sufficient to ensure quality services for the specific group of infants and toddlers. Should a school psychologist, for example, be allowed to provide diagnostic services for infants and toddlers even though he/she may have never professionally dealt with children this young? Is it appropriate for a general practice physician, trained in neither pediatrics nor disabilities, to be empowered to provide services to infants and toddlers? Gallagher and Coleman (1990) queried the ten professional associations to determine whether they planned to ask for something additional in performance or study for those who would work with these young children with special needs and their families. Only one discipline, special education, intended to make some major shifts in credentialing for early childhood intervention, and this only happened in a few states.

The majority of professional associations planned to issue a statement of "best practice" covering desirable characteristics and training for a professional working in this field, while other professions suggested that they might reorganize some of their course requirements to include special material on early childhood. Professions have also felt strong pressure from other special interest groups (aging, AIDS, etc.) to include their particular interests in required professional preparation programs. Professional organizations, therefore, were not eager to develop yet another credential specialty for early childhood.

By holding to the "high standards" for practice as defined by the professional associations, the decision makers have guaranteed a continued severe personnel shortage, because "high standards" translates into advanced degree training, which relatively few persons have completed. A study by Yoder, Coleman, and Gallagher (1990) uncovered enormous personnel shortages in the fields of occupational therapy, physical therapy, and speech/language pathology for services to infants and toddlers with disabilities and clearly indicated that such enormous shortages cannot be substantially narrowed by merely increasing support for existing training programs. What would be required to provide full service is a reconceptualization of how such services should be delivered and by whom. The use of paraprofessionals is one clear alternative of providing quality services.

Also, the call for multidisciplinary programs seems to invade the turf of already-existing, discipline-exclusive programs, and this helps to make such personnel preparation programs difficult to establish voluntarily. There seems to be a need for establishing collaborative structures if any multidisciplinary programs are to become instituted (Gray & Hay, 1986).

What Is the Nature of Services to Be Provided?

Many diverse services may be needed by a family with a child with special needs. These services are unlikely to be the exclusive province of a particular professional discipline or agency. Laws such as the Education for All Handicapped Children Act have recognized the importance of *related services* to the full effectiveness of the educational program designed for the child with special needs (Martin, 1989). One of the major policy questions, therefore, is, "Where is the boundary line that separates 'appropriate related services' from services that fall outside the domain of a particular program?"

This is an especially troubling issue in the implementation of Part H of IDEA because this law strongly stresses the importance of family. The rationale for that emphasis is presented in Chapter 6 of this volume by Bailey and Henderson. For example, should Part H be responsible for the drug treatment of an aunt who lives in the home, or for psychotherapy for the mother because that would presumably improve the mother–child relationship and the mother's effectiveness in parenting? It is likely that the final boundary lines will be established, in each state, based upon a succession of case events that will draw the distinction into sharper and sharper focus.

One of the built-in limitations of Part H is the prohibition of using these funds to pay for health services, with the specific exception of health services that are necessary to help the child maintain himself or herself in an educational setting. For example, an early intervention teacher would be allowed to provide catheterization procedures for a child so that the child could participate in classroom activities. Beyond these narrow exceptions, there would then have to be a blending of financing and cooperative agreements with other programs in order to pick up expenses for health problems that fall outside of Part H boundaries.

What Are the Conditions under Which Services Are Delivered?

The last of the conditions applying to resource allocation would be statements in the legislation or in the regulations and guidelines that put limitations on how the services would be delivered. In the case of the Education for All Handicapped Children Act, one limitation was that the child should be placed in the "least restrictive environment." This did not mean mainstreaming, as it has often been interpreted, but it does suggest that the burden of proof for removing the child from the regular educational setting and placing him or her in a separate educational setting is on the special educator, or the responsible decision maker in that situation.

Under Part H, there is an expectation that services should be delivered in normalized settings with nondisabled children, as elaborated by Hanline and Galant (Chapter 10, this volume). The implication from that policy statement is that major efforts should be made to bring children with disabilities into typical child care facilities. Such a policy creates problems when we find that many child care programs cannot even meet minimum standards for children *without* disabilities (see Whitebook, Howes, & Phillips, 1990). One of the other limitations is that services should be delivered by "qualified personnel." Although that phrase needs to be interpreted by each of the states, it generally refers to personnel who have some established license, certificate, or degree of some sort. The use of paraprofessionals, or noncertified persons, has to be substantially justified. Professional associations have been active in maintaining "high professional standards" and thus creating a familiar paradox: the higher the level of professional qualifications, the greater the actual shortage of personnel to provide such services. Other regulations restrict the use of funds for transportation, service coordination, group therapy, or other needed services.

DESIGNING DIVERSE POLICIES

The question, then, is how to design an "adhocracy" rather than a bureaucracy (Skrtic, 1991). Because it is impossible to predict, in advance, the diversity of an individual case or instance, Part H policy should be organized to allow for clinical or professional judgment that can take into account such diversity.

The Application of Professional Judgment

A specific example would be the requirements for eligibility for services for Part H. It may be that a given child and family, having been referred for possible Part H services, has gone through a complex diagnostic and interview process and the professionals involved in such a process have found it difficult to fit this family into the standard criteria for disability, despite a unanimity among the professionals present that the child and family seem to be eligible under the spirit, if not the letter, of the law.

Under such circumstances, and with due regard for the difficulty of diagnosing disability conditions in infants and toddlers, one might appoint a committee of three professionals. Each would sign off that, in their judgment, the child in question is eligible for the services despite the fact that he/she does not meet the established eligibility criteria. Further regulations may be needed to keep such procedures from running away with the program. Such a restriction might require that no particular program should have more than 10% of its population made up of such special cases, and that all three of the professionals involved in the review process have agreed to sign a paper stating their confidence that the child is, in fact, eligible.

The Missing Professional Services

A second example might well occur at the level of, and type of, personnel providing needed services in a rural area and in some inner city areas. The child and family in question may have the need for an audiological examination, early education intervention programming, and some physical therapy services. We may find, however, that the nearest physical therapist is 150 miles away and can only come to the community a maximum of once a month. Under such circumstances, the IFSP might allow for such services to be provided by a paraprofessional who is in the immediate neighborhood, under the supervision of the distant, qualified physical therapist. The responsibilities for maintaining communication lines and periodic supervisory visits would be held jointly by the physical therapist and the paraprofessional.

Thus, the child and family would not be receiving the full level of professional services, nor the quality of services that might be ideal, but they are getting the full range of services that are available, given the current setting and the availability of professional expertise. Under such circumstances, the team signing off on the IFSP should be reassured that their plan would not be judged as being out of line with the spirit of the Part H provisions.

In other words, there should be an understanding in the administration of the law that exceptions *should* be made whenever a consensus of qualified professional judgement feels it is necessary to take into account a diverse set of circumstances that could not have been anticipated under the original law or the rules and regulations that have been promulgated. Failure to provide this kind of flexibility can only result in a continued rigidification of the rules, such as has happened with Public Law 94-142 (the Education for All Handicapped Children Act). The consequent feelings of many people at the local level will be that the law is being applied inappropriately, or that the law is unable to take account of a diverse set of circumstances that could not have reasonably been anticipated by the original designers of the legislation or the creators of the guidelines and regulations.

If one allows for these exceptions, then, over time, the accumulation of such exceptions may point to flaws in the rules and regulations themselves, which can then be remedied; the exceptions can be used to modify or change some particular aspect of the guidelines and rules. In most instances, however, what we are really recognizing is that no one set of rules can possibly fit the diversity of families, children, and professionals that this law is designed to influence. There is no "one size fits all" in the policy arena.

In the end, such flexibility—allowing for responsible professional judgment to play a role in the decision making when the rules themselves seem to be silent or ambiguous—will keep another undesirable event from occurring. Such flexibility should curtail the desire to write another law, or to amend the current law, in order to take care of the manifest injustice the law has created in specific instances. Allowing for unique cases, or for a particular, unique set of circumstances to be coped with under the current law, with the best human judgment that can be applied will help to maintain services without the feeling that the original intent of the legislation—to help those in need of help—is being thwarted by a set of regulations that ties the hands of those who wish to use the law in its full intent, or for its original purpose.

REFERENCES

Arcia, E., Keyes, L., Gallagher, J., & Herrick, H. (1992). *Potential underutilization of Part H services: An empirical study of national demographic factors.* Chapel Hill, NC: Carolina Policy Studies Program, University of North Carolina at Chapel Hill.

Arcia, E., Serling, J., & Gallagher, J. (1992). *Review of state policies to empower families and reach populations typically underserved.* Chapel Hill, NC: Carolina Policy Studies Program, University of North Carolina at Chapel Hill.

Beder, H. (1984). *Realizing the potential of interorganizational cooperation.* San Francisco, CA: Jossey-Bass.

DiStefano, T. (1984). Interorganizational conflict: A review of an emerging field. *Human Relations, 37,* 351–366.

Fullagar, P. K., Crotser, C., Gallagher, J. J., Loda, F., & Shea, T. (1991). *Provision of services to infants and toddlers with developmental delay: The health perspective* on the role of service coordinators. Chapel Hill, NC: Carolina Policy Studies Program, University of North Carolina at Chapel Hill.

Galaskiewicz, J. (1985). Interorganizational relations. *Annual Review of Sociology, 11*, 281–304.

Gallagher, J. J. (1992). The gifted: A term with surplus meaning. *Journal for the Education of the Gifted, 14*, 353–365.

Gallagher, J., & Coleman, P. (1990). *Professional organizations' role in meeting the personnel demands of P.L. 99-457.* Chapel Hill, NC: Carolina Institute for Child and Family Policy, University of North Carolina at Chapel Hill.

Gallagher, J., Trohanis, P., & Clifford, R. (1989). *Policy implementation and P.L. 99-457.* Baltimore, MD: Paul H. Brookes.

Goggin, M. (1987). *Policy design and the politics of implementation.* Knoxville, TN: University of Tennessee Press.

Gray, B., & Hay, T. (1986). Political limits to interorganizational consensus and change. *Journal of Applied Behavioral Science, 22*, 95–112.

Harbin, G., Gallagher, J., & Terry D. (1991). Define the eligible population: Policy issues and challenges. *Journal of Early Intervention, 15*(1), 13–20.

Harbin, G., & Terry, D. (1990). *Definition of developmentally delayed and at-risk infants and toddlers.* Chapel Hill, NC: Carolina Policy Studies Program, University of North Carolina at Chapel Hill. [Abstract: A policy alert addressing eligibility criteria under Part H. of P.L. 99-457.]

Kaluzny, A. D., Morrisey, J. P., & McKinney, M. M. (1990). Emerging organizational network: The case of the community clinical oncology program. In S. S. Mick & Associates (Eds.), *Innovations in health care delivery.* San Francisco: Jossey-Bass.

Kirk, S., Gallagher, J., & Anastasiow, N. (1993). *Educating exceptional children* (8th ed.). Boston: Houghton-Mifflin.

Martin, E. (1989). Lessons from implementing P.L. 94-142. In J. Gallagher, P. Trohanis, & R. Clifford (Eds.), *Policy implementation and P.L. 99-457* (pp. 19–32). Baltimore, MD: Paul H. Brookes.

Maroney, R. (1986). *Shared responsibility: Families and social policy.* New York: Aldine.

Milner, M. (1980). *Unequal care: A case study of interorganizational relations.* New York: Columbia University Press.

Oliver, C. (1990). Determinants of interorganizational relationships: Integration and future directions. *Academy of Management Review, 15*(2), 241–265.

Skrtic, T. (1991). *Behind special education.* Baltimore, MD: Paul H. Brookes.

Turnbull, H. (1986). *Free appropriate public education.* Denver, CO: Love.

Whitebook, M., Howes, C., & Phillips, D. (1990). *Who cares? Child care teachers and the quality of care in America* (Final Report). Oakland, CA: National Child Care Staffing Study, Child Care Employee Project.

Index